BU5 SO

The 5-Minute

Health

Advisor

Derived from Griffith's 5 Minute Clinical Consult

MARK R. DAMBRO, MD, FAAFP
WITH BRUCE GOLDFARB

The 5-Minute Health Advisor

MARK R. DAMBRO, MD, FAAFP
FORT WORTH, TEXAS
FORMERLY ASSISTANT PROFESSOR OF MEDICINE
AND DIRECTOR OF MEDICAL COMPUTING
UNIVERSITY OF ARIZONA COLLEGE OF MEDICINE
TUCSON, ARIZONA

Consulting Author
BRUCE GOLDFARB

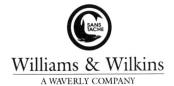

Williams & Wilkins
A WAVERLY COMPANY

BALTIMORE • PHILADELPHIA • LONDON • PARIS • BANGKOK
BUENOS AIRES • HONG KONG • MUNICH • SYDNEY • TOKYO • WROCLAW

Editor: David Charles Retford
Managing Editor: Jennifer Eckhoff
Marketing Manager: Daniell Griffin
Production Coordinator: Marette D. Magargle-Smith
Project Editor: Robert D. Magee
Typesetter: Peirce Graphic Services, Inc.
Printer & Binder: Victor Graphics, Inc.

Copyright © 1997 Williams & Wilkins

351 West Camden Street
Baltimore, Maryland 21201–2436 USA

Rose Tree Corporate Center
1400 North Providence Road
Building II, Suite 5025
Media, Pennsylvania 19063–2043 USA

Accurate indications, adverse reactions and dosage schedules for drugs are provided in this book, but it is possible that they may change. The reader is urged to review the package information data of the manufacturers of the medications mentioned.

Printed in the United States of America

First Edition,

0-683-30440-2

The publishers have made every effort to trace the copyright holders for borrowed material. If they have inadvertently overlooked any, they will be pleased to make the necessary arrangements at the first opportunity.

To purchase additional copies of this book, please call our customer service department at **(800) 638-0672** or fax orders to **(800) 447-8438**. For other book services, including chapter reprints and large quantity sales, ask for the Special Sales department.

Canadian customers should call **(800) 665-1148**, or fax **(800) 665-0103**. For all other calls originating outside of the United States, please call **(401) 528-4223** or fax us at **(410) 528-8550**.

Visit Williams & Wilkins on the Internet: **http://www.wwilkins.com** or contact our customer service department at **custserv@wwilkins.com**. Williams & Wilkins customer service representatives are available from 8:30 am to 6:00 pm, EST, Monday through Friday, for telephone access.

97 98 99 00
2 3 4 5 6 7 8 9 10

Preface to The 5 Minute Health Advisor

The Family Health Advisor is based on the widely used physician's guide, *Griffith's 5 Minute Clinical Consult*. This book has been designed to fit the informed consumer's health care needs, by presenting up-to-date information in an accessible format.

The table of contents covers over 200 common health problems, each explained in a two-page outline that makes the facts easy to find. Each entry is listed alphabetically and contains specific information on diagnosis, options for treatment, recommended medications, and follow-up suggestions. This database can help you communicate more effectively with your doctor and make better choices for your family's health.

This book should not, however, be treated as a license to diagnosis and treat. It is not a guide to evaluate and manage your health independently; these skills take more than data and questions. They require experience, interpretive skills, weighing of conflicting data, judgment and decision making. These skills are not addressed in this book.

This book is a compilation of many people's efforts and time, including the contributing authors and the consultants who review the topics. For this edition, Bruce Goldfarb rewrote the text, taking what was written for a medical audience and redirecting it to you, the health consumer.

My thanks to the staff of Williams and Wilkins for their expertise and cooperation. We hope you like the book and use it wisely.

Contents

Section N

Section O

Section P

Section R

Section S

Section T

Section U

Section V

Section W

Section A

Acetaminophen Poisoning

 ## Basics

DESCRIPTION

- This disorder is marked by liver disease following ingestion of a large amount of acetaminophen (Tylenol).
- Acetaminophen poisoning is most often encountered following a large single ingestion of acetaminophen-containing medications. However, poisoning can occur after ingestion of lesser amounts in susceptible individuals, including those who regularly abuse alcohol, are chronically malnourished, or take medications that affect liver function.

SIGNS AND SYMPTOMS

- Symptoms vary from nausea, vomiting, profuse sweating, and malaise to jaundice, confusion, sleepiness, coma, and death.
- Symptoms develop over the first 24 hours following a large ingestion and may last as long as 8 days.
- Severe symptoms indicate that a large amount of acetaminophen was consumed or that poisoning involves more than one substance.
- Serious liver disease occurs in less than 1% of adults and is very rare in children under 6 years of age.
- Symptoms may develop gradually in susceptible patients following long-term ingestion of smaller amounts of acetaminophen. Such patients may develop liver disease without a history of excessive acetaminophen ingestion.

CAUSES

Accidental or intentional ingestion of acetaminophen or a combination of medications containing acetaminophen.

SCOPE

- There were more than 105,000 cases of ingestion of acetaminophen-containing medications reported by poison control centers in 1995.
- There were 103 total deaths in 1995, one involving a child less than 6 years of age.

MOST OFTEN AFFECTED

- Children and adults of any age.
- About half of poisoning cases involve children under 6 years of age.

RISK FACTORS

- Age younger than 6 years
- Poisoning with other substances
- Psychiatric illness
- History of previous poisoning or suicide attempts
- Regular ingestion of large amounts of alcohol

 ## Diagnosis

WHAT THE DOCTOR LOOKS FOR

- The doctor should consider the ingestion of other poisons, particularly those that affect liver function.
- The doctor will assess the degree of damage to the liver and other organs.

LABORATORY

- Blood tests to measure levels of acetaminophen and other possible poisons
- Blood tests to assess function of liver, heart, and pancreas

 ## Treatment

GENERAL MEASURES

- Contact a regional poison information center for first aid instructions.
- All persons suspected of acetaminophen poisoning should be evaluated at a health care facility.
- Nontoxic accidental ingestion can be managed on an outpatient basis.
- Toxic and intentional ingestion may require hospitalization.
- The person who has been poisoned may be treated by inducing vomiting with syrup of ipecac or have the stomach pumped, which must be performed within 4 hours of ingestion.

- Syrup of ipecac may be given at home if the victim is alert and unable to be seen at a hospital within 1 hour of ingestion.
- Activated charcoal should be given at a hospital.
- Antidote therapy may be effective 36 or more hours after ingestion.

ACTIVITY

Restricted if significant liver damage has occurred

DIET

No special diet except with severe liver damage

 ## Medications

COMMONLY PRESCRIBED DRUGS

- Three classes of medicine:
  - ▶ Ipecac syrup: to induce vomiting
  - ▶ Activated charcoal: to absorb poisons
  - ▶ Acetylcysteine: antidote

CONTRAINDICATIONS

- Ipecac should not be given to persons with decreased responsiveness.
- Some people may have drug allergies.

PRECAUTIONS

- Ipecac therapy may result in severe vomiting.
- To reduce risks, activated charcoal should be given at least 30 minutes to 1 hour after ipecac and never before ipecac.

DRUG INTERACTIONS

Activated charcoal may interfere with antidote.

OTHER DRUGS

N/A

 ## Followup

PATIENT MONITORING

A person should have a psychiatric follow-up after intentional ingestion.

PREVENTION

- Homes with small children should be poison proofed.
- Keep syrup of ipecac in the home first aid kit.
- Keep a list of emergency telephone numbers in a convenient location.

COMPLICATIONS

Complications are rare after recovery from acute poisoning.

WHAT TO EXPECT

- Complete recovery with early therapy.
- Less than 1% of adult patients develop liver failure.
- Liver failure is rare in children younger than 6 years of age.

 ## Miscellaneous

OTHER FACTORS

N/A

PEDIATRIC

Risk of liver damage is decreased in children younger than 6 years of age.

GERIATRIC

Some medications increase risk of liver damage.

OTHERS

N/A

PREGNANCY

Increased incidence of miscarriage

FURTHER INFORMATION

Child Safety: How to keep your home safe for your baby. American Academy of Family Physicians, 8880 Ward Parkway, Kansas City, MO 64114-2797

Acne

 Basics

DESCRIPTION

Acne, also called acne vulgaris, is an inflammatory disorder of the sebaceous glands of the skin, resulting in pimples, boils, and occasionally scarring.

SIGNS AND SYMPTOMS

- Pimples (whiteheads or blackheads)
- Bumps or nodes of the skin
- Scars
- Pimples occur over the forehead, cheeks, and nose and may extend over the central chest and back.

CAUSES

Hormones stimulate the rate of skin growth in the sebaceous gland, blocking the pore. Bacteria stimulates an inflammatory response, resulting in a pimple.

SCOPE

Acne affects virtually 100% of adolescents to some degree. About 15% of people will seek medical advice for acne.

MOST OFTEN AFFECTED

Persons in early to late puberty, although some cases will persist into the 30s and 40s. Males and females are affected with equal frequency, although males tend to be affected more severely.

RISK FACTORS

- Adolescence
- Male gender
- Use of steroids or birth control pills
- Oily cosmetics, including cleansing creams, moisturizers, and oil-based foundations.
- Rubbing or occluding the skin surface, as may occur with sports equipment (helmets and shoulder pads) or holding the telephone or hands against the skin.
- Prescription drugs
- Hair growth disorders
- Hot, humid climate

 Diagnosis

WHAT THE DOCTOR LOOKS FOR

- The doctor will evaluate the condition of the skin.
- Other causes of skin disorders will be considered, such as occupational exposure or drug side effects.

TESTS AND PROCEDURES

Levels of hormone in the blood may be measured in rare cases.

 Treatment

GENERAL MEASURES

- Acne is managed on an outpatient basis.
- Pimples may be treated with surgery or injections.
- Gentle cleansing with a mild soap once or twice a day will control surface oiliness. More frequent washing will further irritate the skin and increase sebum (oil) production.
- Oil-free sun screens: UV light reacts adversely with the medications used to treat acne. Long-term UV exposure causes permanent skin damage. Oil-free sun screens should be used to protect the skin.
- Stress management may be helpful if acne flares with stress.
- There is no cure for acne; treatment only controls the lesions.

ACTIVITY

Full activity. Physical conditioning is important.

DIET

- Good nutrition is important to normal skin health.
- No special diet has been shown to diminish acne. Chocolate and fatty foods do not aggravate acne.

Acne

Medications

COMMONLY PRESCRIBED DRUGS

- Topical medications
  - ▶ Benzoyl peroxide
  - ▶ Tretinoin (retinoic acid, Retin-A, Renova)
  - ▶ Topical erythromycin
  - ▶ Clindamycin (Dalacin T)
- Oral Medications
- Tetracycline
- Erythromycin
- Oral contraceptives
- Isotretinoin (Accutane)

CONTRAINDICATIONS

- Known allergies
- All oral medications could cause severe liver problems.
- Isotretinoin: causes birth defects; not for use in pregnancy or in women of reproductive age who are not using a reliable birth control method.
- Tetracycline: not for use in pregnancy or children younger than 8 years of age

PRECAUTIONS

- Tetracycline: may cause sensitivity to sunlight; sunscreen recommended

DRUG INTERACTIONS

- Tetracycline: avoid antacids, dairy products, and iron
- Erythromycin: Fexofenadine (Allegra) and astemizole
- Some antibiotics may reduce the effectiveness of oral contraceptives.

OTHER DRUGS

N/A

Followup

PATIENT MONITORING

- The doctor should be seen monthly until adequate response is obtained.
- Blood tests should be done before treatment and monthly during treatment.

- Female patients taking isotretinon should have pregnancy tests.

PREVENTION

N/A

COMPLICATIONS

- Severe inflammatory acne with systemic symptoms
- Facial scarring
- Psychological scarring

WHAT TO EXPECT

- Acne gradually improves over time.
- Any treatment takes at least 4 weeks to show results.
- Topical agents cause redness and drying of the skin.

Miscellaneous

OTHER FACTORS

N/A

PEDIATRIC

A mild form of acne, called acne rosacea, can occur in the neonate.

GERIATRIC

N/A

OTHERS

N/A

PREGNANCY

- May result in an acute episode, or remission, of acne
- Isotretinoin causes severe birth defects; effective contraception should be ensured 1 month prior to and 1 month following isotretinoin therapy.
- Erythromycin can be used during pregnancy, but it is less preferable to topical agents.

FURTHER INFORMATION

American Academy of Dermatology, 930 N. Meacham Rd., P.O. Box 4014, Schaumberg, IL 60168-4014, (708) 330-0230

Adenovirus Infections

 Basics

DESCRIPTION

Adenovirus infections are usually self-limited illnesses characterized by fever and inflammation of eyes and the respiratory tract. Adenovirus infections occur in epidemics.

SIGNS AND SYMPTOMS

Vary depending on the type of virus. Most respiratory adenovirus infections cause:
- Headache
- Malaise
- Sore throat
- Cough
- Fever (moderate to high)
- Vomiting
- Diarrhea

CAUSES

One of several types of adenovirus

SCOPE

Adenovirus infections are common in the United States. They are estimated to cause 2–5% of all respiratory infections.

MOST OFTEN AFFECTED

The disease can affect all ages, males and females equally, but it is more common in infants and children.

RISK FACTORS

- Large number of people gathered in a small area (military recruits, college students at the beginning of the school year, day-care centers, community swimming pools, etc.)
- Persons with immune system disorders are at risk for severe disease.

 Diagnosis

WHAT THE DOCTOR LOOKS FOR

- The doctor will perform a physical examination.
- Other similar conditions will be investigated, such as pneumonia, bronchitis, or other respiratory illnesses.

TESTS AND PROCEDURES

- Blood tests to evaluate for signs of infection or inflammation
- Sputum or other body fluids may be cultured for microbiological analysis.
- A chest x-ray may be performed to assess the respiratory system.
- Biopsy (lung or other) may be needed in severe or unusual cases.

 Treatment

GENERAL MEASURES

- Adenovirus is usually treated on an outpatient basis except for severely ill infants.
- Treatment is supportive, aimed at relieving symptoms.
- Adenovirus infections are usually harmless and of short duration.
- Avoid aspirin in children.
- Nasal spray may help relieve nasal congestion.
- Wash hands frequently to avoid transmission of virus.

ACTIVITY

Rest during fever

DIET

No special diet

Medications

COMMONLY PRESCRIBED DRUGS

- Acetaminophen
- Topical corticosteroids for conjunctivitis (pink eye)
- Cough suppressants and/or expectorants

CONTRAINDICATIONS

Read drug product information.

PRECAUTIONS

Read drug product information.

DRUG INTERACTIONS

Read drug product information.

OTHER DRUGS

N/A

 ## Followup

PATIENT MONITORING

Infants with severe pneumonia and conjunctivitis should be seen daily by the doctor until well.

PREVENTION

- Adenovirus vaccine reduces the incidence of acute respiratory disease.
- Frequent hand washing by office personnel and family members reduces the risk of virus transmission.

COMPLICATIONS

- Adenovirus infection causes few if any recognizable long-term problems.

WHAT TO EXPECT

- Adenovirus infection is self-limited, usually without lasting effects.
- Adenovirus can cause severe illness and death in very young persons and in those with immune system disorders.

 ## Miscellaneous

OTHER FACTORS

N/A

PEDIATRIC

Viral pneumonia in infants may be fatal. Aspirin should not be given to children.

GERIATRIC

Complications are more likely among elderly persons.

OTHERS

N/A

PREGNANCY

No special precautions

OTHER INFORMATION

N/A

Alcoholism

 Basics

DESCRIPTION

Alcoholism is an illness characterized by physiological, psychological, and/or social problems associated with persistent and excessive use of alcohol.

SIGNS AND SYMPTOMS

- Behavioral
  - ▶ Psychological and social dysfunction
  - ▶ Marital problems (divorce or separation)
  - ▶ Anxiety, depression, insomnia
  - ▶ Social isolation, frequent moves
  - ▶ Child or spouse abuse
  - ▶ Alcohol-related arrests or legal problems (less likely in women)
  - ▶ Preoccupation with recreational drinking
  - ▶ Repeated attempts to stop or reduce drinking
  - ▶ Loss of interest in nondrinking activities
  - ▶ Employment problems (tardiness, absenteeism, decreased productivity, interpersonal problems at work, frequent job changes)
  - ▶ Blackouts (not remembering what happened during drinking spells)
  - ▶ Complaints by family members or friends about alcohol-related behavior
- Physical
  - ▶ Gastrointestinal: anorexia, nausea, vomiting, abdominal pain, ulcer, pancreatitis, cancer
  - ▶ Cardiovascular: hypertension, irregular heart rhythms, heart disease
  - ▶ Respiratory: pneumonia, bronchitis, and chronic pulmonary disease
  - ▶ Genitourinary: impotence, menstrual irregularities, testicular atrophy
  - ▶ Dermatologic: signs of accidents and trauma, burns (especially cigarette burns), bruises in various stages of healing, poor hygiene
  - ▶ Musculoskeletal: old fractures and fractures in various stages of healing, myopathy
  - ▶ Neurologic: dementia, nerve disease

CAUSES

- Multiple factors, including biological, psychological, and sociocultural
- Evidence suggests a genetic link to alcoholism.

SCOPE

About 10% of men and 3.5% of women are alcoholics in the United States.

MOST OFTEN AFFECTED

- Alcoholism affects all ages.
- Highest prevalence of drinking problems is in the 18-29 age group.
- Slightly more common in men than in women

RISK FACTORS

- Alcohol use
- Use of other psychoactive drugs, including nicotine
- Family history of alcohol abuse
- Young, single male
- Heavy drinking: 5 or more drinks in one sitting, getting drunk at least once per week
- Peer group pressure
- Family or sociocultural background promoting intoxication; accepting it as a norm
- Increased accessibility of alcohol
- Adolescence (alcohol and drug use by peers or parents, delinquency, sociopathy in the parents, poor self-esteem, social nonconformity, and stressful life changes)

Diagnosis

WHAT THE DOCTOR LOOKS FOR

- The person with alcoholism can have a variety of medical and psychiatric disorders.
- The doctor will evaluate the person for the presence of depression, anxiety, or other mental health problems.
- The doctor will perform a physical examination to identify medical problems, such as hypertension, peptic ulcer, heart disease, liver disease, and diabetes.

TESTS AND PROCEDURES

- A variety of blood tests may be performed, including measurement of the blood alcohol level.
- Psychological tests
- X-ray, computed tomography (CT scan) or magnetic resonance imaging (MRI) may be performed to assess structures of the head, chest, and abdomen.
- A sample of liver may be obtained by biopsy for laboratory analysis.

 ## Treatment

GENERAL MEASURES

- Treatment is inpatient or outpatient depending on severity of illness, person's health, and other factors.
- In some cases, detoxification is done as an inpatient, with the remainder of treatment given on an outpatient basis.
- Primary care provider may want to consult an addiction specialist.

ACTIVITY

Fully active as tolerated

DIET

- Well-balanced diet (malnutrition from poor eating habits is common)
- Alcohol interferes with the metabolism of most vitamins.
- Person may have specific vitamin or mineral deficiencies.

Alcoholism

 Medications

COMMONLY PRESCRIBED DRUGS

- For detoxification and management of alcohol withdrawal:
  - ▶ Chlordiazepoxide (Librium)
  - ▶ Diazepam (Valium)
  - ▶ Lorazepam (Ativan)
  - ▶ Phenobarbital
- Detoxification adjuncts:
  - ▶ Beta blockers (propranolol, atenolol)
  - ▶ Clonidine
- To promote sobriety:
  - ▶ Disulfiram (Anabuse)
  - ▶ Naltrexone
- Thiamine

CONTRAINDICATIONS

Do not drink while taking detoxification medications.

PRECAUTIONS

- Medications should be used with caution in individuals with severe liver disease, organic pain, or other conditions.
- Watch for unsteadiness, excessive sleepiness, slurred speech, or other signs of intoxication.

SIGNIFICANT POSSIBLE INTERACTIONS

- Alcohol and benzodiazepines have additive effects.
- Don't mix medication with other sedatives.

OTHER DRUGS

N/A

Followup

PATIENT MONITORING

- Person should be seen daily during detoxification.
- Frequent visits (weekly) after patient completes treatment program
- Less frequent visits as patient becomes established in recovery

PREVENTION

People with a family history of alcoholism or other risk factors may benefit from preventive counseling.

POSSIBLE COMPLICATIONS

- Relapse of drinking
- Nervous system disorders
- Alcoholic dementia
- Increased susceptibility to infection
- Cancer
- Cirrhosis (women sooner than men)

WHAT TO EXPECT

- Alcoholism is a chronic, relapsing disease.
- If untreated, alcoholism is progressive and fatal.

Miscellaneous

OTHER FACTORS

N/A

PEDIATRIC

- Substance abuse has a negative impact on normal maturation and development and attainment of social, educational, and occupational skills.
- Signs and symptoms often include depression, suicidal thoughts or attempts, family disruption, disorderly behavior, violence or destruction of property, poor school or work performance, sexual promiscuity, social immaturity, lack of hobbies or interests, isolation, moodiness.

GERIATRIC

- Alcoholism is often missed in elderly individuals. The signs and symptoms of alcoholism may be different or attributed to a chronic medical problem or dementia.
- The elderly are more sensitive to alcohol effects.

OTHERS

N/A

PREGNANCY

- Alcohol causes birth defects. The greatest damage occurs during the early weeks of fetal development.
- Women should abstain from alcohol when planning conception and throughout pregnancy.

FURTHER INFORMATION

N/A

Alopecia

 ## Basics

DESCRIPTION

Alopecia is defined as the absence of hair from skin areas where it normally is present. There are several forms of alopecia depending on the type of hair loss.

SIGNS AND SYMPTOMS

- Hair loss
- Itching
- Scaling of the scalp
- Broken hairs
- Tapered hair
- Easily removable hairs
- Inflammation

CAUSES

Alopecia has many possible causes, including inherited disease, medication side effects, radiation therapy, infection, and other conditions.

SCOPE

By 50 years of age, 50% of Caucasian males have noticeable male-pattern baldness. Nearly 40% of postmenopausal females show some evidence of hair loss.

MOST OFTEN AFFECTED

The incidence of androgenic alopecia (male-pattern baldness) increases with increasing age. Men are affected more often than women. There is a strong genetic tendency for baldness.

RISK FACTORS

- Family history of baldness
- Physical or psychological stress
- Pregnancy
- Poor nutrition

 ## Diagnosis

WHAT THE DOCTOR LOOKS FOR

The doctor will establish the type of alopecia and search for possible reversible causes.

TESTS AND PROCEDURES

- A variety of blood tests may be ordered, include levels of hormones.
- Hair may be studied microscopically.
- The scalp may be biopsied for microscopic evaluation and other special testing procedures may be performed.

 ## Treatment

GENERAL MEASURES

- Alopecia is managed on an outpatient basis.
- Some forms of alopecia are permanent, while hair grows back in others.
- For male-pattern baldness, 39% of persons report moderate to marked hair growth after using minoxidil (Rogaine) after 12 months.

ACTIVITY

Fully active

DIET

No special diet

Alopecia

 ## Medications

COMMONLY PRESCRIBED DRUGS

- Male-pattern baldness: topical minoxidil (Rogaine)
- Alopecia areata: high-potency topical steroids
- Tinea capitis: griseofulvin or ketoconazole

CONTRAINDICATIONS

Drugs have many interactions; refer to product information.

PRECAUTIONS

- Topical minoxidil: burning and irritation of the eyes, salt and water retention, fast heart rate, chest pain
- Topical steroids: burning and stinging, itching, skin atrophy
- Griseofulvin: sensitivity to light
- Ketoconazole: allergic reactions, liver damage, lowering of sperm count, mental conditions

DRUG INTERACTIONS

Drugs have many interactions; read product information.

OTHER DRUGS

N/A

 ## Followup

PATIENT MONITORING

N/A

PREVENTION

N/A

COMPLICATIONS

N/A

WHAT TO EXPECT

- Recovery varies depending on type of alopecia.
- Recovery from male-pattern baldness depends on treatments.
- Some forms of alopecia have complete recovery and hair growth.

 ## Miscellaneous

OTHER FACTORS

N/A

PEDIATRIC

Tinea capitis is the only common form of alopecia in children.

GERIATRIC

Male-pattern baldness is more common after age 50.

OTHERS

N/A

PREGNANCY

Hair loss after birth is due to altered physiology during pregnancy.

FURTHER INFORMATION

National Alopecia Areata Foundation, 714 C Street, San Rafael, CA 94901

Altitude Illness

 ## Basics

DESCRIPTION

Altitude illness is a medical problem ranging from mild discomfort to fatal illness that may occur on ascent to higher altitude. It can affect anyone, including those who are experienced and fit, and who ascend to more than about 8,000 feet (2438 m). Several factors appear to be important in adaptation to altitude, including how long the ascent takes, how high, and length of stay. Much variation exists between people; in addition, an individual's response may vary from ascent to ascent.

SIGNS AND SYMPTOMS

- Mild to moderately severe symptoms:
  - ▶ Headache
  - ▶ Lack of energy and appetite
  - ▶ Mild nausea
  - ▶ Dizziness
  - ▶ Weakness
  - ▶ Insomnia
- Severe symptoms:
  - ▶ Increased headache
  - ▶ Irritability
  - ▶ Marked fatigue
  - ▶ Shortness of breath with exercise
  - ▶ Nausea and vomiting
  - ▶ Irregular or periodic breathing at night
  - ▶ Difficulty or cessation of breathing
- High altitude pulmonary edema (HAPE) symptoms:
  - ▶ Excessive shortness of breath on exertion
  - ▶ Severe respiratory distress
  - ▶ Shortness of breath at rest
  - ▶ Dry cough and/or wheezing
  - ▶ Increased heart rate and breathing rate
  - ▶ Marked irregular breathing present at night
  - ▶ Gurgling breathing
  - ▶ Frothy cough
  - ▶ Wet crackling sounds in the lungs
  - ▶ Confusion
  - ▶ Coma

- High altitude cerebral edema (HACE) symptoms:
  - ▶ Progressive headache that is unrelieved by mild pain relievers
  - ▶ Lack of coordination
  - ▶ Confusion and bizarre behavior followed by unconsciousness
  - ▶ Other symptoms of moderate altitude sickness, such as dizziness, vomiting, and irritability, are usually present.

CAUSES

The physiology of altitude illness is still not completely understood. The fundamental problem is a decrease in air pressure, resulting in less oxygen delivery to the body.

SCOPE

Unknown

MOST OFTEN AFFECTED

Altitude sickness can affect any age individual, men and women in equal proportion. Young, well-conditioned climbers have a higher incidence of altitude illness, probably because they push themselves more.

RISK FACTORS

- In general, the faster and higher the ascent, the more likely a person will experience symptoms of altitude illness.
- Chronic illness
- Lack of conditioning

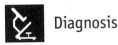
Diagnosis

Treatment

WHAT THE DOCTOR LOOKS FOR

The doctor will consider other respiratory problems, such as pneumonia, respiratory infection, or heart failure.

TESTS AND PROCEDURES

- A variety of blood tests may be performed.
- Arterial blood may be obtained to measure blood gasses.
- A chest X-ray may be done to evaluate the respiratory system.
- An electrocardiogram (EKG) may be done to monitor heart function.

GENERAL MEASURES

- Severe cases of altitude sickness may require hospitalization.
- Treatment is tailored to fit the severity of disease and may be limited by the environment.
- Definitive treatment is to descend to a lower altitude. Dramatic improvement accompanies even modest reductions in altitude (as little as 1,000 feet).
- Giving oxygen helps relieve symptoms.
- Descent is rarely needed for mild cases. Drink fluids, eat a light diet, and curtail activity.
- For severe symptoms, the victim should be immediately evacuated to a lower altitude and given continuous oxygen.
- A portable hyperbaric chamber is another effective and practical alternative for severe symptoms when descent is not possible.

ACTIVITY

Rest until symptoms clear.

DIET

Increased intake of fluids, a light diet, and avoidance of alcohol

Altitude Illness

 Medications

COMMONLY PRESCRIBED DRUGS

- Aspirin or codeine to relieve headache
- Antibiotics, if infection is present
- Dexamethasone or acetazolamide
- Corticosteroids

CONTRAINDICATIONS

Read drug product information.

PRECAUTIONS

Read drug product information.

DRUG INTERACTIONS

Read drug product information.

OTHER DRUGS

N/A

Followup

PATIENT MONITORING

- For mild cases, no followup is needed.
- Persons with more severe cases should be followed by doctor until symptoms subside.
- Person with underlying cardiopulmonary or cardiovascular disease should be followed by doctor as needed.

PREVENTION

- Staged ascent with appropriate acclimatization
- Sleeping elevation: "Climb high and sleep low" is a prudent practice for anyone going above 12,000 feet (3656 m).
- Adequate hydration: Dehydration makes altitude sickness worse.
- Good physical conditioning
- Consider carrying a supply of oxygen.
- Some drugs can prevent or lessen the symptoms of altitude sickness.

COMPLICATIONS

- Without treatment, severe illness can cause motor and sensory problems, seizures, and coma.
- May progress to respiratory distress

WHAT TO EXPECT

- Mild to moderate altitude sickness resolves over 1 to 3 days. Climbers may resume ascent once symptoms subside.
- People with severe symptoms can expect complete recovery if there is no underlying disease. They should not resume ascent.
- Problems are more likely among people who have had one or more attacks.

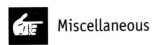 ## Miscellaneous

OTHER FACTORS

N/A

PEDIATRIC

Children younger than 6 years of age are more susceptible to altitude sickness than adults.

GERIATRIC

Elderly persons are more likely to have chronic conditions (coronary artery disease, congestive heart failure, chronic obstructive pulmonary disease) that may become worse at altitudes of 6000 to 8000 feet (1829-2438 m).

OTHERS

Women in premenstrual phase are more vulnerable to altitude sickness.

PREGNANCY

N/A

FURTHER INFORMATION

N/A

Alzheimer's Disease

 ## Basics

DESCRIPTION

Alzheimer's disease is a degenerative mental disease characterized by progressive brain deterioration and dementia. It usually occurs after age 65. The diagnosis is made after ruling out treatable disorders with similar characteristics. The usual course of Alzheimer's disease is progressive and chronic.

SIGNS AND SYMPTOMS

- Anxiety
- Confusion
- Delusions
- Dementia
- Depression
- Impaired speech
- Intellectual decline
- Lack of concern, interest
- Occupational dysfunction
- Personality changes
- Recent memory loss
- Restlessness
- Sleep disturbances
- Social withdrawal
- Weight loss
- Late signs: seizures, muscle spasm, incontinence

CAUSES

Unknown

SCOPE

Nearly 4 million people in the United States have Alzheimer's disease, which strikes about 40% of individuals over age 85.

MOST OFTEN AFFECTED

Persons 50–90 years of age. About half of individuals with Alzheimer's disease have a family history of the illness. Women are affected slightly more often than men.

RISK FACTORS

- Aging
- Head trauma
- Low education level
- Down syndrome
- Positive family history

 ## Diagnosis

WHAT THE DOCTOR LOOKS FOR

- The doctor will obtain a medical history and perform a thorough medical examination.
- Other conditions with similar symptoms should be investigated, such as Parkinson's disease and drug interactions.

TESTS AND PROCEDURES

- A number of blood tests may be performed to help rule out other causes of dementia.
- An electrocardiogram (EKG) may be done to assess heart function.
- An electroencephalogram (EEG) may be done to monitor brain activity.
- X-ray, computed tomography (CAT scan), or magnetic resonance imaging (MRI) may be done to evaluate internal structures.
- A sample of cerebrospinal fluid may be obtained for chemical and microscopic analysis.
- Psychological tests may be administered.

 ## Treatment

GENERAL MEASURES

- Management of the person with Alzheimer's disease is usually done on an outpatient basis, with adult day care or nursing home care when need.
- Management is primarily supportive.
- Other medical conditions should be identified and treated.
- Exercises to reduce restlessness
- The person may benefit from occupational therapy or music therapy.
- Challenging the mind slows the rate of deterioration.
- Make sure the person's home environment is safe and secure.
- Consider adult day care, nursing home as needed.
- Plan advance directives (residential, medical preferences) as early as possible.
- Prepare durable power of attorney.
- Person with Alzheimer's disease or family may benefit from referral to:
  - ▶ Visiting nurse
  - ▶ Social worker

▶ Physical therapist
▶ Occupational therapist
▶ Lawyer
▶ Support groups
▶ Alzheimer's special care group

ACTIVITY

To whatever extent possible

DIET

No special diet

 ## Medications

COMMONLY PRESCRIBED DRUGS

• No specific drug therapy is available for halting the disease.
• As few drugs as possible should be used. Persons with Alzheimer's disease tolerate drugs poorly.
• No drugs are helpful for wandering, restlessness, fidgeting, uncooperativeness, hoarding, irritability.
• Depression: selective serotonin reuptake inhibitors or trazodone (Desyrel)
• Insomnia: trazodone, zolpidem (Ambien), or temazepam (Restoril)
• Moderate anxiety/restlessness: benzodiazepines
• Psychosis, severe aggressive agitation: butyrophenones or phenothiazines
• Severe aggressive agitation: carbamazepine (Tegretol) and propranolol (Inderal)
• Memory enhancement in mild to moderate disease: tacrine (Cognex), donepezil (Aricept)
• Nonsteroidal anti-inflammatory drugs (NSAIDs) and estrogen replacement therapy (ERT) for women are related to lower incidence and slower progression of Alzheimer's disease.

CONTRAINDICATIONS

Read drug product information.

PRECAUTIONS

Read drug product information.

DRUGS INTERACTIONS

Drugs have many interactions; read drug product information.

OTHER DRUGS

N/A

 ## Followup

PATIENT MONITORING

• The person with Alzheimer's disease should be seen by the doctor as often as necessary to manage nutrition, health, and drug therapy and to support family care givers.
• Periodic mental status testing may be helpful.
• Care giver should be closely monitored to avoid burnout.

WHAT TO EXPECT

• Alzheimer's disease is a progressive disease with a poor outcome.
• A person with Alzheimer's has an average of 8 to 10 years survival.

PREVENTION

• None known for patient
• In near future, family members may seek genetic screening.

COMPLICATIONS

• Behavioral: hostility, agitation, wandering, uncooperativeness
• Medical: infection, dehydration, drug toxicity, malnutrition, falls
• Family or care giver burnout
• Depression occurs in one-third of patients.
• Suicide: in early stages, especially if depression present

 ## Miscellaneous

OTHER FACTORS
N/A

PEDIATRIC
N/A

GERIATRIC
Alzheimer's disease is a frequent and serious problem in this age group.

OTHERS
N/A

PREGNANCY
N/A

FURTHER INFORMATION
Alzheimer's Association, 70 E. Lake Street, Suite 600, Chicago, IL, (312) 853-3060

Amenorrhea

 ## Basics

DESCRIPTION

Amenorrhea is the absence of menstrual periods.

SIGNS AND SYMPTOMS

- The absence of menstrual periods
- Milky discharge from the nipple
- Temperature intolerance
- Symptoms of early pregnancy
- Signs of excess male hormone

CAUSES

- Congenital disorders
- Pregnancy, breast-feeding
- Hormone disorders
- Chemotherapy or hormone therapy
- Numerous other possible causes

SCOPE

About 3.3% of adult women have amenorrhea.

MOST OFTEN AFFECTED

Females between menarche and menopause

RISK FACTORS

- Overtraining (e.g., long-distance runner, ballet dancer)
- Eating disorders
- Psycho-social crisis

 ## Diagnosis

WHAT THE DOCTOR LOOKS FOR

- The doctor will evaluate for possible causes of amenorrhea.
- One of the most common causes of amenorrhea is pregnancy.

TESTS AND PROCEDURES

- Several blood tests may be performed to assist with diagnosis.
- Pregnancy test should be performed.
- Internal structures may be assessed with ultrasound or X-ray imaging.
- The doctor may visually inspect internal organs by laparoscopy.

 ## Treatment

GENERAL MEASURES

- Amenorrhea is usually managed on an outpatient basis.
- Treatment depends on the cause of the amenorrhea.
- Not all cases require treatment, especially if amenorrhea is temporary.
- Surgery may be required if amenorrhea is due to an intact hymen.
- Use appropriate contraceptive, as fertility returns before menses.

ACTIVITY

No restrictions

DIET

Correct overweight or underweight by dietary management.

 ## Medications

COMMONLY PRESCRIBED DRUGS

- Progesterone replacement: medroxyprogesterone (Provera)
- Estrogen replacement: conjugated estrogen (Premarin)
- Hormonal therapies will not correct underlying problem. Other drugs might be required to treat specific conditions.
- Hormonal replacement therapy is recommended after 6 months of amenorrhea, regardless of cause.

CONTRAINDICATIONS

- Pregnancy
- Blood clots
- Previous heart attack or stroke
- Estrogen-dependent malignancy
- Severe liver disease

PRECAUTIONS

- Diabetes
- Seizure disorder
- Migraine headache
- Smoker over age 35

DRUG INTERACTIONS

Barbiturates, phenytoin, rifampin, corticosteroids, theophyllines, tricyclics, oral anticoagulants

OTHER DRUGS

Oral contraceptives for hormonal replacement

 ## Followup

PATIENT MONITORING

- Followup depends on the cause and the treatment chosen.
- Hormonal replacement may be discontinued after 6 months to assess whether spontaneous menstruation resumes.

PREVENTION

Maintenance of proper body mass index (BMI)

COMPLICATIONS

- Estrogen deficiency symptoms, e.g., hot flushes, vaginal dryness
- Osteoporosis

WHAT TO EXPECT

Depends on the underlying cause. In many cases, amenorrhea spontaneously resolves in time.

 ## Miscellaneous

OTHER FACTORS

N/A

PEDIATRIC

N/A

GERIATRIC

N/A

OTHERS

N/A

PREGNANCY

One of the primary causes of amenorrhea

FURTHER INFORMATION

Society for Menstrual Cycle Research, 10559 N. 104th Place, Scottsdale, AZ 85258, (602) 451-9731

Anaphylaxis

 Basics

DESCRIPTION

Anaphylaxis is an acute, systemic allergic reaction following exposure to an allergen in a sensitized person.

SIGNS AND SYMPTOMS

- Itching, flushing, rash, swelling
- Cough, difficult breathing
- Runny nose, congestion, noisy breathing
- Difficulty swallowing
- Nausea, vomiting, diarrhea, cramps, bloating
- Rapid heart rate, low blood pressure, shock, fainting
- Malaise, shivering
- Dilated pupils

CAUSES

- Allergic reaction following exposure to allergen
- Other anaphylaxis-like syndromes may have other causes.
- Some important causes of anaphylaxis are:
  - ▶ Antibiotics (e.g., penicillin)
  - ▶ Blood products
  - ▶ Diagnostic chemicals
  - ▶ Exercise
  - ▶ Foods (e.g., peanuts, nuts, fish, shellfish, cow milk, eggs, soybean)
  - ▶ Insect stings (e.g., honeybees, wasps, kissing bugs, deer flies)
  - ▶ Latex rubber (condoms, gloves, catheters)
  - ▶ Vaccines

SCOPE

- The incidence of anaphylaxis is unknown.
- Between 20,000 and 50,000 cases of anaphylaxis occur per year in United States.
- There are 3-7 anaphylaxis deaths per 10,000 people annually.

MOST OFTEN AFFECTED

Anaphylaxis affects all ages, males and females in equal proportion. Some allergies have a genetic predisposition.

RISK FACTORS

Previous anaphylaxis; history of allergies or asthma

 Diagnosis

WHAT THE DOCTOR LOOKS FOR

- Signs and symptoms of allergic reactions
- Other conditions with similar signs should be investigated.

TESTS AND PROCEDURES

- Blood tests will be done to look for signs of inflammation or infection.
- Arterial blood may be obtained.

 Treatment

GENERAL MEASURES

- Treatment depends on the severity of the allergic reaction.
- Severe reaction requires first aid. Seek hospital care as quickly as possible.
- Maintain airway, breathing, and circulation as needed.
- If sting or bite is on arm or leg, apply constrictive band between sting and body (do not apply too tightly and loosen if uncomfortable).
- Individuals with swelling, rash, or mild breathing problems may be released from hospital when symptoms resolve; they are then managed on an outpatient basis.
- Moderate to severe anaphylaxis requires hospitalization, possibly mechanical breathing.
- Allergist may be consulted if the cause of anaphylaxis is unclear.
- Individuals with anaphylaxis from insect stings may benefit from desensitization immunotherapy.

ACTIVITY

Bed rest until anaphylaxis clears and patient is stable

DIET

Nothing by mouth until acute symptoms are controlled

Medications

COMMONLY PRESCRIBED DRUGS

- Epinephrine
- Antihistamine: diphenhydramine
- Cimetidine
- Corticosteroids
- Bronchodilators: inhaled beta-2 agonists, aminophylline

CONTRAINDICATIONS

Read drug product information.

PRECAUTIONS

Read drug product information.
Read drug product information.

OTHER DRUGS

N/A

 ## Followup

PATIENT MONITORING

The person with acute anaphylaxis should be followed closely during treatment and for several hours after symptoms resolve. Symptoms can recur for up to 72 hours.

PREVENTION

- Avoid drugs, foods that trigger allergic reaction.
- Carry a prefilled epinephrine syringe (bee sting kit); avoid areas where insect exposure is likely. Avoid wearing things that attract insects (e.g., perfumes, bright-colored clothing).
- Carry/wear medical alert identification about anaphylaxis-causing substance or event.

WHAT TO EXPECT

- Anaphylaxis has a good outcome if treated immediately.
- The outcome is worse if medical care is delayed more than 30 minutes.
- Of individuals with anaphylaxis of unknown cause, 60% will not experience another episode after 2.5 years; most others have a decrease in the number of episodes.
- Allergy to one species of legume (e.g., peanuts) or one type of seafood (e.g., shrimp) does not mean that an allergy to all products in that category exists.

COMPLICATIONS

Inadequate oxygenation, cardiac arrest, death

 ## Miscellaneous

OTHER FACTORS

N/A

PEDIATRIC

N/A

GERIATRIC

N/A

OTHERS

N/A

PREGNANCY

N/A

FURTHER INFORMATION

- Asthma & Allergy Foundation of America, 1717 Massachusetts Avenue, Suite 305, Washington, DC 20036, (800) 7-Asthma
- American Allergy Association, P.O. Box 7273, Menlo Park, CA 94026, (415)322-1663
- Medic-Alert Foundation, Turlock, CA 95381-1009

Anemia, Pernicious

 ## Basics

DESCRIPTION

Pernicious anemia is a disorder due to vitamin B12 deficiency. Usual course is slow but progressive.

SIGNS AND SYMPTOMS

- Anorexia, weight loss
- Confusion
- Dementia
- Depression
- Dizziness
- Enlarged liver
- Heart failure
- Increased skin pigmentation
- Lack of coordination
- Numbness or tingling in extremities
- Pallor
- Prematurely gray-haired
- Rapid heartbeat, palpitations
- Ringing in ears (tinnitus)
- Shortness of breath upon exertion
- Sore tongue
- Weakness

CAUSES

- Digestive disorder
- Metabolic disorder
- Immune system disorder

SCOPE

Unknown

MOST OFTEN AFFECTED

This disorder primarily affects older adults, 60 years of age or older. It occurs equally among males and females.

RISK FACTORS

- Vegetarian diet without B12 supplementation
- Digestive disease, surgery
- Drugs side effect
- Chronic pancreatitis
- Alcoholism

 ## Diagnosis

WHAT THE DOCTOR LOOKS FOR

- The doctor will take a history and perform a thorough physical examination.
- Other causes of similar signs and symptoms should be investigated, such as neurological disorder, liver disorders, hypothyroidism, bleeding, or alcoholism.
- The doctor will evaluate for the presence of other conditions associated with pernicious anemia.

TESTS AND PROCEDURES

- A number of blood tests may be performed to assist in diagnosis.
- A sample of bone marrow may be obtained for analysis.
- Cerebrospinal fluid may be obtained for analysis.
- Cells from the digestive system may be microscopically analyzed.
- The digestive system may be visually inspected by endoscopy.

 ## Treatment

GENERAL MEASURES

- Pernicious anemia is managed on an outpatient basis.
- The underlying disorder leading to pernicious anemia must be identified and treated.
- Treatment must be continued for life.

ACTIVITY

No limitations

DIET

Emphasize meat, animal protein foods, and legumes unless contraindicated.

Anemia, Pernicious

 Medications

COMMONLY PRESCRIBED DRUGS

Vitamin B12 (cyanocobalamin)

CONTRAINDICATIONS

None

PRECAUTIONS

Do not take folic acid supplements without vitamin B12. Folic acid without B12 vitamin may cause neurological problems.

DRUG INTERACTIONS

N/A

OTHER DRUGS

None

 Followup

PATIENT MONITORING

- Monthly injections of vitamin B12
- Endoscopy every 5 years to rule out gastric cancer

PREVENTION

Monitoring by primary care provider will help assure early detection and treatment of anemia.

WHAT TO EXPECT

- Pernicious anemia is reversible with vitamin B12.
- Neurologic effects of pernicious anemia are not reversible with vitamin B12.
- People with pernicious anemia have an increased risk of developing gastric cancer. Endoscopy should be done about every 5 years even if free of symptoms.

COMPLICATIONS

- Neurological problems may be permanent if pernicious anemia is not treated within 6 months of the onset of symptoms.
- Gastric polyps
- Stomach cancer

 Miscellaneous

OTHER FACTORS

N/A

PEDIATRIC

- Juvenile pernicious anemia occurs in older children and is the same in most respects as in adults.
- Congenital pernicious anemia is usually evident before 3 years of age.

GERIATRIC

Pernicious anemia is more common among the elderly and is often associated with immune system disorders, depression, and dementia.

OTHERS

N/A

PREGNANCY

N/A

FURTHER INFORMATION

N/A

Anemia, Sickle Cell

 Basics

DESCRIPTION

Sickle cell anemia is a chronic inheritable blood disorder, marked by moderately severe chronic anemia, periodic acute episodes of painful "crises," and increased susceptibility to infections.

SIGNS AND SYMPTOMS

- Often no symptoms in the early months of life.
- After 6 months of age, the earliest symptoms are pallor and symmetric, painful swelling of the hands and feet.
- Chronic anemia
- Painful "crises" in bones, joints, abdomen, back, and viscera
- Increased susceptibility to infections
- Delayed physical/sexual maturation, especially among boys
- Many multisystem complications, especially in later childhood and adolescence

CAUSES

- Genetic defect in hemoglobin
- Sickle red blood cells are inflexible and oddly shaped. They increase the thickness of blood and block smaller blood vessels.
- Chronic anemia

SCOPE

Sickle cell anemia affects about 1 in 500 black Americans; 8–10% black Americans carry the sickle trait.

MOST OFTEN AFFECTED

An inheritable disorder, primarily affecting blacks. Males and females are affected equally.

RISK FACTORS

- Dehydration
- Infection
- Fever
- Cold
- Strenuous physical exercise
- Severe infections
- Folic acid deficiency
- Exposure to certain drugs

 Diagnosis

WHAT THE DOCTOR LOOKS FOR

- Other types of anemia
- Other causes of acute pain in bones, joints, and abdomen

TESTS AND PROCEDURES

- Several blood tests may be performed to assist in diagnosis
- Radiological imaging may be performed, including chest X-ray, computed tomography (CAT scan), magnetic resonance imaging (MRI), and bone scan.

 Treatment

GENERAL MEASURES

- Sickle cell anemia is usually managed on an outpatient basis.
- General health care maintenance should include assessment of growth/development, regular immunizations, vision/hearing screening, and regular dental care.
- Hospitalization is required for most crises and complications.
- Infections should be promptly treated with antibiotics.
- Transfusion may be required for severe crises.
- Maintaining good hydration is important to health.

ACTIVITY

- Bed rest with crises. Otherwise, activity level as tolerated.
- Activity may be limited by chronic anemia and poor muscular development.

DIET

Well-balanced diet with folic acid supplementation

Medications

COMMONLY PRESCRIBED DRUGS

- Painful crises (mild, outpatient): non-narcotic analgesics (ibuprofen, acetaminophen)
- Painful crises (severe, hospitalized): morphine, meperidine (Demerol), acetaminophen-codeine, ibuprofen
- Antibiotics
- Penicillin to prevent infection is controversial but often recommended.

CONTRAINDICATIONS

None

PRECAUTIONS

Avoid high-dose estrogen oral contraceptives.

DRUG INTERACTIONS

None

OTHER DRUGS

- Other nonsteroidal anti-inflammatory drugs (NSAIDs)
- Folic acid supplements

Followup

PATIENT MONITORING

- The doctor should be seen as frequently as needed depending on the severity of crises and complications.
- Temperature of 101 F (38.3 C) or above requires immediate medical attention.
- Counseling, tutoring, and/or vocational training may be needed.

PREVENTION

Avoid conditions that precipitate sickling (dehydration, cold, infection, fever).

COMPLICATIONS

- Bone disease
- Cardiovascular disease
- Liver disease
- Persistent erection (priapism)
- Hematuria/hyposthenuria
- Eye disease
- Respiratory disease
- Infections

WHAT TO EXPECT

- Sickle cell anemia is a life-long condition.
- In the second decade of life, the number of crises diminish but complications become more frequent.
- Some patients die in childhood of stroke or infection.
- Most persons with sickle cell anemia live to early-mid adulthood; few live more than 50 years of age.
- Common causes of death are infections, blood clots, or renal failure.

Miscellaneous

OTHER FACTORS

N/A

PEDIATRIC

- Some signs and symptoms are seen only in infants and young children.
- The frequency of complications and tissue damage increases with age.
- Psychological complications of adolescents: body-image and sexual identity problems, interrupted schooling/career training, restriction of activities, stigma of chronic disease, low self-esteem, fear of future

GERIATRIC

N/A

OTHERS

N/A

PREGNANCY

- Usually complicated and hazardous, especially in the third trimester and delivery.
- Fetal death rate is 35-40%.
- Blood transfusion in third trimester reduces maternal morbidity and fetal death.

FURTHER INFORMATION

N/A

Angina

 Basics

DESCRIPTION

Angina is defined as chest pain and other symptoms that result when the oxygen demand of the heart exceeds the supply. Also called angina pectoris.

SIGNS AND SYMPTOMS

- Pressure or heaviness in the center of the chest, brought on by exercise, emotional stress, meals, cold air, or smoking, and relieved by rest or nitroglycerine medication
- Pain may radiate to neck, lower jaw, teeth, shoulders, inner aspects of the arms, or back.
- Individuals with angina may describe their pain with a clenched fist over the sternum.
- Shortness of breath on exertion may be the only symptom.

CAUSES

- Atherosclerosis of the coronary arteries (hardening of the arteries)
- Heart disease
- Disease of blood vessels

SCOPE

Angina is the presenting symptom of coronary artery disease in 38% of men and 61% of women.

MOST OFTEN AFFECTED

It is most common in middle-aged and older men and postmenopausal women. Males are affected more often than females.

RISK FACTORS

- Family history of premature coronary artery disease (CAD)
- High cholesterol levels
- High blood pressure
- Smoking
- Diabetes mellitus
- Male gender
- Advanced age

 Diagnosis

WHAT THE DOCTOR LOOKS FOR

- Other possible causes of chest pain should be investigated, such as digestive disorders, respiratory disease, or anxiety.
- The doctor will evaluate for other conditions known to be associated with angina, such as high blood cholesterol level or high blood pressure.

TESTS AND PROCEDURES

- Blood tests, urinalysis
- An electrocardiogram (EKG) may show evidence of disease.
- Special imaging procedures may be done to assess heart function, including radionuclide scintigraphy, stress echocardiography, stress thallium, and coronary angiography.
- Exercise stress testing may be done to evaluate heart function.

 Treatment

GENERAL MEASURES

- The person's symptoms should be brought under control.
- The person with angina should be hospitalized if symptoms are unstable.
- The goal of treatment is to restore adequate levels of oxygen to the heart.
- Quit smoking.
- Minimize emotional stress.

ACTIVITY

- Physical activity as tolerated after consulting physician
- Exercise program after physician's approval

DIET

Low-fat, low-cholesterol diet

Angina

 Medications

COMMONLY PRESCRIBED DRUGS

- Aspirin
- To slow heart rate, ease demand: beta-blockers such as atenolol, metoprolol, propranolol
- Acute anginal episodes: nitroglycerin. The dose may be repeated 2-3 times over a 10-15 minute time period; if the patient does not experience relief, he or she should be instructed to seek medical attention immediately.
- Long-acting nitrates (e.g., skin patches)
- Calcium antagonists: verapamil, nifedipine, amlodipine
- Cholesterol-lowering drugs: pravastatin, lovastatin, and others
- Heparin: blood thinner; for those hospitalized with unstable angina

CONTRAINDICATIONS

Read drug product information.

PRECAUTIONS

Read drug product information.
Significant possible interactions: Read drug product information.

OTHER DRUGS

Cholesterol-lowering drugs are often given to individuals with an unfavorable lipid profile.

 Followup

PATIENT MONITORING

- The doctor should be seen with a frequency that depends on the severity of symptoms.
- Individuals with unstable angina should be hospitalized for observation and treatment.

PREVENTION

- Stop smoking; adhere to a low-fat, low-cholesterol diet; establish a regular aerobic exercise program.
- Cholesterol-lowering drugs

COMPLICATIONS

Heart conditions: heart muscle damage, irregular heartbeat, heart failure, cardiac arrest

WHAT TO EXPECT

- The outcome of angina is variable, depending on the extent of disease as well as heart function.
- The annual death rate is 3-4%.

 Miscellaneous

OTHER FACTORS

N/A

PEDIATRIC

N/A

GERIATRIC

The elderly may be very sensitive to the side effects of medications (e.g., beta-blockers and depression).

OTHERS

N/A

PREGNANCY

- Other causes of chest pain should be excluded.
- Requires close management by obstetrician and cardiologist as pregnancy will make symptoms worse and interfere with treatment

FURTHER INFORMATION

American Heart Association, 7320 Greenville Avenue, Dallas, TX 75231, (214) 373-6300

Animal Bites

 ## Basics

DESCRIPTION

Animal bites include bite wounds from dogs, cats, and other animals (including humans).

SIGNS AND SYMPTOMS

- Bite wounds can be tears, punctures, scratches, avulsions, or crush injuries.
- Dog bites
  - ▶ Most commonly occur on the hands (up to 68% of bites).
  - ▶ Occur on the face in up to 29% of cases, the lower extremities in 10%
  - ▶ Do not commonly occur on the trunk
- Cat bites
  - ▶ Most commonly involves the hands, followed by lower extremities, face and trunk.
  - ▶ Are more likely to become infected because of puncture wound

CAUSES

- Most bite wounds are from a domestic pet known to the victim, commonly a large dog.
- Human bites are often the result of one person striking another in the mouth with a clenched fist.

SCOPE

- There are about 1,200 dog bites per 100,000 persons in the United States annually.
- There are about 160 cat bites per 100,000 persons.
- Snake bites are relatively rare in the United States, with 15 nonvenomous bites per 100,000 persons and 3 venomous bites per 100,000 persons annually.
- About half of all people will experience an animal bite at some time in their life.

MOST OFTEN AFFECTED

Bites can occur in any age group but are more likely to occur among children. They are more common among males than females.

RISK FACTORS

- Dog bites are more common in the early afternoon, especially during warm weather.
- Cat bites more common in the morning.
- Clenched fist injuries are frequently associated with the use of alcohol.

 ## Diagnosis

WHAT THE DOCTOR LOOKS FOR

The diagnosis of animal bite is straightforward. Of primary concern to the doctor is judging the risk from the injury and resulting infection.

TESTS AND PROCEDURES

- Routine blood tests
- Fluid from the wound may be cultured for microbiological analysis.
- If bite wound is near a bone or joint, an X-ray may be taken.
- In human bite wounds from clenched fist injuries, X-rays may be taken of the hands.

 ## Treatment

GENERAL MEASURES

- Animal bites are managed in the outpatient setting unless the person has a serious infection requiring intravenous antibiotics, close observation, or surgery.
- Elevate the injured extremity to prevent swelling.
- The hand should be splinted if it is injured.

 ## Medications

COMMONLY PRESCRIBED DRUGS

- Antibiotics
- Pain relievers: acetaminophen, ibuprofen

CONTRAINDICATIONS

Penicillin-derived antibiotics should not be used in people with penicillin allergy.

PRECAUTIONS

Read drug product information.
Significant possible interactions: Antibiotics may decrease effectiveness of oral contraceptives.*OTHER DRUGS*
N/A

 # Followup

PATIENT MONITORING

- Bite victim should be rechecked within 24 to 48 hours.
- The doctor may be seen daily for treating active infections.

PREVENTION

Children should be instructed to use caution around animals.

COMPLICATIONS

Complications from bites can include arthritis, osteomyelitis, extensive soft tissue injuries with scarring, infection, bleeding, and death.

WHAT TO EXPECT

Wounds should steadily improve and close over within 7 to 10 days.

 # Miscellaneous

OTHER FACTORS

N/A

PEDIATRIC

No special precautions

GERIATRIC

- Serious injury from any bite wound is more common among individuals older than 50 years of age, those with wounds in the upper extremities, or those with puncture wounds.
- The risk of infection is increased in individuals older than 50 years of age.

OTHERS

N/A

PREGNANCY

No special precautions

FURTHER INFORMATION

N/A

Anxiety

 Basics

DESCRIPTION

Anxiety is a common, acute or chronic, fearful emotion with associated physical symptoms. Types of anxiety disorders include:
- Acute situational anxiety: response to recent stressful event; usually transient
- Adjustment disorder with anxious mood: reaction following psychosocial that lasts up to 6 months
- Generalized anxiety disorder: persistent anxiety lasting more than 6 months
- Panic disorder: recurrent unexpected attacks of anxiety
- Post-traumatic stress disorder: recurrent flash-backs or nightmares of catastrophic event by survivors, often associated with panic attacks and major depression
- Phobias: intense fear of an object or situation (simple phobia) or of public embarrassment (social phobia)
- Obsessive-compulsive disorder: persistent unwanted and disturbing thoughts and recurrent behavioral patterns (e.g., hand washing) that interfere with daily life

SIGNS AND SYMPTOMS

Patterns vary with the type of anxiety; not all signs and symptoms are present in each case.
- Unrealistic or excessive anxiety or worry
- Sense of impending doom
- Nervousness
- Rapid heart rate, palpitations
- Hyperventilation, choking sensation
- Sighing respiration
- Nausea or abdominal distress
- Tingling sensation in extremities
- Excessive sweating
- Dizziness or syncope
- Flushing
- Muscle tension
- Tremor
- Restlessness
- Chest tightness, pressure
- Headache, backaches, muscle spasm

CAUSES

- Panic disorder and obsessive compulsive disorder are associated with genetic factors.
- Psychosocial stressors commonly trigger anxiety disorders.

SCOPE

Anxiety is the most common psychiatric disorder in the United States, affecting about 40 million persons.

MOST OFTEN AFFECTED

Mainly adults, highest among 20-to-45 year age group. Females are affected more often than males. There is evidence for a genetic cause of anxiety.

RISK FACTORS

- Social and financial problems
- Medical illness
- Family history
- Lack of social support

Diagnosis

WHAT THE DOCTOR LOOKS FOR

The doctor will investigate the variety of medical conditions that can cause anxiety-like symptoms, including cardiovascular, respiratory, neurological, hormonal, and nutritional disorders; alcohol or drug use; or other conditions.

TESTS AND PROCEDURES

- Blood tests, urinalysis, chest X-ray, electrocardiogram (EKG)
- An electroencephalogram (EEG) may be done to assess brain activity.
- Psychological testing may be performed.

 ## Treatment

GENERAL MEASURES

- Anxiety is managed on an outpatient basis.
- The doctor should do a thorough work-up to identify the cause and type of anxiety disorder.
- Other substance abuse should be identified and treated.
- Counseling or psychotherapy along with medications
- Regular exercise program
- Biofeedback in selected cases

ACTIVITY

Fully active

DIET

No special diet

Anxiety

 Medications

COMMONLY PRESCRIBED DRUGS

- Acute situational anxiety:
  - ▶ Short-term (up to 1 month) treatment with benzodiazepines: alprazolam (Xanax), clonazepam (Klonopin), lorazepam (Ativan), diazepam (Valium)
- Adjustment disorder with anxiety mood:
  - ▶ Benzodiazepines
- Generalized anxiety disorder:
  - ▶ Azapirones: buspirone (BuSpar)
- Panic disorder:
  - ▶ Tricyclic antidepressants (TCAs): imipramine (Tofranil)
  - ▶ Serotonin reuptake inhibitors (SRIs): fluoxetine (Prozac), sertraline (Zoloft) paroxetine (Paxil)
- Obsessive-compulsive disorder:
  - ▶ Clomipramine (Anafranil)
  - ▶ SRIs: fluoxetine (Prozac), sertraline (Zoloft), paroxetine (Paxil)

CONTRAINDICATIONS

- Benzodiazepines: first-trimester pregnancy, acute alcohol intoxication with depressed vital signs, acute glaucoma, sleep apnea, history of personality disorder, or substance abuse. Long-term use should be avoided.
- Buspirone: concurrent monoamine oxidase (MAO) inhibitor use
- TCAs: acute myocardial infarction (heart attack)

PRECAUTIONS

Drugs used for anxiety have numerous precautions; read drug product information.

DRUG INTERACTIONS

- Benzodiazepines: cimetidine, disulfiram, oral contraceptives, ethanol, levodopa, rifampin
- Buspirone: MAO inhibitors
- TCAs: amphetamines, barbiturates, guanethidine, clonidine, epinephrine, ethanol, norepinephrine, MAO inhibitors, propoxyphene
- SRIs: MAO inhibitors

OTHER DRUGS

- Generalized anxiety disorder: short-term use of benzodiazepine or TCAs
- Panic disorder: TCAs, SRIs, benzodiazepines, MAO inhibitors
- Obsessive-compulsive disorder: fluoxetine (Prozac), sertraline (Zoloft), paroxetine (Paxil)

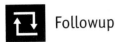

Followup

PATIENT MONITORING

- The doctor should be seen on a regular basis.
- Associated depression should be noted if it develops and treated.
- Drug therapy should be evaluated.

PREVENTION

- Manage stress to the extent possible.
- Learn relaxation techniques or meditation.

COMPLICATIONS

- Impaired social/occupational functioning
- Drug dependence (benzodiazepines)
- Cardiac rhythm disturbances (TCAs)

WHAT TO EXPECT

- With proper treatment, excellent results can be expected, especially with short-term anxiety disorders, including panic disorder.
- Obsessive-compulsive disorder and post-traumatic stress disorder are more difficult to treat, often requiring longer-term psychotherapy and medication.

Miscellaneous

OTHER FACTORS

N/A

PEDIATRIC

Reduced dosage of medications

GERIATRIC

Reduced dosage of medications

OTHERS

N/A

PREGNANCY

- Benzodiazepines: These drugs are contraindicated in first-trimester pregnancy and should be used with caution later in pregnancy and during lactation. They may cause lethargy and weight loss in nursing infants; avoid breast feeding if taking benzodiazepines.
- TCAs: There is some evidence of fetal risk, especially in first trimester.
- SRIs: Taper and discontinue, if possible, in first trimester; they may be used later in pregnancy.

FURTHER INFORMATION

- American Academy of Family Physicians Foundation, P.O. Box 8418, Kansas City, MO 64114, (800) 274-2237, ext. 4400
- National Institute of Mental Health (NIMH)—National Anxiety Awareness Program, 9000 Rockville Pike, Bethesda, MD 20892

Appendicitis, Acute

 Basics

DESCRIPTION

Acute appendicitis is the acute inflammation of the vermiform appendix. It must be treated promptly by surgical removal to avoid rupture of the appendix, which can be life-threatening.

SIGNS AND SYMPTOMS

- Abdominal pain around the navel that later moves to the right lower quadrant of the abdomen. Pain is lessened by flexing the thigh.
- Anorexia (almost 100%)
- Nausea (90%)
- Mild vomiting (75%)
- Severe constipation
- Mild diarrhea
- Sequence of symptom appearance in 95% of persons: anorexia, then abdominal pain, then vomiting
- Slight temperature elevation
- Slightly fast heartbeat

CAUSES

Obstruction of the appendix opening in the digestive tract

SCOPE

Acute appendicitis affects about 10 out of 100,000 persons. About 1 in 15 persons (7%) will have acute appendicitis at some point in their life. It is the most common acute surgical condition of the abdomen.

MOST OFTEN AFFECTED

- Between the ages of 10 and 30, appendicitis is more common in males than females.
- Among those over age 30, males and females are affected in equal numbers.

RISK FACTORS

- Adolescent males
- Family member with a history of appendicitis
- Abdominal tumors

 Diagnosis

WHAT THE DOCTOR LOOKS FOR

- The doctor will perform a thorough physical examination, including checking for several classic signs of appendicitis.
- A rectal digital exam may be done to assess the appendix.
- Other conditions that may cause similar symptoms should be investigated, such as urologic causes, inflammatory bowel disease, colonic disorders, and gynecologic diseases.

TESTS AND PROCEDURES

- Blood tests, urinalysis
- Imaging may be done to assist in diagnosis, including ultrasound, X-ray of the abdomen, barium enema, and computed tomography (CT scan).
- Internal organs may be visually inspected by laparoscopy.

 Treatment

GENERAL MEASURES

Acute appendicitis is usually managed by inpatient surgery.

ACTIVITY

- Walking soon after surgery
- Return to full activity by 4 to 6 weeks

DIET

Regular diet with return of bowel function, usually within 24 to 48 hours after surgery

 Medications

COMMONLY PRESCRIBED DRUGS

Antibiotics: cefoxitin (Mefoxin), cefotetan (Cefotan)

CONTRAINDICATIONS

Documented allergy to specific antibiotic

PRECAUTIONS

Read drug product information.

DRUG INTERACTIONS

Read drug product information.

OTHER DRUGS

- Metronidazole (Flagyl)
- Ampicillin-sulbactam (Unasyn)
- Ticarcillin-clavulanate (Timentin)

 Followup

PATIENT MONITORING

- The doctor should be seen at 2 and 6 weeks after surgery.
- Contact the physician if anorexia, nausea, vomiting, abdominal pain, fever, or chills develop after surgery.

PREVENTION

N/A

COMPLICATIONS

- Wound infection
- Abdominal abscess
- Intestinal problems

WHAT TO EXPECT

- Young adults who have nonruptured appendicitis generally have a good course of recovery.
- Risks of complications increase with age and presence of ruptured appendix.

 Miscellaneous

OTHER FACTORS

N/A

PEDIATRIC

- Rare in infancy
- Higher fever, more vomiting
- May return to full activities earlier

GERIATRIC

Patients over 60 years of age account for 50% of deaths from acute appendicitis.

OTHERS

N/A

PREGNANCY

N/A

FURTHER INFORMATION

N/A

Arteriosclerotic Heart Disease

 Basics

DESCRIPTION

Arteriosclerosis, also called "hardening of the arteries" or coronary artery disease, involves the thickening of the arterial wall that, along with loss of elasticity of the artery, progressively blocks the coronary arteries supplying the heart. The process is chronic, developing over many years, and is the most common cause of cardiovascular disability and death. High levels of cholesterol and low-density lipoproteins in the bloodstream are involved in the development of arteriosclerosis.

SIGNS AND SYMPTOMS

- May not cause symptoms, even in advanced stages
- Chest pain
- Difficulty breathing
- Easier to breathe sitting up
- Shortness of breath during sleep
- Rapid or irregular heartbeat
- Swelling of the ankles

CAUSES

- Deposits of fats and cholesterol within blood vessels (atherosclerosis)
- Narrowing of coronary arteries
- Blood clot formation
- Lesions within the blood vessels

SCOPE

Arteriosclerotic heart disease is common in the United States. It is responsible for 35% of deaths among men 35-50 years of age. The death rate among persons 55-64 years of age is about 1%.

MOST OFTEN AFFECTED

Peak symptoms are seen in men 50-60 years of age, women 60-70 years of age. Men are affected more often than women. The tendency to develop arteriosclerotic heart disease is inheritable.

RISK FACTORS

- High levels of cholesterol and fats in the bloodstream

- Smoking
- Family history of premature arteriosclerosis
- Obesity
- High blood pressure
- Stress
- Sedentary life style
- Increasing age
- Male gender
- Postmenopausal women
- Diabetes mellitus

 Diagnosis

WHAT THE DOCTOR LOOKS FOR

The physician will take a history and perform a thorough physical examination, particularly listening to the heart and lungs.

TESTS AND PROCEDURES

- Blood tests
- Chest X-ray
- An electrocardiogram (EKG) may be done to assess the heart's electrical activity.
- An exercise stress test may be done to measure how the heart responds while working.
- Special imaging procedures may be done to evaluate the heart and related structures, such as a stress thallium test, angiography, and echocardiography.

 Treatment

GENERAL MEASURES

- Arteriosclerotic heart disease is managed on an outpatient basis except for episodes of acute ischemia (decreased oxygen supply to the heart) that require hospitalization.
- Prevention of further progression of the disease:
  - ▶ Stop smoking
  - ▶ Treatment of high cholesterol (diet, drugs)
  - ▶ Control of blood pressure
  - ▶ Diabetes mellitus treated early and adequately
  - ▶ Exercise

- ▶ Aspirin to prevent blood clots
- ▶ Stress reduction
- ▶ Diet changes
- ▶ Weight loss
- ▶ Estrogen replacement therapy (ERT) in postmenopausal women
- Treatment of complications: angina, heart attack, heart failure, stroke, etc.

ACTIVITY

Exercise may be helpful in preventing and treating heart disease.

DIET

- Low-fat (20-30 grams of fat/day total intake) diet
- Weight-loss diet, if obesity a problem
- Increase soluble fiber

 ## Medications

COMMONLY PRESCRIBED DRUGS

- Aspirin: one 325 mg tablet per day unless contraindicated, to prevent blood clots from forming in the coronary arteries. Do not take daily aspirin without a doctor's permission.
- Cholesterol-lowering agents: cholestyramine, colestipol, nicotinic acid, gemfibrozil, probucol, pravastatin (Pravachol), lovastatin (Mevacor), fluvastatin (Lescol)

CONTRAINDICATIONS

Read drug product information.

PRECAUTIONS

Read drug product information.

DRUG INTERACTIONS

Read drug product information.

OTHER DRUGS

- Ticlopidine: prevents clots

 ## Followup

PATIENT MONITORING

- Health status should be monitored regularly.
- Preventive programs (weight loss, smoking cessation)

PREVENTION

See General measures.

COMPLICATIONS

- Heart attack (myocardial infarction)
- Irregular heartbeat
- Heart failure
- Angina pectoris
- Sudden death

WHAT TO EXPECT

The outcome of arteriosclerotic heart disease varies. In many cases, the outcome is favorable. Many risk factors can be changed and improved.

 ## Miscellaneous

OTHER FACTORS

N/A

PEDIATRIC

Preventive measures can begin early (proper nutrition, exercise, weight control, etc.).

GERIATRIC

The greatest incidence of arteriosclerotic heart disease is among the elderly.

OTHERS

N/A

PREGNANCY

Arteriosclerotic heart disease is practically nonexistent in pregnant women.

FURTHER INFORMATION

American Heart Association, 7320 Greenville Avenue, Dallas, TX 75231, (214) 373-6300

Arthritis, Osteo

 Basics

DESCRIPTION

Osteoarthritis (OA) is the most common form of joint disease. It involves progressive loss of cartilage and changes of the joint and bone.

SIGNS AND SYMPTOMS

- Joint pain that develops slowly
- Pain following use of a joint
- Stiffness, especially in the morning and after sitting
- Joint enlargement
- Decreased range of motion
- Crackling sensation in joint

CAUSES

Multiple factors are implicated in the cause of OA.

SCOPE

- About 60 million Americans suffer from OA at any one time.
- OA affects 33% to almost 90% in people older than 65 years of age.

MOST OFTEN AFFECTED

- Persons over 40 years of age
- OA is the leading cause of disability in people older than 65 years of age.
- Male and females affected in equal proportions

RISK FACTORS

- Age over 50
- Obesity
- Prolonged occupational or sports stress
- Injury to a joint

 Diagnosis

WHAT THE DOCTOR LOOKS FOR

- The doctor will perform a thorough physical examination.

- Other causes of similar symptoms should be investigated, such as other forms of arthritis, cancer, or bone disorders.

TESTS AND PROCEDURES

- Blood tests
- A sample of joint fluid may be obtained for analysis.
- X-rays may be taken of the affected joints.

 Treatment

GENERAL MEASURES

- OA is managed in the outpatient setting.
- Weight reduction if obese
- General fitness program
- Heat (local, tub baths, etc.)
- Physical therapy to maintain or regain joint motion and muscle strength.
- Protect joints from overuse (e.g., cane, crutches, walker, neck collar, elastic knee support).
- Surgery may be required for advanced disease.

ACTIVITY

As active as tolerated

DIET

No special diet

 Medications

COMMONLY PRESCRIBED DRUGS

- Pain relief: acetaminophen, ibuprofen, salsalate, choline-magnesium salicylate
- Other nonsteroidal anti-inflammatory drugs (NSAIDs)
- Narcotic painkillers: codeine, oxycodone, propoxyphene

CONTRAINDICATIONS

NSAIDs are relatively contraindicated for individuals with kidney disease, heart failure, hypertension, peptic ulcer, or allergy to NSAIDs or aspirin.

PRECAUTIONS

Drugs used to treat OA have many precautions. Read drug product information.

DRUG INTERACTIONS

- NSAIDs reduce effectiveness of ACE inhibitors and diuretics.
- Aspirin and NSAIDs may increase effects of anticoagulants.
- Aspirin may interfere with diabetes medication.
- Aspirin and other NSAIDs should not be taken together.

OTHER DRUGS

- Drug therapy should be tailored to symptoms and changed if not effective.
- Anti-inflammatory drugs: magnesium salicylate, choline salicylate
- Capsaicin cream is a topical application that relieves pain. It is most effective in small joints of the hand. It may cause a local burning sensation.

 ## Followup

PATIENT MONITORING

- The doctor should be seen regularly to monitor health status and drug therapy.
- Tests should be periodically done to detect gastrointestinal bleeding caused by NSAIDs.

PREVENTION

N/A

COMPLICATIONS

- Side effects of medication
- Infection or accelerated cartilage loss

WHAT TO EXPECT

- OA tends to be progressive.
- Early in disease, pain is relieved by rest.
- As disease develops, pain may occur at rest and at night.
- Joint enlargement occurs later due to bony enlargement.
- Spurs may form, especially at joint margins, as disease progresses.

 ## Miscellaneous

OTHER FACTORS

N/A

PEDIATRIC

N/A

GERIATRIC

- Becomes increasingly common with age
- Almost universal in persons over 65 years of age

OTHERS

N/A

PREGNANCY

NSAIDs pose some risk to the fetus during pregnancy; however, they may be taken while breast-feeding.

FURTHER INFORMATION

American Academy of Family Physicians Foundation, P.O. Box 8418, Kansas City, MO 64114, (800) 274-2237, ext. 4400

Arthritis, Rheumatoid (RA)

 ## Basics

DESCRIPTION

Rheumatoid arthritis (RA) is a chronic, systemic, inflammatory disease of unknown cause that tends to involve the joints. The disease also causes effects throughout the body, including the nervous system, heart, and other internal organs.

SIGNS AND SYMPTOMS

- Joints
  - ▶ Most often involved are wrists, knees, elbows, shoulders, ankles, and feet
  - ▶ Swelling
  - ▶ Sensation of heat
  - ▶ Deformity
  - ▶ Morning stiffness
  - ▶ Pain
- Fatigue
- Depression
- Malaise
- Anorexia
- Anemia
- Swollen glands
- Eye disease

CAUSES

Immune disorder; cause unknown

SCOPE

- RA affects 0.3-1.5% of the population.
- Women are affected twice as often as men, although men tend to show more signs of systemic disease.
- Prevalence in Native Americans is 3.5-5.3%.

MOST OFTEN AFFECTED

Persons 30-60 years of age. RA tends to run in families.

RISK FACTORS

- Genetic factors
- Family history
- Native American ethnicity
- Female gender, 20-50 years of age

 ## Diagnosis

WHAT THE DOCTOR LOOKS FOR

- The doctor will perform a thorough physical examination.
- Other possible cause of similar signs and symptoms will be investigated, such as bone disorders, infection, or inflammatory diseases.

TESTS AND PROCEDURES

- Blood tests to look for signs of infection and inflammation
- A sample of joint fluid may be obtained for analysis
- X-rays may be taken to monitor progress of the disease
- Special imaging procedures may be done to assist in diagnosis, including arthrography, bone scan, computed tomography (CT scan), and magnetic resonance imaging (MRI).

 ## Treatment

GENERAL MEASURES

- RA is managed on an outpatient basis except for complicating emergencies or orthopedic procedures.
- The emphasis of therapy is on exercise and mobility and general health care.
- Special emphasis should be placed on reduction of joint stress and physical and occupational therapy.

ACTIVITY

- Full activity is encouraged, but heavy work and vigorous exercise during acute episodes should be avoided.
- Hydrotherapy or water exercise is effective.

DIET

No special diet

Medications

COMMONLY PRESCRIBED DRUGS

- Early disease or acute/chronic inflammation: aspirin or other nonsteroidal anti-inflammatory drugs (NSAIDs)
- Severe disease: corticosteroids
- Persistent disease activity:
  - ▶ Steroid injections
  - ▶ Antimalarials: hydroxychloroquine (Plaquenil)
  - ▶ Gold: auranofin
  - ▶ Sulfasalazine
  - ▶ Penicillamine (d-penicillamine)
  - ▶ Methotrexate

CONTRAINDICATIONS

Depends on drugs used. Read drug product information.

PRECAUTIONS

Some drugs require careful monitoring of disease activity and signs of drug toxicity.

DRUG INTERACTIONS

- Many drugs interfere with NSAIDs, including antacids, anticoagulants, diabetes medication, blood pressure medication, and numerous others.
- Read drug product information.

OTHER DRUGS

N/A

 Followup

PATIENT MONITORING

- The doctor should be seen regularly for evaluation of RA and the effectiveness of therapy.
- Blood tests should be repeated periodically.

PREVENTION

- Oral contraceptive may decrease risk of RA.

COMPLICATIONS

- Joint destruction

- Skin disorders
- Heart disease
- Respiratory disease
- Other medical disorders
- Complications induced by treatment

WHAT TO EXPECT

The usual course of RA has been a progressive decline in function. Proper medical, surgical, and physiotherapeutic interventions can significantly improve the outcome.

 Miscellaneous

OTHER FACTORS

N/A

PEDIATRIC

N/A

GERIATRIC

- Onset in geriatric population is less common.
- Elderly have less tolerance to medication and increased incidence of side effects.

OTHERS

N/A

PREGNANCY

- Labor/delivery pose no serious problems, unless the mother has severe joint disease (e.g., hips).
- More than 75% of RA patients experience improvement during pregnancy. The cause of improvement unclear. Relapse invariably occurs within 6 months after delivery.
- No increased number of birth defects have been reported due to RA itself.

FURTHER INFORMATION

American Rheumatism Association, (800) 282-7023

Asthma

 Basics

DESCRIPTION

Asthma, also called reactive airway disease, is marked by mild to severe obstruction of flow through the airway. Symptoms range from coughing to difficulty breathing and usually have a sudden onset.

- The clinical hallmark of asthma is wheezing, but some patients may complain primarily of only a cough.
- Acute symptoms are caused by the narrowing of large and small airways due to spasm of bronchial smooth muscle, swelling and inflammation of airway tissues, and the production of mucus.

SIGNS AND SYMPTOMS

- Wheezing
- Cough
- Difficulty breathing
- Symptoms that become periodically acute
- Attacks during sleep
- A bluish discoloration of the skin around the eyes, lips, and nail beds.
- Increased heart rate

CAUSES

- Allergies to pollens, molds, house dust, mites, animal dander, feather pillows
- Other factors: smoke and other pollutants, infection, sinusitis, aspirin, exercise, gastroesophageal reflux, sleep

SCOPE

- There are 10 million new cases of asthma each year. However, lack of a uniform definition of asthma leads to confusion about the diagnosis.
- Asthma affects 7-19% of children
- Asthma is a leading cause of missed school days, about 7.5 million days annually.

MOST OFTEN AFFECTED

- Asthma can occur at any age, but primarily affects young adults (16-30 years of age).
- Half of asthma cases occur in children younger than 10 years of age.
- Asthma is more common in males during childhood until puberty and is more common in females among adults.
- Asthma and allergies tend to run in families. Search for an asthma gene is presently underway.

RISK FACTORS

- Family history of asthma
- Viral infection of the lower respiratory tract during infancy

 Diagnosis

WHAT THE DOCTOR LOOKS FOR

- The doctor will evaluate breathing status and the severity of symptoms.
- The doctor will rule out possible causes related to the heart, such as congestive heart failure or mitral valve prolapse.
- Other causes of breathing difficulty include infection, cystic fibrosis, or a foreign body in the airway.
- May be associated with sinusitis or irritation of the esophagus due to reflux (heartburn)

TESTS AND PROCEDURES

- Blood tests may be done to determine the presence of inflammation or infection.
- The levels of salt in the sweat of a child with chronic asthma should be measured to make sure he or she does not have cystic fibrosis.
- In severe cases, arterial blood may be drawn to measure levels of oxygen and carbon dioxide.
- A chest x-ray may be performed to assess the respiratory system.
- Pulmonary function tests may be performed to evaluate breathing and detect reversible airway obstruction.
- Allergy testing may be done to identify causes of asthma.
- Exercise tolerance testing may be done to assess the impact of physical activity.
- Patients may be given peak flow meters for self-assessment of breathing status.

 Treatment

GENERAL MEASURES

- Asthma is usually treated on an outpatient basis.
- A person may be hospitalized if asthma is not relieved by medication.
- Sources of irritants at the home and workplace should be eliminated.
- Anti-inflammatory drugs, such as cromolyn sodium and inhaled steroids, are used to prevent the development of symptoms.
- Dosages of beta-agonist drugs are increased in response to symptoms.
- The person with asthma may be treated for allergies.
- Education about asthma and its management is essential for well-being.

ACTIVITY

A person with asthma should have no restrictions on activity if diagnosed early and properly treated.

DIET

No special diet

 Medications

COMMONLY PRESCRIBED DRUGS

- Five major classes of drugs are used:
  ▶ Cromoglycate and nedocromil
  ▶ Steroids (beclomethasone, prednisone)
  ▶ Beta-agonists (albuterol, bitolterol, salmeterol)
  ▶ Methylxanthines (theophylline)
  ▶ Anticholinergics (atropine, ipratropium bromide)
- Mild asthma (brief wheezing once or twice a week):
  ▶ Intermittent use of beta-agonist by nebulizer or metered dose inhaler (MDI)
  ▶ Oral beta-agonist or theophylline may be prescribed.
- Moderate asthma: (weekly symptoms interfering with sleep or exercise, occasional visits to an emergency department, peak flow rate 60-80% of predicted)
  ▶ Regular maintenance schedule
  ▶ Inhaled steroids (beclomethasone diproprionate)
  ▶ Cromolyn sodium four times a day or nedocromil twice a day may be prescribed.
  ▶ If asthma is not controlled with inhaled steroid, the doctor may prescribe slow-release xanthines by mouth or inhaled ipratropium bromide.
  ▶ Acute episodes are treated with inhaled beta-agonists and steroids.

Asthma

- Severe asthma: (frequent symptoms affecting activity, nocturnal symptoms, frequent hospital stays, peakflow rate less than 60% predicted)
  - ▶ Cromolyn sodium and ipratropium
  - ▶ Inhaled steroids; some patients may need oral steroids every other day.
  - ▶ Theophylline is often useful, particularly for nighttime symptoms.
- Acute episode—outpatient management
  - ▶ Inhaled beta-agonist (albuterol)
  - ▶ Short course of steroids
  - ▶ Observation for at least 1 hour
- Delivery systems
  - ▶ Children younger than 2 years of age: nebulizer or MDI with valved spacer and mask
  - ▶ Children 2-4 years of age: MDI and valved spacer
  - ▶ Over 5 years of age: MDI or powder inhaler
- Hospital management
  - ▶ Intravenous (IV) steroids
  - ▶ Other medications may be given by inhalation or IV if symptoms do not improve.
  - ▶ In rare cases, mechanical ventilation may be needed to support breathing.

CONTRAINDICATIONS

- Sedatives
- Beta-adrenergic blocking drugs should be avoided.

PRECAUTIONS

Chronic use of beta-agonists can result in harmful effects. Use only when experiencing symptoms of asthma. Chronic asthma may require chronic use of beta-agonists.

DRUG INTERACTIONS

Some antibiotics increase levels of theophylline.

OTHER DRUGS

- Ketotifen
- H1-antagonists
- Troleandomycin (TAO)
- Methotrexate
- Immune globulin, intravenous (IVIG)
- Furosemide (Lasix)

Followup

PATIENT MONITORING

- The person with asthma may be given a device to monitor peak flow rates while at home. The patient should keep a record to track trends and report if flow drops below 70% of baseline.
- The patient should have blood drawn periodically for testing, including arterial blood for blood gases and pH.
- The doctor may order a test called oximetry that measures the oxygen-carrying ability of blood.
- The patient should be tested for tuberculosis annually.

PREVENTION

- Management of asthma by the patient is essential. A person with asthma should:
  - ▶ Understand medication, inhalers, nebulizers, peak flow meters
  - ▶ Monitor his or her symptoms and peak flows
  - ▶ Have written guidelines prepared by a doctor
  - ▶ Have pre-arranged action plan for an acute episode
- If symptoms are severe, control triggering factors: pollutants, exercise, mites, molds, animal dander.
- Have flu shots every year.
- Avoid the use of aspirin.
- Avoid sulfites and tartrazine (food additives).

COMPLICATIONS

- Collapsed lung, pneumothorax, or other lung conditions.
- Respiratory failure; mechanical ventilation may be needed to support breathing.
- Death

WHAT TO EXPECT

- In most cases, the outcome is excellent with attention to general health and use of medications to control symptoms.
- Less than 50% of children with asthma "outgrow it."
- If the response to treatment is poor, the doctor should review the diagnosis and compliance with therapy before prescribing stronger drugs.

Miscellaneous

OTHER FACTORS

N/A

PEDIATRIC

Half of new cases of asthma occur in children younger than 10 years of age.

GERIATRIC

It is unusual for an initial episode of asthma to occur in an elderly person.

OTHERS

N/A

PREGNANCY

- About 50% of asthma patients have no change in symptoms during pregnancy, 25% seem to improve, and 25% have worse symptoms.
- It is important to prevent stress during pregnancy.
- Avoid medications that are contraindicated during pregnancy.

FURTHER INFORMATION

- American Lung Association, 1740 Broadway, New York, NY 10019, (212)315-8700
- Asthma and Allergy Foundation of America, 1125 15th St., NW, Washington, DC 20005, (800)7-ASTHMA, (800)727-8462

Attention Deficit Hyperactivity Disorder

 Basics

DESCRIPTION

Attention deficit hyperactivity disorder (ADHD), also called hyperactivity, is a behavior problem marked by a short attention span, low frustration tolerance, impulsivity, distractibility, and usually, hyperactivity. ADHD can result in poor school performance, difficulty in peer relationships, and parent/child conflict.

SIGNS AND SYMPTOMS

- Fidgets
- Difficulty remaining seated
- Easily distracted
- Can't wait turn
- Blurts out answers before question is complete
- Difficulty following instructions
- Difficulty sustaining attention
- Shifts from one uncompleted task to another
- Difficulty playing quietly
- Talks excessively
- Interrupts others
- Doesn't seem to be listening
- Loses things
- Engages in physically dangerous activities without considering consequences

CAUSES

Multiple factors

SCOPE

ADHD affects about 5% of school-aged children.

MOST OFTEN AFFECTED

- Onset before 7 years old
- Lasts into adolescence and adulthood
- 50% can be diagnosed by age 4
- May affect more than one family member
- Males affected 4-6 times more often than females

RISK FACTORS

- Poor prenatal health (preeclampsia, drug and alcohol use, smoking)
- Associated with, but not caused by, other conditions:
  - ▶ Learning disabilities

- ▶ Tourette's syndrome
- ▶ Mood disorders
- ▶ Conduct disorder

 Diagnosis

WHAT THE DOCTOR LOOKS FOR

- The doctor will obtain a history and perform a thorough physical examination of the patient.
- Other possible causes of the behavior will be investigated, such as learning disability or hearing/vision disorder.

TEST AND PROCEDURES

- Laboratory testing rarely needed
- Lead level in the blood may be measured.
- Behavioral or psychological testing may be performed.

 Treatment

GENERAL MEASURES

- ADHD is managed in the outpatient setting.
- Doctor and parents must work closely with teachers and other school officials.
- Avoid unproved therapies.
- Reinforce good behavior with rewards and attention.
- Make eye contact with each request.
- Keep child on one task at a time.
- Administer time-out (brief) for problems.
- Stop behavior before it escalates.
- Find things the child is good at and emphasize these tasks.
- Some families benefit from "anger training," "social training," and family therapy.
- Keep realistic expectations during growth stages (newborn to adulthood).
- Discuss pros and cons of drug therapy with doctor.
- Parents may need help dealing with feelings (guilt, shame, anxiety, exhaustion, and blame).
- At school:
  - ▶ Keep work sessions short.
  - ▶ Make sure rules are clear.

Attention Deficit Hyperactivity Disorder

▶ Consequences for unacceptable behavior must be immediate.

▶ Reinforce good behavior.

▶ Teachers should coordinate homework with parent (child may not bring home messages).

ACTIVITY

• Allow for increased activity in safe environment.
• Children with ADHD often respond well to water play/bathtubs.

DIET

• No dietary changes have been proven to help ADHD.
• Parents can experiment with nonharmful diets by eliminating sugar, dyes, additives.

COMMONLY PRESCRIBED DRUGS

• Methylphenidate (Ritalin)
• Pemoline (Cylert)
• Dosage should start low and be increased as needed.
• Some physicians give "holidays" off drugs in the summer, and a few patients can have weekend "holidays."
• Some children experience withdrawal (tearfulness, agitation) after a missed dose.

PRECAUTIONS

Don't crush sustained-release tablets.

DRUG INTERACTIONS

N/A

OTHER DRUGS

• Dextroamphetamine (Dexedrine)
• Clonidine
• Tricyclics

 Followup

PATIENT MONITORING

• Person with ADHD and family should be tested regularly.
• The doctor should be seen at least every 3 months to monitor medication.

PREVENTION

• Children are at risk for abuse, depression, and social isolation.
• Parents need regular support and advice.
• Establish contact with teacher each school year.

COMPLICATIONS

• Medications can cause headaches, abdominal pain, growth delay.
• Untreated ADHD can lead to failing in school, parental abuse, social isolation, poor self-esteem.

WHAT TO EXPECT

• ADHD lasts through school years and into adulthood.
• The condition becomes easier to control with increasing age.
• Encourage career choices that allow autonomy and mobility.
• There is no increased incidence of delinquency unless other conditions exist (e.g., conduct disorder).

 Miscellaneous

OTHER FACTORS

N/A

PEDIATRIC

N/A

GERIATRIC

N/A

OTHERS

N/A

PREGNANCY

Avoid stimulants in pregnancy.

FURTHER INFORMATION

N/A

Section B

Balanitis

 Basics

DESCRIPTION

Balanitis is the inflammation of the glans penis.

SIGNS AND SYMPTOMS

- Penile pain
- Difficult or painful urination
- Infection
- Reddening
- Swelling of the prepuce (foreskin)
- Ulcers or plaques

CAUSES

- Allergic reaction (condom latex, contraceptive jelly)
- Fungal and bacterial infections
- Drug side effects
- Other medical causes

SCOPE

N/A

MOST OFTEN AFFECTED

Adult males

RISK FACTORS

- Presence of foreskin (uncircumcised)
- Oral antibiotics in male infants can predispose to infection.

 Diagnosis

WHAT THE DOCTOR LOOKS FOR

- The doctor will perform a physical examination and consider other possible causes of similar signs and symptoms.
- The doctor will check for known associated conditions, such as diabetes mellitus.

TESTS AND PROCEDURES

- Blood tests
- Cells or fluid may be analyzed in the laboratory.

 Treatment

GENERAL MEASURES

- Balanitis is managed in the outpatient setting.
- Warm compresses or sitz baths may relieve symptoms.
- Practice good hygiene.
- Circumcision may be considered as preventive measure.
- Avoid substances that trigger an allergic reaction.

ACTIVITY

No limitations

DIET

No special diet

 Medications

COMMONLY PRESCRIBED DRUGS

- Antifungal drugs: clotrimazole (Lotrimin), nystatin (Mycostatin)
- Antibacterial drug: bacitracin, neomycin-polymyxin B-bacitracin (Neosporin), cephalosporin, sulfa drugs
- Topical steroids

CONTRAINDICATIONS

Read drug product information.

PRECAUTIONS

Read drug product information.

DRUG INTERACTIONS

Read drug product information.

OTHER DRUGS

N/A

Followup

PATIENT MONITORING

- The doctor should be seen every 1–2 weeks until the cause of balanitis has been identified.
- Persistent inflammation may require biopsy to rule out cancer.

PREVENTION

- Proper hygiene
- Avoidance of allergy-triggering substances
- Circumcision

COMPLICATIONS

- Narrowing or scarring of the urinary opening
- Cancerous changes from chronic irritations
- Urinary tract infections

WHAT TO EXPECT

Balanitis should resolve with identification of the cause and appropriate treatment.

 Miscellaneous

OTHER FACTORS

N/A

PEDIATRIC

Oral antibiotics predispose infants to infection.

GERIATRIC

Condom-type urinary catheters can lead to balanitis.

OTHERS

N/A

PREGNANCY

N/A

FURTHER INFORMATION

N/A

Basal Cell Carcinoma

 ## Basics

DESCRIPTION

Basal cell carcinoma is a slow-growing malignant cancer of the skin. Tumors rarely spread but are capable of local tissue destruction.

SIGNS AND SYMPTOMS

- Basal cell carcinoma begins as a small, smooth-surfaced, well-defined lump on skin.
- The affected area is pink to red in color, with a pearly translucent border.
- Area may be covered with blood vessels.
- May be pigmented to varying degrees
- A crusting ulcer develops as the lesion grows.

CAUSES

Sun exposure

SCOPE

Approximately 400,000 cases occur each year in the United States.

MOST OFTEN AFFECTED

More common in fair-skin blondes and redheads. Generally affects individuals over 40 years of age, but the incidence of basal cell carcinoma is increasing in younger populations. It is more common in males than females, although the incidence is increasing in females.

RISK FACTORS

- Chronic sun exposure
- Light complexion
- Tendency to sunburn
- Male gender, although risk is increasing in women due to lifestyle changes, such as the use of tanning salons

 ## Diagnosis

WHAT THE DOCTOR LOOKS FOR

The diagnosis is confirmed by biopsy, in which a small sample of tissue is obtained by needle or surgical procedure. The tissue sample is then examined microscopically for the presence of cancer cells.

TESTS AND PROCEDURES

A sample of tissue will be examined microscopically.

 ## Treatment

GENERAL MEASURES

- Basal cell carcinoma is treated on an outpatient basis unless the lesion is extensive.
- Lesions may be surgically removed or treated with freezing or electrical devices.
- The type of treatment selected depends on the location, extent, and nature of the lesion.
- Radiation therapy may be used on patients unable to tolerate minor surgery, such as the elderly. It may also be used to preserve tissue, such as near lips and eyelids.

ACTIVITY

No restrictions on physical activity except to avoid overexposure to sun

DIET

No special diet

Medications

COMMONLY PRESCRIBED DRUGS

Topical antibiotic medication may be prescribed for the first 24–48 hours after skin cancer is removed by surgery.

CONTRAINDICATIONS

N/A

PRECAUTIONS

N/A

DRUG INTERACTIONS

N/A

OTHER DRUGS

N/A

Followup

PATIENT MONITORING

The patient is usually seen in the doctor's office or clinic every month for the first 3 months after treatment, then twice a year for 5 years and once a year thereafter.

PREVENTION

- Reduce the risk of skin cancer with the use of sunscreen lotion.
- Wear hats, long-sleeve shirts when outdoors in bright sunlight.
- Avoid excessive tanning.
- Examine the skin regularly to detect changes in moles, freckles, and other spots.

COMPLICATIONS

- The lesion could recur, which usually happens within 5 years if at all.
- The lesion could spread, which rarely occurs.

WHAT TO EXPECT

- Between 90 to 95% of people who receive proper treatment are cured.
- Most recurrences happen within 5 years.
- About 36% of patients will develop a new basal cell carcinoma lesion within 5 years.

Miscellaneous

OTHER FACTORS

N/A

PEDIATRIC

Rare in children

ELDERLY

More common among the elderly

OTHERS

N/A

PREGNANCY

N/A

FURTHER INFORMATION

N/A

Bed Wetting

 Basics

DESCRIPTION

Enuresis is involuntary urination. Nocturnal enuresis, or bed-wetting, is involuntary urination during sleep more than once a month in girls older than 5 and in boys older than 6 years of age.

SIGNS AND SYMPTOMS

- Inability to keep from urinating while asleep at least once per month.
- Some children may be withdrawn and shy; some may show aggressive behaviors.
- Stress factors such as family discord, significant life events, and psychosocial or emotional problems may be present.

CAUSES

- Hormone disorder
- Reduced bladder capacity
- Food allergies may influence bladder capacity.
- Infection
- Other urinary tract disorders

SCOPE

Enuresis affects about 10% of children.

MOST OFTEN AFFECTED

Enuresis affects 40% of 3-year olds, 10% of 6-year olds, 3% of 12-year olds, and 1% of 18-year olds. It is more common in males than females. It may be an inheritable trait.

RISK FACTORS

- History of enuresis in one or both parents
- First-born child

 Diagnosis

WHAT THE DOCTOR LOOKS FOR

- The doctor will perform a physical examination to rule out causes of enuresis, such as infection, diabetes, or other disorders.

TESTS AND PROCEDURES

- Urinalysis and culture
- Pregnancy test, if indicated
- The volume of the bladder may be measured by urinating into a measuring cup.
- Imaging that may be performed includes ultrasound, intravenous pyelogram, and voiding cystourethrogram.
- X-rays of the spine may be obtained.

 Treatment

GENERAL MEASURES

- Enuresis is managed in the outpatient setting.
- Counseling and behavior modification
- Encourage daytime fluids and less frequent urination to help increase bladder size.
- Discourage any fluids during the 2 hours prior to bedtime.
- Protect the bed from urine by covering the mattress with plastic, have the child wear extra thick underwear (not diapers), and put a towel on the bed in the area of the child's bottom.
- Encourage the child to take responsibility for the problem.
- Encourage the child to get up to urinate during the night, but parents should not awaken the child to urinate.

Bed Wetting

- When enuresis occurs, the child should rinse pajamas and underwear and the towel.
- Do not punish the child for wet nights, but act sympathetically.
- Heap praise on the child for dry nights. A calendar for gold stars or happy faces can be used as an incentive.
- Bladder stretching exercises may be helpful.
- Self-awakening or hypnotherapy programs may be helpful.
- Bed-wetting alarms have the greatest rate of success (70%) and the lowest rate of relapse (30%).

ACTIVITY

No restrictions

DIET

No fluids for 2 hours prior to bedtime

 ## Medications

COMMONLY PRESCRIBED DRUGS

Tricyclic antidepressants: imipramine, desipramine

CONTRAINDICATIONS

Read drug product information.

PRECAUTIONS

Imipramine is one of the leading causes of childhood drug-related deaths in the United States, usually from unintentional overdose; read drug product information.

DRUG INTERACTIONS

Read drug product information.

OTHER DRUGS

Desmopressin (DDAVP)

 ## Followup

PATIENT MONITORING

The doctor should be seen as often as necessary.

PREVENTION

No preventive measures are known.

COMPLICATIONS

Urinary tract infection

WHAT TO EXPECT

- Enuresis is a self-limited problem.
- Most children overcome the problem between ages 6 and 10, and in only very few cases does the problem persist beyond 16 years of age.
- By age 4.5 years, 12% of children will not have complete urinary control. These 12% convert to complete control at a rate of 15% per year. By puberty, only 2–3% have not achieved complete control.

 ## Miscellaneous

OTHER FACTORS

N/A

PEDIATRIC

N/A

GERIATRIC

N/A

OTHERS

N/A

PREGNANCY

N/A

FURTHER INFORMATION

N/A

Bell's Palsy

 ## Basics

DESCRIPTION

Bell's palsy is the paralysis or weakness of facial muscles, usually only on one side, resulting from the inflammation of the facial nerve.
- May be a complication of zoster (shingles)
- The development of Bell's palsy on both sides of the face is highly unusual. Other possible explanations should be considered, such as Guillain-Barré syndrome and chronic meningitis.

SIGNS AND SYMPTOMS

- Total or partial paralysis of the muscles on one side of the face
- Mild numbness on the affected side
- One-sided ear ache
- Loss of flavor perception
- Excessive production of tears, or dry eye, on one side
- Develops suddenly, within hours or days

CAUSES

- Inflammation of the facial nerve
- Infection, usually viral
- Exposure to cold
- Cause may be unknown

SCOPE

Bell's palsy affects about 25 in 100,000 persons.

MOST OFTEN AFFECTED

Affects all ages, but it is most common among individuals over 30 years of age. Males and females are affected equally often. Bell's palsy tends to run in families.

RISK FACTORS

- Age over 30 years
- Exposure to a cold environment

 ## Diagnosis

WHAT THE DOCTOR LOOKS FOR

- The doctor will evaluate the extent of facial paralysis and related signs and symptoms.
- Other causes of signs and symptoms, including infection, cancer and nerve conditions, should be considered as possible explanations for the symptoms.
- The patient should be observed for corneal abrasions caused by dry eye.

TESTS AND PROCEDURES

- A sample of cerebrospinal fluid (CSF) may be obtained by spinal tap. Analysis of CFS may reveal signs of inflammation or infection.
- Magnetic resonance imaging (MRI) may be done to make sure a lesion or tumor is not affecting the nerves or bone.
- A test known as electromyography may be performed to measure and record the electrical activity of facial muscles.
- Tests may be done to evaluate the conduction of impulses along the nerve.
- The doctor may test the blink reflex by tickling or stimulating the eyelashes.

 ## Treatment

GENERAL MEASURES

- Typically managed on an outpatient basis
- Surgery is rarely performed.
- Cover the eye on the affected side with a patch.
- Lubricating drops may be prescribed if the eye is dry.

ACTIVITY

No limitations on physical activity. Caution should be used when performing activities that require keen depth perception.

DIET

No special diet

Medications

COMMONLY PRESCRIBED DRUGS

A course of steroids should begin immediately after onset of Bell's palsy. There is little benefit in starting steroids after 4 days.

CONTRAINDICATIONS

Pre-existing infections, such as tuberculosis

PRECAUTIONS

Steroids should be used with caution in pregnancy, peptic ulcer disease, and diabetes.

DRUG INTERACTIONS

May interact with vaccines

OTHER DRUGS

N/A

 ## Followup

PATIENT MONITORING

- The patient should be evaluated once a month for 6 to 12 months.
- The eye should be examined for signs of corneal abrasion.

PREVENTION

N/A

COMPLICATIONS

- Steroids may unmask infection, such as tuberculosis.
- Steroids may cause psychological disturbances.
- Corneal abrasion and ulceration

WHAT TO EXPECT

Recovery of function may be partial or complete, and in some cases there is no recovery at all. Patients with partial nerve loss typically fully recover. Patients with total nerve loss usually partially recover and may have long-term complications such as tearing or spasm of facial muscles.

 ## Miscellaneous

OTHER FACTORS

N/A

PEDIATRIC

N/A

GERIATRIC

N/A

OTHERS

N/A

PREGNANCY

Steroids should be used cautiously if the patient is pregnant. Primary care provider should consult with the patient's obstetrician.

FURTHER INFORMATION

N/A

Blepharitis

 Basics

DESCRIPTION

Blepharitis is an inflammation of the edge of the eyelid. It occurs as an ulcerous form or nonulcerous form. It commonly occurs as a combination of both forms.

SIGNS AND SYMPTOMS

- Ulcerous (staph) blepharitis
  - ▶ Itching
  - ▶ Excessive tearing
  - ▶ Burning sensation
  - ▶ Light sensitivity
  - ▶ Usually worse in morning
  - ▶ Recurring stye
  - ▶ Ulcerations at the base of eyelashes
  - ▶ Broken, sparse, misdirected eyelashes
- Nonulcerous (seborrheic) blepharitis
  - ▶ Reddening at the edge of the eyelid
  - ▶ Dry flakes, oily skin on lid edge and/or lashes
  - ▶ Dandruff of scalp, eyebrows
  - ▶ Sometimes reddening or flaking of skin on the nose and lips
- Mixed blepharitis (seborrheic with associated staph)
  - ▶ Most common type of blepharitis
  - ▶ Symptoms and signs of both staph and seborrheic present

SCOPE

Common; blepharitis is the most common eye disease in the United States.

MOST OFTEN AFFECTED

Adults, males and females in equal proportion

CAUSES

- Sebaceous gland dysfunction
- Bacterial (Staphylococcus) infection
- Dermatitis

RISK FACTORS

- Infection
- Dermatitis
- Rosacea
- Diabetes mellitus
- Immune system disorders

 Diagnosis

WHAT THE DOCTOR LOOKS FOR

The doctor will assess the eye and consider other similar conditions.

TESTS AND PROCEDURES

- Blood tests may be done to assist in diagnosis.
- Fluid or cells from the affected area may be analyzed in the laboratory.

 Treatment

GENERAL MEASURES

- Blepharitis is managed in an outpatient setting.
- Wash affected area with cleanser at least once daily.
- If infection is suspected, topical antibiotic should be applied with cotton-tipped swab.
- Clean lids and apply ointment nightly in mild cases, up to 4 times daily in severe cases.
- Discontinue soft contact lenses until condition clears.
- Chronic blepharitis requires referral to ophthalmologist for evaluation.

ACTIVITY

No restrictions

DIET

No restrictions

Medications

COMMONLY PRESCRIBED DRUGS

- Topical antibiotic: bacitracin, erythromycin ointment
- In some cases, oral antibiotics: tetracycline

CONTRAINDICATIONS

- Allergy to medication
- Tetracycline: not for use in pregnancy or children younger than 8 years of age

PRECAUTIONS

Tetracycline may cause photosensitivity; sunscreen is recommended.

DRUG INTERACTIONS

- Tetracycline: avoid antacids, dairy products, and iron
- Antibiotics may reduce the effectiveness of oral contraceptives.

OTHER DRUGS

Quinolones may be helpful for persistent or recurrent blepharitis.

 ## Followup

PATIENT MONITORING

The doctor should be seen every 2 months.

PREVENTION

Follow treatment guidelines.

COMPLICATIONS

- Stye
- Scarring of eyelid
- Misdirection of eyelashes
- Corneal infection

WHAT TO EXPECT

- Blepharitis is a chronic condition, prone to recurrence if hygiene is not maintained after antibiotic treatment is discontinued.
- Long-term eyelid hygiene is required to control blepharitis.

 ## Miscellaneous

OTHER FACTORS

N/A

PEDIATRIC

N/A

GERIATRIC

N/A

OTHERS

N/A

PREGNANCY

N/A

FURTHER INFORMATION

N/A

Breast Cancer

 Basics

DESCRIPTION

Breast cancer is malignant neoplasm of the breast. Breast cancers are classified as noninvasive (in situ) or invasive (infiltrating). Approximately 70% of all breast cancers have a component of invasion.

SIGNS AND SYMPTOMS

- Palpable lump (55%)
- Abnormal mammogram without a palpable mass (35%)
- Change in the color or texture of breast skin
- Dimpling of breast skin
- Nipple retraction
- Breast enlargement
- Lump in the armpit
- Bone pain (rare)

CAUSES

Unknown

SCOPE

- One in eight women in the United States will develop breast cancer within a lifetime.
- 150,000 new cases are diagnosed annually, and 50,000 women die.

MOST OFTEN AFFECTED

Women 30–80 years of age, with a peak at ages 45–65. More common in females, although 1% occurs in males. About 20% of women have a family history of breast cancer. A breast cancer gene has been identified that affects about 1 in 400 women.

RISK FACTORS

- Family history of breast cancer
- Early menarche, late menopause, no births, or first full-term pregnancy after age 30
- Women with a history of breast cancer or previous breast biopsies revealing atypical changes
- Other risk factors may include estrogen use, high dietary fat, high alcohol use

Diagnosis

WHAT THE DOCTOR LOOKS FOR

- The doctor will perform a thorough physical examination.
- Other diseases with similar signs and symptoms will be investigated, such as abscess and other benign breast conditions.
- If cancer is identified, the doctor will "stage" the disease, i.e., determine the extent of involvement.

TESTS AND PROCEDURES

- Several blood tests may be done to assist in diagnosis, particularly those to assess liver function and hormone activity.
- Chest X-ray
- Specialized radiological imaging that may be done includes mammography, ultrasound, bone scan, liver imaging, computed tomography (CT scan).
- Tissue may be obtained by biopsy for analysis in the laboratory.

 ## Treatment

GENERAL MEASURES

- Persons with breast cancer are usually treated by a team consisting of a medical oncologist, a surgeon, and a radiation oncologist.
- Treatment of breast cancer involves period of hospitalization for surgery and other treatment.
- The decision to treat with hormone therapy or chemotherapy is complex. Premenopausal women tend to respond more to cytotoxic (cell-killing) chemotherapy, and postmenopausal women tend to obtain greater benefit from hormone therapy.
- Treatment of early disease:
  - ▶ Local control measures
  - ▶ Modified radical mastectomy or lumpectomy followed by radiation
  - ▶ The optimal treatment is unclear.
- Treatment of locally advanced breast cancer:
  - ▶ Combination chemotherapy and radiation therapy prior to mastectomy
- Treatment of metastatic cancer (cancer that has spread to adjacent lymph nodes)
  - ▶ Measures to provide symptom improvement
  - ▶ Combinations of chemotherapy, hormone therapy, or radiation therapy

ACTIVITY

Minimal activity restrictions during treatment

DIET

No proven relationship exists between breast cancer and diet.

Breast Cancer

 Medications

COMMONLY PRESCRIBED DRUGS

- Chemotherapy
- Hormone therapy: tamoxifen, medroxyprogesterone, and aminoglutethimide
- Combination chemotherapy: cyclophosphamide, methotrexate, fluorouracil,
anthracyclines, taxanes

CONTRAINDICATIONS

N/A

PRECAUTIONS

Monitoring for infection is important for
patients receiving chemotherapy.

SIGNIFICANT POSSIBLE INTERACTIONS

Drug interactions are common and depend on
the combinations used. The oncologist will
provide information about drug interactions.

OTHER DRUGS

- Chemotherapy agents: vinblastine, cisplatin,
thiotepa, mitomycin, etoposide, and paclitaxel (Taxol)
- Ondansetron (Zofran), dronabinol (Marinol),
metoclopramide (Reglan), and others for
nausea control.

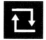 Followup

PATIENT MONITORING

- Regular followup physical examinations by the
doctor are important to detect relapses.
- Up to 60% of patients with invasive disease
will have a relapse within 5 years despite
initial therapy.

PREVENTION

- Decreasing dietary fat or alcohol has not been
shown to alter breast cancer risk.
- The synthetic anti-estrogen drug tamoxifen
may be a useful preventive agent in high-risk
women (such as those with a family history).
- Perform a monthly breast self-examination to
detect lumps, skin, or nipple changes.
- Clinical breast examination (breast examina-
tion by a doctor) should be part of the
gynecological examination.
- Mammography:
  - ▶ In women over 50 years of age, mammog-
    raphy screening can reduce breast cancer
    deaths by 30%.
  - ▶ All women over 35 years of age should
    have baseline screening mammogram.
  - ▶ Mammography should be repeated every
    1–2 years between the ages of 40–49 and
    annually after age 50.

COMPLICATIONS

- Post-operative: lymphedema, wound infection, limited shoulder motion
- Chemotherapy: nausea, vomiting, hair loss, bladder irritation, inflamed mouth, fatigue, and menstrual abnormalities
- Tamoxifen: hot flashes, menstrual irregularities including menopause, vaginal discharge, skin rashes, possibly uterine cancer
- Irradiation: skin reaction, rib fracture, swelling of the arm, pulmonary disease, and rarely second breast cancer

WHAT TO EXPECT

- 10-year survival rates:
  - ▶ Noninvasive: 95%
  - ▶ Stage I occult: 90%
  - ▶ Stage II: 40%
  - ▶ Stage III: 15%
  - ▶ Stage IV (metastatic): 0%

 Miscellaneous

OTHER FACTORS

N/A

PEDIATRIC

Breast cancer occurs rarely in children.

GERIATRIC

There is a higher percentage of hormone-positive tumors among the elderly. These cancers are responsive to hormone therapy, and thus disease-free survival may be improved.

OTHERS

N/A

PREGNANCY

Breast cancer occurs infrequently during pregnancy.

FURTHER INFORMATION

N/A

Breast Feeding

 Basics

DESCRIPTION

- Advantages
  - ▶ Babies who are breast-fed have fewer respiratory, gastrointestinal, and ear infections.
  - ▶ Breast milk is an ideal food. It is easily digestible, nutrients are well-absorbed, and breast-fed babies have less constipation.
  - ▶ Increased contact between mother and baby
  - ▶ Economical, portable, easy to meet needs quickly
  - ▶ Breast-feeding may decrease incidence of allergies in childhood.
  - ▶ Mothers often find it more convenient than bottle-feeding.
  - ▶ More rapid and complete recovery from pregnancy
- Contraindications
  - ▶ Human immunodeficiency virus (HIV) infection; active tuberculosis
  - ▶ Drugs of abuse will pass into human milk.
- Technique
  - ▶ Mother should get in comfortable position, usually sitting or reclining with baby's head in crook of mother's arm (side-lying position is often useful following C-section delivery).
  - ▶ Mother should bring baby to her, not lean toward baby, in order to avoid stress on back.
  - ▶ Baby's belly and mother's belly should face each other or touch (belly-to-belly).
  - ▶ Mother initiates the rooting reflex by tickling baby's lips with nipple or finger. As baby's mouth opens wide, mother guides her nipple to back of her baby's mouth while pulling the baby closer. This will ensure that the baby's gums are sucking on the areola, not the nipple.

SCOPE

About 56% of new mothers breast-feed in the early postpartum period and 21% were breast-feeding at 5-6 months.

MOST OFTEN AFFECTED

Females 16–45 years of age

SIGNS AND SYMPTOMS

N/A

CAUSES

N/A

RISK FACTORS

N/A

 Diagnosis

WHAT THE DOCTOR LOOKS FOR

N/A

TESTS AND PROCEDURES

N/A

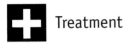 Treatment

GENERAL MEASURES

See Patient Education

ACTIVITY

No restrictions

DIET

- Adequate calorie and protein intake while nursing
- Drink plenty of fluids.
- Continue prenatal vitamins.
- Fluoride supplement unnecessary

PATIENT EDUCATION

- Consider plans after birth, e.g., if returning to work. It is possible to nurse part-time after returning to work. Some mothers wean (stop breast-feeding) the week before returning to work.
- For some mothers, an occasional supplemental bottle can be used.
- Colostrum (a fluid that appears before milk that is rich in antibodies) is present in breast at birth but may not be seen.
- Milk will not come in before third day after birth.
- Frequent nursing (at least 9 or more times in 24 hours) will lead to milk coming in sooner and in greater quantities.

- Allow baby to determine duration of each feeding; baby will lose weight the first few days and may not get back to birth weight until day 10.
- Immediately after birth, baby should stay in mother's room, as much as possible, to encourage on-demand feeding.
- Signs of adequate nursing:
  ▶ Breasts become hard before and soft after feeding
  ▶ Six or more wet diapers in 24 hours
  ▶ Baby satisfied; appropriate weight gain (average 1 ounce per day in first few months)
  ▶ Anticipate growth spurts around 10 days, 6 weeks, 3 months, and 4–6 months. Baby will nurse more often at these times for several days. More frequent feedings will increase milk production to allow for further adequate growth.
  ▶ Supplemental baby vitamins are unnecessary unless the baby has very limited exposure to sun (If this is so, then the baby needs vitamin D).

Breast Feeding

- Weaning
  - ▶ Breast milk alone is adequate food for first 6 months.
  - ▶ Solids may be introduced at 4 to 6 months.
  - ▶ For mothers going to work, start switching the baby to bottle-feeding during the hours mother will be gone about a week ahead of time. Do this by eliminating a breast-feed every few days and substituting pumped breast milk or formula, preferably given by another caregiver.
  - ▶ To increase the likelihood that baby will take a bottle occasionally, introduce it at 3 to 4 weeks and give once or twice a week.

 Medications

COMMONLY PRESCRIBED DRUGS

N/A

CONTRAINDICATIONS

N/A

PRECAUTIONS

N/A

DRUG INTERACTIONS

N/A

OTHER DRUGS

N/A

 Followup

PATIENT MONITORING

Mother and baby should be seen by the doctor within a few days of hospital discharge if she is a first-time breast-feeder.

PREVENTION

N/A

COMPLICATIONS

- Clogged ducts
  - ▶ Sore lump in 1 or both breasts without fever
  - ▶ Use moist hot packs on lump prior to and during nursing.
  - ▶ More frequent nursing on affected side
  - ▶ Use good technique.
- Mastitis (infection of the breast duct)
  - ▶ Sore lump in 1 or both breasts plus fever and/or redness on skin overlying lump
  - ▶ Use moist hot packs on lump prior to and during nursing.
  - ▶ More frequent nursing on affected side
  - ▶ Antibiotics
  - ▶ Mastitis can make a person quite ill.
  - ▶ Other possible sources of fever should be ruled out, such as uterine or kidney disorders. Get increased rest, use acetaminophen (Tylenol) as necessary.
  - ▶ Fever should resolve within 48 hours. If it does not, type of antibiotic may be changed. Lump should also resolve. If it continues, minor surgery may be required to drain abscess.

- Milk supply inadequate
  - ▶ Check baby's weight gain.
  - ▶ Review technique, frequency, and duration of nursing.
  - ▶ Supplementing with formula decreases breast milk production.
- Sore nipples
  - ▶ Check technique.
  - ▶ Take baby off the breast by breaking the suction with a finger in the mouth.
  - ▶ Air-dry nipples after each nursing.
  - ▶ Do not use breast creams
  - ▶ Do not wash nipples with soap and water.
- Engorgement
  - ▶ Usually develops after milk first comes in (day 3 or 4).
  - ▶ Signs are warm, hard, sore breasts.
  - ▶ To resolve, offer baby more frequent nursing.
  - ▶ May have to hand-express a little milk to soften areola enough to let baby latch on.
  - ▶ Nurse long enough to empty breasts.
  - ▶ Generally resolves within a day or two.
- Flat or inverted nipples
  - ▶ When stimulated, inverted nipples will retract inward, flat nipples remain flat.
  - ▶ Nipple shells, a doughnut-shaped insert, can be worn inside the bra during the last month of pregnancy to gently force the nipple through the center opening of the shell.
  - ▶ Babies can nurse successfully even if the shell does not correct the problem before birth. A lactation consultant or La Leche League member may be a good resource in this situation.

WHAT TO EXPECT

A healthy baby

 ## Miscellaneous

OTHER FACTORS

N/A

PEDIATRIC

N/A

GERIATRIC

N/A

OTHERS

N/A

PREGNANCY

N/A

FURTHER INFORMATION

N/A

Bronchitis, Acute

 Basics

DESCRIPTION

Acute bronchitis is an inflammation of the airway resulting from a respiratory tract infection. It is generally self-limited with complete healing and full return of function.

SIGNS AND SYMPTOMS

- Follows respiratory tract infection, such as a common cold (runny nose, malaise, chills, slight fever, sore throat, back and muscle pain)
- Cough: initially dry and unproductive, then productive
- Fever
- Fatigue, aching muscles
- Spitting up blood
- Burning sensation in chest
- Difficulty breathing (sometimes)
- Wheezing or noisy breathing

CAUSES

- Viral or bacterial infection
- Less often, infection by fungi or other microbe

SCOPE

Acute bronchitis is common in the United States.

MOST OFTEN AFFECTED

All ages are affected by acute bronchitis, males and females equally.

RISK FACTORS

- Chronic lung diseases
- Chronic sinusitis
- Allergies
- Enlarged tonsils and adenoids in children
- Immune system disorders
- Air pollutants

- Elderly
- Infants
- Smoking
- Second-hand smoke
- Alcoholism
- Reflux esophagitis
- Tracheostomy
- Environmental changes

 Diagnosis

WHAT THE DOCTOR LOOKS FOR

- The doctor will take a history and perform a thorough physical examination.
- Other conditions with similar signs and symptoms will be investigated, such as influenza (flu), pneumonia, or asthma.

TESTS AND PROCEDURES

- A number of blood tests may be performed to assist in diagnosis.
- Arterial blood may be obtained.
- CBC (blood count) may be obtained.
- Fluids may be cultured for microbiological analysis.
- Chest X-ray
- Pulmonary function tests may be done to assess the respiratory system.

 Treatment

GENERAL MEASURES

- Acute bronchitis is usually managed on an outpatient basis unless the person is elderly or the bronchitis is complicated by severe underlying disease.
- Rest
- Steam inhalations
- Vaporizers
- Antibiotics, if bacterial infection suspected
- Maintain adequate hydration.
- Stop smoking.

ACTIVITY

Rest until fever subsides

DIET

Increased fluids (up to 3 to 4 liters per day) if fever present

Medications

COMMONLY PRESCRIBED DRUGS

- Amantadine if influenza A is suspected; most effective if started within 24 to 48 hours of development of symptoms.
- Decongestants if accompanied by sinus condition
- Fever-reducing pain reliever, such as aspirin (do not give to children) or acetaminophen.
- Antibiotics: amoxicillin, trimethoprim-sulfamethoxazole (TMP-SMX), cephalosporin, doxycycline, clarithromycin
- Cough suppressant for troublesome cough
- Bronchodilators (aerosols/steroids)

CONTRAINDICATIONS

- Doxycycline should not be used during pregnancy.

PRECAUTIONS

Read drug product information.

SIGNIFICANT POSSIBLE INTERACTIONS

Read drug product information.

OTHER DRUGS

- Other antibiotics
- Antiviral drugs

Followup

PATIENT MONITORING

The doctor should be seen as necessary depending on the nature of the disease and the person's health status.

PREVENTION

- Avoid smoking.
- Control underlying risk factors (asthma, sinusitis, reflux).
- Avoid exposure.

COMPLICATIONS

- Pneumonia
- Acute respiratory failure

WHAT TO EXPECT

- Usually, there is complete healing with good return of function.
- Bronchitis can be serious in elderly or debilitated patients.
- Cough may persist for several weeks after initial improvement.
- May result in reactive airway disease or other serious conditions (rare)

Miscellaneous

OTHER FACTORS

N/A

PEDIATRIC

- Bronchitis among children usually occurs in association with other upper and lower respiratory tract conditions.
- Some children seem to be more susceptible than others. If attacks of bronchitis recur, child should be further evaluated.
- If acute bronchitis is caused by respiratory syncytial virus, it may be fatal.

GERIATRIC

Bronchitis can be a serious illness among the elderly, particularly if part of influenza.

OTHERS

N/A

PREGNANCY

N/A

FURTHER INFORMATION

American Lung Association, 1740 Broadway, New York, NY 10019, (212) 315-8700

Bulimia

Basics

DESCRIPTION

Bulimia nervosa is defined as body dissatisfaction. Persons with bulimia nervosa engage in repeated binge eating, with or without purging by self-induced vomiting, laxatives, or diuretics. An alternative pattern is binging followed by sharply restricted diet and/or vigorous exercise.

SIGNS AND SYMPTOMS

- Person may switch back and forth between binging and purging.
- Onset may be related to stress.
- Affected person may be average weight or even somewhat obese; most are slightly below average weight but have frequent fluctuations in weight.
- Denial of problem
- Eating high-calorie foods during binge
- Claim to feel fat even when thin
- Preoccupation with weight control
- Food collection and hoarding
- Drug and/or alcohol abuse
- Diet pill, diuretic, laxative, ipecac, and thyroid medication abuse
- Calories used up through vigorous exercise, especially running, aerobics
- Diabetic patients often withhold insulin.
- Depressed mood and self-depreciation following binges
- Relief and increased ability to concentrate following binges
- Vomiting (may be effortless)
- Abdominal pain
- Salivary gland swelling
- Eroded teeth
- Scarred hands

CAUSES

Unknown; thought to be largely emotional

SCOPE

About 2% of females suffer from bulimia nervosa. True incidence is unknown because it is a secretive disease. It is more common among university women.

MOST OFTEN AFFECTED

Bulimia nervosa is most common among adolescents and young adults, more often seen in females than males.

RISK FACTORS

- Impulsiveness
- Low self-esteem
- Pressure to achieve; high self-expectations
- Acceptance of the culturally condoned ideal of slimness
- Ambivalence about dependence/independence
- Stress due to multiple responsibilities, tight schedules, competition
- Unstable body image, perceptual distortions
- High risk: ballet dancers, models, cheerleaders, athletes

Diagnosis

WHAT THE DOCTOR LOOKS FOR

- The doctor will take a history and perform a thorough physical examination.
- Other medical problems should be identified, such as gastrointestinal disorders.
- Any mental health issues should be identified and addressed.

TESTS AND PROCEDURES

- A number of blood tests may be done to assist in diagnosis.
- The function of the gastrointestinal system may be evaluated.
- An electrocardiogram (EKG) may be done to assess heart activity.
- Psychological testing may be performed.

Treatment

GENERAL MEASURES

- Most patients can be treated as outpatients.
- A person may require hospitalization if she or he is suicidal; if there is evidence of marked electrolyte imbalance or marked dehydration; or if there has been no response to outpatient therapy.

ACTIVITY

- Monitor excess activity.
- Playful, pleasurable activities are important.

DIET

- Goal is a balanced diet with adequate calories and a normal eating pattern. Affected person needs support in eliminating preoccupation with calories, weight, purging.
- Feared foods should be gradually introduced.

 ## Medications

COMMONLY PRESCRIBED DRUGS

- Medication is indicated for patients who are severely depressed or who have not responded to an adequate trial of therapy.
- Tricyclic antidepressants (TCAs), monoamine oxidase inhibitors (MAOs), serotonin reuptake inhibitors (SRIs).

CONTRAINDICATIONS

Read drug product information.

PRECAUTIONS

Read drug product information.

DRUG INTERACTIONS

Read drug product information.

OTHER DRUGS

- If there is an underlying bipolar disorder, patients may benefit from lithium (Eskalith).
- Opiate antagonist such as naltrexone (Trexan) to suppress consumption of sweet and high fat foods.
- Metoclopramide (Reglan) or cisapride before each meal and at bedtime for after-meal abdominal discomfort.

 ## Followup

PATIENT MONITORING

The person with bulimia nervosa should see the doctor as often as necessary to monitor health status and disease activity.

PREVENTION

- Maintain rational attitude about weight.
- Moderate overly high self-expectations.
- Enhance self-esteem.
- Diminish stress.

COMPLICATIONS

- Suicide
- Drug and alcohol abuse
- Potassium depletion, irregular heart rhythm, cardiac arrest

WHAT TO EXPECT

- The outcome of treatment is highly variable; bulimia nervosa tends to wax and wane.
- The illness may spontaneously remit.
- People who stay in therapy tend to improve.

Miscellaneous

OTHER FACTORS

N/A

PEDIATRIC

N/A

GERIATRIC

N/A

OTHERS

Infrequently diagnosed in men or in older women

PREGNANCY

- Poor nutritional status may affect fetus.
- Binging and purging may increase or decrease during pregnancy.

FURTHER INFORMATION

N/A

Burns

 ## Basics

DESCRIPTION

Burns are tissue injuries caused by heat, chemicals, electricity, or irradiation. The extent of injury (depth of burn) reflects the intensity of heat and the duration of exposure.

SIGNS AND SYMPTOMS

- First-degree burn (superficial layers of the skin)
  - ▶ Reddening of affected tissue
  - ▶ Skin blanches with pressure.
  - ▶ Skin may be tender.
- Second-degree burn (varying degrees of skin, with blister formation)
  - ▶ Skin is red and blistered.
  - ▶ Skin is very tender.
- Third-degree burn (destruction of the full thickness of skin and underlying tissues)
  - ▶ Burned skin is tough and leathery.
  - ▶ Skin is not tender.

CAUSES

- Open flame and hot liquid (most common)
- Caustic chemicals or acids
- Electricity
- Excess sun exposure

SCOPE

- Between 2 and 5 million Americans receive burns requiring assistance annually. One million people require hospitalization for burn injuries each year, and 12,000 people die.
- Burns are the leading cause of accidental death in children

MOST OFTEN AFFECTED

Burns affect all age groups and both genders in equal proportions.

RISK FACTORS

- Hot water heaters set too high
- Work place exposure to chemicals, electricity, or radiation
- Young children and elderly adults with thin skin are more susceptible to injury.
- Carelessness with burning cigarettes
- Inadequate or faulty electrical wiring

 ## Diagnosis

WHAT THE DOCTOR LOOKS FOR

- The doctor will perform a physical examination, measuring the depth of burn and percentage of body surface area affected.
- The doctor will diagnose and treat other associated conditions, such as smoke inhalation.

TESTS AND PROCEDURES

- A number of blood tests may be done to assist in diagnosis and treatment.
- Chest X-ray
- Arterial blood may be obtained to measure blood gasses.
- An electrocardiogram (EKG) may be done to evaluate the heart's activity.
- Urinalysis
- Bronchoscopy may be necessary to evaluate the respiratory tract.

 ## Treatment

GENERAL MEASURES

- Initiate first aid.
- Remove all rings, watches, etc., from injured extremities to avoid tourniquet effect.
- Remove clothing and cover all burned areas with dry sheet.
- Cool burned skin with water.
- Do not apply ice to burn site.
- Flush area of chemical burn (for approximately 2 hours).
- Serious burns require hospitalization.
- Surgery may be required.

ACTIVITY

Early mobilization is the goal of treatment.

DIET

High-protein, high-calorie diet when bowel function resumes; nasogastric tube feedings may be required in early postburn period.

Medications

COMMONLY PRESCRIBED DRUGS

- Morphine
- Silver sulfadiazine (Silvadene) topically to burn site
- Cimetidine, ranitidine, famotidine, or nizatidine for stress ulcer prevention in severely burned patients

CONTRAINDICATIONS

Specific drug allergies

PRECAUTIONS

N/A

DRUG INTERACTIONS

Read drug product information.

OTHER DRUGS

- Third-degree burn: mafenide (Sulfamylon)
- Silver nitrate 0.5%
- Povidone-iodine (Betadine)

 ## Followup

PATIENT MONITORING

The doctor should be seen as often as necessary according to the extent of burn and treatment.

PREVENTION

- Use sunscreen when out of doors.
- Keep electrical cords and outlets in the home safe.
- Isolate household chemicals.
- Use low-temperature setting for hot water heater.
- Household smoke detectors with special emphasis on maintenance
- Prepare household evacuation plan.
- Store and use flammable substances properly.
- Skin grafts and healing skin are highly sensitive to sun exposure and heat.

COMPLICATIONS

- Gastroduodenal ulcer
- Skin cancer developing in old burn site
- Burn wound sepsis
- Pneumonia
- Decreased mobility with possibility of future flexion contractures

WHAT TO EXPECT

- First-degree burn: complete resolution
- Second-degree burn: healing in 10 to 14 days (deep second-degree burns will probably require skin graft)
- Third-degree burn: skin graft required
- Length of hospital stay and need for intensive care depends on extent of burn, smoke inhalation, and age.
- 50% survival rates: with 62% of body burned in ages 0–14 years, with 63% burn in ages 15–40, with 38% burn in ages 40–65, and with 25% burn in patients over age 65.
- 90% of survivors can be expected to return to work.

 ## Miscellaneous

OTHER FACTORS

N/A

PEDIATRIC

Child abuse should be considered with hot water burns in children.

GERIATRIC

The outcome is poorer for elderly persons with severe burns.

OTHERS

N/A

PREGNANCY

N/A

FURTHER INFORMATION

N/A

Bursitis

 Basics

DESCRIPTION

Bursitis is inflammation of a bursa, a fluid-filled sac that serves as a cushion between tendons and bones. Bursae are located in areas subject to friction, such as where tendons pass over bone. Bursae essentially lubricate the area with fluid. Common sites of bursae are the shoulder, elbow, and knee.

SIGNS AND SYMPTOMS

- Pain and tenderness of the affected area
- Decreased range of motion
- Redness of the skin
- Swelling
- Crackling or popping noise when moving

CAUSES

- The cause of bursitis is often unknown.
- Bursitis may be acute or chronic.
- There are many types of bursitis, including in-flammatory, infectious, traumatic, and gouty.

SCOPE

Bursitis is common in the United States.

MOST OFTEN AFFECTED

Individuals 15–50 years of age, males more often than females. Traumatic bursitis is more common in patients younger than 35 years of age.

RISK FACTORS

Repeated vigorous physical training or a sudden increase in level of activity (e.g., "weekend warriors"). Improper or overzealous stretching can cause injury.

 Diagnosis

WHAT THE PHYSICIAN LOOKS FOR

- The physician evaluates the patient to determine the presence, type, and severity of bursitis.
- Conditions with signs and symptoms similar to bursitis include tendinitis, strains and sprains, gout, rheumatoid arthritis, osteoarthritis.
- Bursitis may be associated with tendinitis, sprains and strains, stress fractures.

TESTS AND PROCEDURES

- Blood tests will help discriminate bursitis from other conditions.
- X-ray may show deposits of calcium within the affected bursa.
- Computed tomography (CT scan) or magnetic resonance imaging (MRI) may be performed to evaluate the affected area.
- Fluid from the affected bursa may be withdrawn by needle to look for signs of in-flammation or infection.
- If the pain is located in the chest or left arm, the doctor may order an electrocardiogram (EKG) to make sure the pain is not being caused by a cardiac condition.

 Treatment

GENERAL MEASURES

- Usually treated on an outpatient basis, with only difficult cases referred to a specialist
- Conservative therapy includes rest, ice, gentle compression, and elevation of the affected area.
- Invasive therapy includes the withdrawal of fluid from the bursa, injection of steroids.
- Treatment may include physical therapy and the application of moist heat.
- A splint or sling may be used to protect and support the affected arm or leg.
- Antibiotic is prescribed if bursitis is caused by infection.
- In severe cases, the bursa may be removed by surgery.

ACTIVITY

Rest and elevation of affected arm or leg

DIET

Changes to the diet may be recommended if bursitis is related to obesity or the formation of mineral deposits.

 ## Medications

COMMONLY PRESCRIBED DRUGS

- Nonsteroidal antiinflammatory drugs (NSAIDs) or aspirin
- Steroids or stronger pain-killing drugs may be injected if needed.
- Antibiotic may be prescribed if bursitis is caused by infection.

CONTRAINDICATIONS

Read drug product information.

PRECAUTIONS

Read drug product information.

DRUG INTERACTIONS

Read drug product information.

OTHER DRUGS

- Topical analgesic or capsaicin creams may be used for symptomatic relief of bursitis.
- Oral steroids may be prescribed.

 ## Followup

PATIENT MONITORING

- The patient should stop taking nonsteroidal antiinflammatory drugs (NSAIDs) as soon as possible to avoid side effects (e.g., ulcers).
- Some patients may require repeated injections of steroid and analgesic, although usually no more than three.

PREVENTION

- Appropriate warm-up and cool-down routines can help prevent the symptoms of bursitis.
- Don't overdo physical activity.
- Get adequate rest between work-outs.
- Perform exercises to increase range of motion.
- Maintain high level of fitness and general good health.

COMPLICATIONS

- Acute bursitis may lead to chronic bursitis.
- Long-lasting limitation of range of motion

WHAT TO EXPECT

- Most bouts of acute bursitis heal without long-term effects.
- Repeated bouts of acute bursitis may lead to chronic bursitis.
- The affected bursae may need to be repeatedly drained of fluid or ultimately surgically removed.

 ## Miscellaneous

OTHER FACTORS

N/A

PEDIATRIC

Other causes of signs and symptoms of bursitis should be investigated.

ELDERLY

Bursitis is more common among the elderly.

OTHERS

N/A

PREGNANCY

N/A

FURTHER INFORMATION

N/A

Section C

Candidiasis

 Basics

DESCRIPTION

Candidiasis is an infection with *Candida albicans* (a fungus) or a related species. Candidiasis affecting the skin causes lesions or a rash between the fingers or toes, ingrown or inflamed hair follicles, inflammation of the penis, a rash at the armpits or other folds of skin, inflammation or infection of the nails, or diaper rash. Infections may also affect mucous membranes, such as the mouth or vagina. The most serious form of the illness is acute systemic candidiasis.

SIGNS AND SYMPTOMS

- Fever
- Malaise
- Rapid heart rate
- Low blood pressure
- Altered mental status
- Skin rash

CAUSES

- Most Candida infections are due to *Candida albicans.* Other species of Candida are important causes of disease.
- Candida species grow on mucous membranes, and most infections are acquired from the Candida growing on these membranes.
- Human-to-human transmission of Candida can occur (e.g., through sexual contact).

SCOPE

Candidiasis affects at least 120,000 persons annually in the United States.

MOST OFTEN AFFECTED

Persons of all ages are susceptible to candidiasis. Premature infants are at particularly high risk. Males and females are affected equally often.

RISK FACTORS

- White blood cell disorders
- Antibiotic therapy
- Indwelling intravenous access devices
- Dialysis

 Diagnosis

WHAT THE DOCTOR LOOKS FOR

The doctor will evaluate for other causes of similar signs and symptoms, such as bacterial infection or immune sytem disorder.

TESTS AND PROCEDURES

- Blood or cells from a lesion may be micro-scopically analyzed.
- Imaging of internal organs may be done by liver scan, ultrasound, or computed tomogra-phy (CT scan) to assist in diagnosis.

 Treatment

GENERAL MEASURES

- Candidiasis is usually managed on an inpatient basis.
- Fluids and electrolytes may need to be given.
- Medication and mechanical breathing support may be required in seriously ill patients.

ACTIVITY

As tolerated

DIET

No special diet

Medications

COMMONLY PRESCRIBED DRUGS

Antifungal drugs: fluconazole, amphotericin B

CONTRAINDICATIONS

The safety of amphotericin B during pregnancy has not been established.

PRECAUTIONS

Amphotericin B is highly toxic. Acute reactions commonly occur at the beginning of therapy.

DRUG INTERACTIONS

Fluconazole: Potentially important drug interactions may occur in patients receiving oral diabetes medication, anticoagulants, phenytoin, cyclosporine, rifampin, theophylline, terfenadine, or astemizole. Read drug product information for other interactions.

OTHER DRUGS

Other antifungal drugs

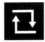 ## Followup

PATIENT MONITORING

- Blood tests may be required as often as twice weekly.
- The doctor should be seen as often as necessary depending on the person's health status.

PREVENTION

N/A

COMPLICATIONS

- Kidney disease
- Eye disease
- Heart disease
- Arthritis or other joint/bone disease
- Respiratory disease
- Central nervous system infection

WHAT TO EXPECT

The overall mortality rate for patients with serious candidiasis infection is 40–75%.

 ## Miscellaneous

OTHER FACTORS

N/A

PEDIATRIC

N/A

GERIATRIC

N/A

OTHERS

N/A

PREGNANCY

N/A

FURTHER INFORMATION

N/A

Carbon Monoxide Poisoning

 Basics

DESCRIPTION

Carbon monoxide poisoning results from the inhalation of carbon monoxide (CO). CO is produced by incomplete combustion of wood, gas, or other material. Inhalation of CO prevents hemoglobin in red blood cells from carrying oxygen.

SIGNS AND SYMPTOMS

- Headaches
- Ringing or buzzing in ear (tinnitus)
- Nausea
- Dizziness
- Weakness
- Confusion
- Lethargy or sleepiness
- Fainting
- Chest pain
- Fast or irregular heart rate
- Cardiac dysrhythmias
- Uncoordination
- Seizures
- Coma
- Cardiopulmonary arrest

CAUSES

CO inhalation

SCOPE

CO poisoning is responsible for about 3,800 deaths and 10,000 injuries annually.

MOST OFTEN AFFECTED

CO affects all age groups and both genders.

RISK FACTORS

- Cigarette smoke
- Smoke inhalation
- Closed space with faulty furnaces or stoves
- Coal mining
- Inhalation of car exhaust
- Paint strippers
- Solvent manufacturing

 Diagnosis

WHAT THE DOCTOR LOOKS FOR

- The doctor will perform a complete physical examination.
- Other possible toxic exposure will be considered, such as cyanide poisoning.
- The doctor will look for other associated injuries, such as burns.

TESTS AND PROCEDURES

Blood tests to measure the level of CO

 Treatment

GENERAL MEASURES

- Provide emergency care as needed.
- Remove the person from the source of CO.
- Provide rescue breathing and cardiopulmonary resuscitation (CPR) if needed.
- People with mild CO poisoning can be treated in the emergency room.
- People with moderate or severe CO poisoning require hospitalization.

ACTIVITY

Rest until CO levels are reduced and symptoms ease.

DIET

N/A

Medications

COMMONLY PRESCRIBED DRUGS

Oxygen; a hyperbaric chamber may be used for severe cases.

CONTRAINDICATIONS

N/A

PRECAUTIONS

N/A

DRUG INTERACTIONS

N/A

OTHER DRUGS

N/A

 Followup

PATIENT MONITORING

- CO levels and blood gases may be measured.
- The doctor should be seen as often as needed based on symptoms.

PREVENTION

- Make sure furnaces, stoves, and fireplaces are properly maintained.
- People who work in high-risk occupations should have adequate ventilation.

COMPLICATIONS

- Heart attack
- Brain damage

WHAT TO EXPECT

Most survivors recover completely.

 Miscellaneous

OTHER FACTORS

N/A

PEDIATRIC

N/A

GERIATRIC

Complications are more common among the elderly.

OTHERS

N/A

PREGNANCY

CO poisoning affects the fetus. CO poisoning can cause significant birth defects depending on the developmental stage.

Carpal Tunnel Syndrome

 Basics

DESCRIPTION

Carpal tunnel syndrome is the compression of the median nerve as it passes through the carpal tunnel in the wrist and hand. The tunnel contains flexor tendons and the median nerve. Symptoms tend to affect the dominant hand, but over one-half of people with carpal tunnel syndrome have symptoms in both hands.

SIGNS AND SYMPTOMS

- Tingling or prickling sensations in the fingers
- Burning pain in the fingers, particularly at night
- Loss of sensation in the fingers
- Symptoms usually relieved by shaking or rubbing the hands
- Arm pain
- During waking hours, symptoms occur when driving the car, reading the newspaper, and occasionally when using the hands repetitively.
- Symptoms usually affect the thumb, index and middle finger, although the entire hand may be affected.
- Weakness of the hand while performing tasks such as opening a jar

CAUSES

- Disorders affecting the musculoskeletal system in the area of the wrist, such as injury or arthritis
- Often associated with hypothyroidism and diabetes, which also occur more often during pregnancy
- Other diseases

SCOPE

Carpal tunnel syndrome is a common nerve disorder.

MOST OFTEN AFFECTED

Carpal tunnel syndrome primarily affects individuals between 40 and 60 years of age and it affects females 3–6 times more often than it does males. It may affect more than one member of a family.

RISK FACTORS

Jobs that involve repetitive motion of the wrist may influence the development of carpal tunnel syndrome. However, there is no universal agreement that carpal tunnel syndrome is job-related.

 Diagnosis

WHAT THE DOCTOR LOOKS FOR

- The doctor will look for signs that are diagnostic of carpal tunnel syndrome.
- Other conditions that can cause similar conditions should be identified and treated.

TESTS AND PROCEDURES

- Blood tests
- Studies of muscle and nerve (electromyography) may be performed.
- X-rays may be done of the wrist and arm.

 Treatment

GENERAL MEASURES

- Carpal tunnel syndrome is usually managed in the outpatient setting.
- Splinting the wrist may provide significant relief of symptoms.
- Surgery may be necessary, usually as an outpatient under local anesthesia.

ACTIVITY

As tolerated

DIET

No special diet

Medications

COMMONLY PRESCRIBED DRUGS

- Nonsteroidal anti-inflammatory agents: ibuprofen, naproxen
- Steroids

CONTRAINDICATIONS

Gastrointestinal intolerance

PRECAUTIONS

N/A

DRUG INTERACTIONS

Read drug product information.

ALTERNATIVE DRUGS

N/A

 Followup

PATIENT MONITORING

- Patients treated with wrist splints and other symptomatic measures should see the doctor for a followup within 4 to 12 weeks to assess treatment.
- Patients who receive surgery rarely experience recurrence of the disorder. Routine followup once the incision has healed is not necessary.

PREVENTION

Take a break once an hour when doing repetitive work involving hands.

COMPLICATIONS

- Infection after surgery (rare)
- Nerve injury

WHAT TO EXPECT

- Untreated, the condition may lead to numbness and weakness in the hand, atrophy of hand muscles, and permanent loss of function of the extremity.
- Surgery is effective in about 95% of cases.

 Miscellaneous

OTHER FACTORS

N/A

PEDIATRIC

N/A

GERIATRIC

N/A

OTHERS

N/A

PREGNANCY

May occur in pregnancy

FURTHER INFORMATION

American Academy of Family Physicians Foundation, P.O. Box 8418, Kansas City, MO 64114, (800)274-2237, ext.4400

Cataract

 Basics

DESCRIPTION

A cataract is a clouding of the lens of the eye. It is the single largest cause of blindness in the world, blinding an estimated 17 million people at any point in time.

SIGNS AND SYMPTOMS

- Blurred vision and distortion or "ghosting" of images
- Visual problems in bright light or night driving (glare)
- Falls or accidents
- Injuries (e.g., hip fracture)

CAUSES

- Age
- Numerous other causes

SCOPE

Cataracts affect 5% of people 52–62 years of age and 46% of people 75–85 years of age. Ninety-two percent of people 75–85 years of age have some degree of visual impairment.

MOST OFTEN AFFECTED

Cataracts affect males and females with equal frequency. Some forms of cataract may be inherited.

RISK FACTORS

- Aging
- Predisposing diseases

 Diagnosis

WHAT THE DOCTOR LOOKS FOR

- The doctor will perform a thorough examination of the eyes, looking for clouding of the lens as well as other eye conditions.
- Special visual tests may be performed.
- Because cataracts develop gradually, the person may not be aware of how it has changed his or her lifestyle. The doctor may note cataracts when the patient is unaware of problems.
- The doctor will also look for other diseases known to be associated with cataract, such as diabetes.

 Treatment

GENERAL MEASURES

- Cataracts are treated by surgical removal and replacement of the affected lens.
- Cataract surgery may be done in an outpatient setting, or hospitalization may be required.
- An evaluation will be performed before surgery, including blood tests and an electrocardiogram (EKG).
- A second opinion by another ophthalmologist (eye specialist) may be indicated before surgery.

ACTIVITY

N/A

DIET

N/A

PATIENT EDUCATION

N/A

Cataract

 ## Medications

COMMONLY PRESCRIBED DRUGS

There is no medication at present to prevent or slow the progression of cataracts.

CONTRAINDICATIONS

N/A

PRECAUTIONS

N/A

DRUG INTERACTIONS

N/A

OTHER DRUGS

N/A

 ## Followup

PATIENT MONITORING

- As cataract develops, an ophthalmologist may change a patient's eyeglass prescription to maintain vision. When these changes are no longer practical or successful, surgery is recommended.
- Following surgery, eyeglasses may be required to maximize vision. Eyes are tested several weeks after surgery.

PREVENTION

- Sunglasses that filter ultraviolet rays may slow the development of cataract, but this is not proven by scientific studies.
- Antioxidants (vitamins C, E, etc.) may be helpful, but not proven.

COMPLICATIONS

Blindness

WHAT TO EXPECT

The outcome is good after cataract surgery if the patient has no other eye disease.

 ## Miscellaneous

OTHER FACTORS

N/A

PEDIATRIC

Congenital cataracts can occur in newborns; outcome is poor.

GERIATRIC

Ninety-two percent of people over age 75 have cataracts.

OTHERS

N/A

PREGNANCY

N/A

FURTHER INFORMATION

N/A

Cervical Dysplasia

 Basics

DESCRIPTION

Cervical dysplasia is defined as precancerous changes in the tissue of the cervix, often associated with infection by human papilloma virus (warts). The changes may involve partial or full thickness of the tissue.

SIGNS AND SYMPTOMS

- Often no symptoms
- Occasionally associated with genital warts
- Occasionally occurs with sexually transmitted diseases, e.g., chlamydia, gonorrhea

CAUSES

Cervical dysplasia is strongly linked to infection by human papilloma viruses, the virus that causes genital warts.

SCOPE

The scope has been difficult to assess. Cervical dysplasia has been found in 3,600 per 100,000 women 27–28 years of age.

MOST OFTEN AFFECTED

The average age for noninvasive cancer of the cervix is 28 years. Cervical dysplasia probably can be expected to occur at younger ages.

RISK FACTORS

- Multiple pregnancies and births before 20 years of age
- Multiple sexual partners
- Early age in first sexual intercourse
- Warts elsewhere in the body
- Cigarette smoking
- Prostitution
- Lower socio-economic status

 Diagnosis

WHAT THE DOCTOR LOOKS FOR

- The doctor will perform a physical examination of the lower reproductive tract.
- Other diseases of the cervix will be investigated, such as cancer and genital warts.

TESTS AND PROCEDURES

- A sample of cervical tissue may be examined microscopically, called a Pap smear.
- The lower reproductive tract may be visually examined by colposcopy.
- Other special tests may be performed, such as cervicography and speculoscopy.
- A sample of cervical tissue may be obtained by biopsy.

 Treatment

GENERAL MEASURES

- Cervical dysplasia is managed in an outpatient setting.
- Outpatient surgery may be performed.

ACTIVITY

4 weeks of pelvic rest after biopsy

DIET

No restrictions

Medications

COMMONLY PRESCRIBED DRUGS

- Treatment is primarily surgical and aimed at removing the abnormal tissue.
- Fluorouracil (Efudex) vaginal cream is used as supplemental therapy.

CONTRAINDICATIONS

Allergy to 5-fluorouracil

PRECAUTIONS

- If the hand is used to apply 5-fluorouracil, wash hand immediately afterward.
- Avoid getting 5-fluorouracil in the eyes, nose, or mouth.

DRUG INTERACTIONS

N/A

OTHER DRUGS

N/A

Followup

PATIENT MONITORING

- The doctor should be seen every 4 months during the first year after treatment for repeat Pap smears, then every 6 months thereafter.
- For less serious cases, the doctor may repeat Pap smear annually.

PREVENTION

- Monogamy of both sexual partners
- Use of condom during intercourse if unable to practice monogamy
- Abstain from smoking
- Annual Pap smear to detect changes early

COMPLICATIONS

- Some cases of severe dysplasia will develop into cancer.
- Possible complications of biopsy include:
  - ▶ Bleeding
  - ▶ Infection
  - ▶ Infertility
  - ▶ Incomplete removal of affected tissue
  - ▶ Recurrence of dysplasia
  - ▶ Other cervical disorders

WHAT TO EXCPECT

- The outcome of cervical dysplasia is generally excellent.
- The condition may persist if it is not completely removed.
- The condition may come back.

Miscellaneous

OTHER FACTORS

N/A

PEDIATRIC

Very rare among children

GERIATRIC

Less frequent among the elderly

OTHERS

Cervical dysplasia is usually a problem for women in the reproductive age group. The median age is 28 years for severe dysplasia. For less severe cervical dysplasia, the median ages tend to be much lower.

PREGNANCY

- Dysplasia may get worse during pregnancy.
- Dysplasia does not require definitive treatment during pregnancy.
- Dysplasia by itself is not an indication for cesarean section.

FURTHER INFORMATION

N/A

Chickenpox

 ## Basics

DESCRIPTION

Chickenpox, also called varicella, is a common, highly contagious disease marked by the development of blisters on the skin and mucous membranes.

- The virus that causes chickenpox (varicella zoster virus) is spread directly by breathing air or contact with blisters, or indirectly through contact with freshly soiled articles.
- Outbreaks of chickenpox tend to occur from January to May.
- Incubation period is 14–16 days (range is 11–21 days).
- Patients are infectious from 24 hours before onset of the rash until the final lesions have crusted.
- Most people acquire chickenpox during childhood and develop long immunity.
- A vaccination can prevent chickenpox.

SIGNS AND SYMPTOMS

- Symptoms that develop before appearance of the rash include fever, malaise, lack of appetite, and mild headache.
- The chickenpox rash is characterized by crops of "teardrop" blisters on reddened bases.
- Blisters erupt in successive crops.
- The individual blisters form from a pimple-like lesion.
- Eventually, the blisters begin to crust over.
- The rash causes intense itching.
- Rash usually begins on trunk, then spreads to face and scalp.
- Rash does not usually affect the arms or legs.
- Blisters may be present on mucous membranes, such as the mouth and vagina.

CAUSES

Infection by the varicella zoster virus

SCOPE

Chickenpox is common in the United States.

MOST OFTEN AFFECTED

Chickenpox has a peak incidence among children 5 to 9 years of age, but it can occur at any age. Males and females are affected equally as often.

RISK FACTORS

- No prior history of chickenpox
- Lack of vaccination
- Immune system disorders

 ## Diagnosis

WHAT THE DOCTOR LOOKS FOR

- The doctor will perform a physical examination to rule out other similar-appearing conditions, such as herpes, impetigo, or scabies.

TESTS AND PROCEDURES

- Blood tests to look for signs of infection
- Virus may be isolated from tissue culture and examined by electron microscopy.
- Specialized tests may be done to analyze the genetic material of a virus.

 ## Treatment

GENERAL MEASURES

- Chickenpox is managed in the outpatient setting except when complicating emergencies occur.
- Treatment involves providing support and relief of symptoms.
- Good hygiene is important to prevent infection of blisters.

ACTIVITY

As tolerated. Children may return to school when lesions have scabbed over, temperature is normal, and sense of well being has returned.

DIET

No special diet

 ## Medications

COMMONLY PRESCRIBED DRUGS

- Fever-reducing drugs, such as acetaminophen
- Aspirin should be avoided because of its link to Reye's syndrome.

- Local and/or systemic anti-itching agents
- Acyclovir: This antiviral drug decreases duration of fever and shortens time of viral shedding. It is recommended for adolescents, adults, and high-risk patients. It is most helpful if given early in the disease.

CONTRAINDICATIONS

Drug allergies

PRECAUTIONS

Possible kidney disease with acyclovir

DRUG INTERACTIONS

N/A

OTHER DRUGS

Other antiviral drugs

 ## Followup

PATIENT MONITORING

- Usually no followup is needed for mild cases.
- If complications occur, intensive supportive care may be required.

PREVENTION

- People who have been exposed to chickenpox and who are susceptible to it (i.e., have not been vaccinated or have never had it) are considered infectious for 21 days.
- Varicella zoster virus vaccine (Varivax) is a vaccine against chickenpox. It is made from live, attenuated (changed in the laboratory to be non-disease-causing) varicella zoster virus.
- Vaccine recipients should avoid contact with individuals with immune system disorders and pregnant women who have never had chickenpox and their newborns for up to 6 weeks after vaccination.
- Varicella zoster immune globulin (VZIG) can also protect against chickenpox, but it is not as effective as Varivax. VZIG is given to individuals who should not receive Varivax (e.g., people with immune system disorders).

COMPLICATIONS

- Secondary bacterial infection
- Pneumonia
- Encephalitis
- Reye's syndrome
- Skin bruising
- Inflammation of the lymph nodes
- Inflammation of the kidney

WHAT TO EXPECT

- In the healthy child, chickenpox is rarely a serious disease and recovery is complete.
- The illness provides long immunity.
- A second illness is rare.
- The virus may remain latent in the body and may be reactivated later, causing herpes zoster (shingles).
- Deaths rarely occur from complications.

 ## Miscellaneous

OTHER FACTORS

N/A

PEDIATRIC

- Neonates born to mothers who develop chickenpox 5 days before or 2 days after delivery are at risk for serious disease.

GERIATRIC

- Infection is more severe than in children.
- Latent virus may reactivate and cause shingles.

OTHERS

N/A

PREGNANCY

- The risk of infection across the placenta following maternal infection is 25%.
- Birth defects are seen in 5% of newborns infected during the first or second trimester of pregnancy.
- There is an increased risk of pneumonia or other complications in women infected during pregnancy

FURTHER INFORMATION

N/A

Child Abuse

 Basics

DESCRIPTION

- Abuse may be emotional, psychological, or physical.
- Sexual abuse is any contact or interaction between a child and another person in which the child is sexually exploited for the gratification or profit of the perpetrator. Offenders can be juveniles.
- Neglect occurs when those responsible for meeting the basic needs of a child fail to do so.

SIGNS AND SYMPTOMS

- Nonspecific symptoms of abuse include:
  - ▶ Behavior regression
  - ▶ Anxiety, depression
  - ▶ Sleep disturbances, night terrors
  - ▶ Increased sex play
  - ▶ School problems
  - ▶ Self-destructive behaviors
- Physical abuse:
  - ▶ May be no physical signs
  - ▶ Skin markings (lacerations, burns, bruises)
  - ▶ Bruises with definite shapes (coat hangers, belt buckles)
  - ▶ Circular bruises on trunks or limbs (finger pressure points)
  - ▶ Bites
  - ▶ Cigarette burns on palms, arms, or legs
  - ▶ Immersion injuries
  - ▶ Oral injury
  - ▶ Ear injury
  - ▶ Eye injury
  - ▶ Abdominal injury
  - ▶ Fractures
  - ▶ Head injury
- Sexual abuse:
  - ▶ Unequivocal signs are found in only a small number of children (2–8%).
  - ▶ Abuse often consists of fondling, rubbing, and other contacts that are not likely to produce injuries.
  - ▶ Unexplained vaginal injuries or bleeding
  - ▶ Pregnancy
  - ▶ Sexually transmitted diseases

- ▶ Reddening of tissues
- ▶ Anal injury
- ▶ May be no physical signs
- Neglect:
  - ▶ Child may be small, scrawny, dirty, with rashes
  - ▶ Fearful or too trusting
  - ▶ Clinging to or avoiding mother
  - ▶ Flat or balding area on the back of the head
  - ▶ Abnormal development or growth

SCOPE

There are more than 1 million cases of child abuse annually in the United States.

MOST OFTEN AFFECTED

The most common age of abused children is 7 years old. Males and females are affected in equal proportion.

CAUSES

Not well-defined

RISK FACTORS

- May be many risk factors for child abuse
- Poverty (5 times greater risk)
- Parental substance abuse
- Lower educational status
- Maternal history of abuse
- Unwanted pregnancy

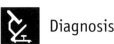 Diagnosis

WHAT THE DOCTOR LOOKS FOR

- The doctor will perform a thorough physical examination, paying particular attention to other possible causes of signs, such as accidental injury, bleeding disorders, or medical diseases.

TESTS AND PROCEDURES

- Urinalysis, culture
- Blood tests
- X-rays
- In cases of suspected sexual abuse, special tests may be done to detect semen or sexually transmitted disease.
- Photographs

Treatment

GENERAL MEASURES

- Acute episodes, especially of sexual abuse, are often best managed in an emergency room equipped for collecting forensic specimens and maintaining "chain of evidence."
- Children with moderate to severe injuries, unstable physical condition, or acute psychological trauma may be hospitalized.
- If not hospitalized, a child should be sent to another relative or placed in foster care should the suspected abuser live with the child.
- Counseling is imperative.
- Reporting to child protective authorities is mandatory.
- After initial evaluation, child victim of sexual abuse should be referred to sexual assault center.
- Do not use negative terms such as "ruined," "violated," or "dirty" in reference to the child. The child's emotional reaction to abuse will be profoundly influenced by the responses of adult caretakers.

ACTIVITY

As allowed by doctor

DIET

As allowed by doctor

Medications

COMMONLY PRESCRIBED DRUGS

Antibiotics for sexually transmitted diseases

CONTRAINDICATIONS

Read drug product information.

PRECAUTIONS

Read drug product information.

DRUG INTERACTIONS

Read drug product information.

OTHER DRUGS

"Morning-after" contraceptive drugs

Followup

PATIENT MONITORING

The child must be referred to the appropriate state protective services and followed as closely as necessary.

PREVENTION

Early detection and intervention whenever possible

COMPLICATIONS

Long-term physical and psychological damage

WHAT TO EXPECT

Without intervention, child abuse is a recurrent and escalating phenomenon.

Miscellaneous

OTHER FACTORS

N/A

PEDIATRIC

N/A

GERIATRIC

N/A

OTHERS

N/A

PREGNANCY

N/A

FURTHER INFORMATION

N/A

Chlamydial Sexually Transmitted Diseases

 Basics

DESCRIPTION

The most common sexually transmitted disease (STD) in the United States is infection by the bacteria *Chlamydia trachomatis*. Chlamydial STD often has no symptoms and is difficult to diagnose. The infection has serious consequences, and its transmission is difficult to control.

SIGNS AND SYMPTOMS

- In both genders: inflammation of the urinary or reproductive tract
- Most women infected with *Chlamydia trachomatis* have no symptoms.
- In women: inflammation of the cervix with production of mucus, pelvic inflammatory disease (PID)
- In infants: conjunctivitis (pink eye), airway or gastrointestinal disorders

CAUSES

Infection by *Chlamydia trachomatis*

SCOPE

Chlamydial infection affects 3–5% of the general population and up to 20% of individuals who seek treatment at STD clinics.

MOST OFTEN AFFECTED

Males and females 15–25 years of age

RISK FACTORS

- Sexual promiscuity
- Lower socioeconomic groups
- Youth

 Diagnosis

WHAT THE DOCTOR LOOKS FOR

The doctor will examine the urinary and reproductive organs and will look for signs of other STDs (syphilis, gonorrhea).

TESTS AND PROCEDURES

Cells from the urinary or reproductive tract may be cultured and analyzed in the laboratory.

 Treatment

GENERAL MEASURES

- Chlamydial infection is managed in the outpatient setting.
- HIV counseling and testing should be offered.
- Sex partners should be evaluated and treated.

ACTIVITY

Abstain from sexual activity until the infection is treated.

DIET

N/A

 Medications

COMMONLY PRESCRIBED DRUGS

Antibiotics: doxycycline, azithromycin, erythromycin, tetracycline, ceftriaxone, cefoxitin, quinolone

CONTRAINDICATIONS

Tetracycline should not be used during pregnancy or by children younger than 8 years of age.

PRECAUTIONS

Tetracycline may cause light sensitivity; sunscreen recommended.

DRUG INTERACTIONS

- Tetracycline: avoid antacids, dairy products, and iron.
- Antibiotics may reduce the effectiveness of oral contraceptives; barrier method is recommended.
- Erythromycin plus Fexofenadine (Allegra) may cause heart rhythm disturbances.

OTHER DRUGS

Other antibiotics

 ## Followup

PATIENT MONITORING

- The doctor may be seen for retesting weeks to months after treatment.
- Sexual partners need to be evaluated and treated to prevent passage of the disease back and forth between partners.
- Contact the doctor if symptoms persist or return.

PREVENTION

- Practice safe sex, such as barrier protection (condoms).
- It is important to finish the entire course of antibiotics.

COMPLICATIONS

- Males
  - ▶ Temporary infertility
  - ▶ Scarring of urethra
- Females
  - ▶ Tubal infertility
  - ▶ Tubal pregnancy
  - ▶ Chronic pelvic pain

WHAT TO EXPECT

The outcome of chlamydial infection is good with early and complete therapy.

 ## Miscellaneous

OTHER FACTORS

N/A

PEDIATRIC

N/A

GERIATRIC

N/A

OTHERS

After the onset of sexual activity, incidence drops off with age.

PREGNANCY

Infection during pregnancy may affect the fetus.

FURTHER INFORMATION

American Academy of Family Physicians Foundation, P.O. Box 8418, Kansas City, MO 64114, (800) 274-2237, ext. 4400

Cholera

 Basics

DESCRIPTION

Cholera is an acute infectious disease caused by the bacteria *Vibrio cholerae*. Characteristics include severe diarrhea with extreme fluid and electrolyte depletion, vomiting, muscle cramps, and prostration.

SCOPE

Cholera is rare in the United States. It is endemic in India, Southeast Asia, Africa, Middle East, Southern Europe, Oceania, and South and Central America. The few cases of cholera in the United States have occurred in returning travelers or have been associated with food brought into the country illicitly.

MOST OFTEN AFFECTED

Affects all ages, males and females equally

SIGNS AND SYMPTOMS

- Abdominal discomfort, lack of appetite
- Apathy, lethargy, malaise, listlessness
- Cyanosis
- Dehydration
- Vomiting
- Severe diarrhea that eventually turns gray in color with flecks of mucus; called "rice-water diarrhea" because the mucus flecks resemble grains of rice.
- Profuse sweating
- Rapid or irregular heart rate
- Fever
- Shock
- Weakness

CAUSES

Infection by *Vibrio cholerae*

RISK FACTORS

- Traveling or living in areas where cholera is endemic
- Exposure to contaminated food or water
- Person-to-person transmission (rare)

 Diagnosis

WHAT THE DOCTOR LOOKS FOR

The doctor will investigate other possible causes of severe diarrhea and dehydration.

TESTS AND PROCEDURES

- Blood tests
- A sample of stool may be cultured for laboratory analysis.
- X-rays of the chest and abdomen

 Treatment

GENERAL MEASURES

- Mild cases of cholera are managed in the outpatient setting.
- Moderate or severe cases of cholera may require hospitalization.
- Rehydration therapy: oral fluids for mild to moderate cases, intravenous (IV) fluids for severe dehydration

ACTIVITY

Bed rest until symptoms resolve and strength returns

DIET

Small, frequent meals when vomiting stops and appetite returns

Medications

COMMONLY PRESCRIBED DRUGS

- Oral fluids: Pedialyte, Rehydralyte, Resol, Ricelyte
- IV fluids
- Antibiotics: doxycycline (Vibramycin), tetracycline, trimethoprim, sulfamethoxazole (SMX-TMP, Bactrim, Septra), furazolidone (Furoxone)

CONTRAINDICATIONS

- Tetracycline should not be used during pregnancy or by children younger than 8 years of age.
- Do not drink alcohol when taking furazolidone.

PRECAUTIONS

- Tetracycline may cause sensitivity to sunlight; sunscreen recommended.

SIGNIFICANT POSSIBLE INTERACTIONS

- Tetracycline: avoid antacids, dairy products, and iron

OTHER DRUGS

N/A

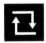 Followup

PATIENT MONITORING

The doctor should be seen often until symptoms resolve.

PREVENTION

- Use precautions in endemic areas: purify water, select food carefully (i.e., do not eat raw shellfish)
- Vaccination

POSSIBLE COMPLICATIONS

- Hypovolemic (low fluid volume) shock
- Chronic gallbladder infection
- Up to 50% death rate with untreated shock

WHAT TO EXPECT

- Clinical course is 3–5 days.
- Prompt oral or IV treatment can be lifesaving.
- Antibiotic treatment reduces duration and infectivity of disease.
- Mortality rate is less than 1% with appropriate supportive care.
- The risk of death increases with untreated shock.

 Miscellaneous

OTHER FACTORS

N/A

PEDIATRIC

- Breast-feeding protects against cholera.
- Vaccine is not recommended for children younger than 6 months of age.

GERIATRIC

N/A

OTHERS

N/A

PREGNANCY

N/A

FURTHER INFORMATION

- Centers for Disease Control. Traveler's Information Hotline: (404) 332-4559 (available 24 hours via a touch-tone telephone)
- International Association for Medical Assistance to Travelers, 417 Center St., Lewiston, NY 14092, (716) 754-4883

Chronic Fatigue Syndrome

 Basics

DESCRIPTION

Chronic fatigue syndrome (CFS) is characterized by profound fatigue and multiple physical and emotional symptoms, lasting at least 6 months, and which are severe enough to reduce or impair daily activity.

SIGNS AND SYMPTOMS

- Fatigue
- Unexplained general muscle weakness
- Pain or ache of muscles or joints
- Forgetfulness, inability to concentrate
- Confusion
- Mood swings, irritability, depression
- Low-grade fever (37.5-38.6°C)
- Prolonged fatigue lasting 24 hours after exercise
- Headaches
- Sensitivity to light
- Difficulty sleeping, night sweats
- Allergies
- Vertigo
- Swollen or painful glands
- Shortness of breath
- Chest pain
- Nausea
- Weight loss or gain
- Hot flushes
- Palpitations
- Gastrointestinal complaints
- Rash

CAUSES

Unknown

SCOPE

Chronic fatigue syndrome affects about 10 out of 100,000 persons in the United States.

MOST OFTEN AFFECTED

Young adults, females slightly more often than males

RISK FACTORS

Unknown

 Diagnosis

WHAT THE DOCTOR LOOKS FOR

The doctor will conduct a history and perform a thorough physical examination to identify and treat other potential causes of fatigue, such as infection, chronic inflammation, immune system disorders, or cancer.

TESTS AND PROCEDURES

- A number of blood tests may be ordered.
- Urinalysis, chest x-ray

 Treatment

GENERAL MEASURES

- Chronic fatigue syndrome is managed in the outpatient setting.
- As the cause of CFS is unknown and no specific therapy has shown consistent results, mainstay of therapy is supportive care.
- While not a cure, a program of moderate exercise (with rest periods during acute episodes), a healthy diet, stress reduction, and support groups or counselling are likely to be helpful.
- Alternative therapies (chiropractic, homeopathy, acupuncture, enforced rest) are helpful for some, but have not been proven to work. However, they may be worth trying.

ACTIVITY

As tolerated, but strenuous exercise tends to make symptoms worse in most persons with CFS.

DIET

No restrictions

Medications

COMMONLY PRESCRIBED DRUGS

- None
- Ampligen, essential fatty acid therapy, intra-venous (IV) immune globulin, vitamin B12, and bovine liver extract (LEFAC) have been used experimentally.
- Relief of symptoms with nonsteroidal anti-in-flammatory drugs (NSAIDs) and antidepressants

CONTRAINDICATIONS

Read drug product information.

PRECAUTIONS

Read drug product information.

DRUG INTERACTIONS

Read drug product information.

OTHER DRUGS

N/A

 ## Followup

PATIENT MONITORING

The doctor should be seen as often as necessary.

PREVENTION

Unknown

COMPLICATIONS

- Depression
- Socio-economic problems (e.g., inability to work)

WHAT TO EXPECT

- CFS is indolent, and waxes and wanes over time.
- Generally very slow improvement over months or years

 ## Miscellaneous

OTHER FACTORS

N/A

PEDIATRIC

CFS has been reported in children.

GERIATRIC

CFS has been reported in elderly persons.

OTHERS

N/A

PREGNANCY

N/A

FURTHER INFORMATION

- CFS Association, 3521 Broadway, Suite 222, Kansas City, MO 64111, (816)931-4777
- CFIDS Association. P.O. Box 220398, Charlotte, NC 28222-0398.
- International Chronic Fatigue Syndrome Society. P.O. Box 230108, Portland, OR 97223

Chronic Obstructive Pulmonary Disease and Emphysema

 Basics

DESCRIPTION

The term chronic obstructive pulmonary disease (COPD) encompasses several pulmonary diseases, including chronic bronchitis, asthma, cystic fibrosis, and emphysema. COPD usually refers to a mixture of chronic bronchitis and emphysema.
- Symptoms of chronic bronchitis include increased mucus production and recurrent cough.
- Emphysema involves the destruction of deep airway tissue.

SIGNS AND SYMPTOMS

- Chronic bronchitis
  - ▶ Cough
  - ▶ Sputum production
  - ▶ Frequent infections
  - ▶ Difficulty breathing
  - ▶ Swelling around the feet and ankles
  - ▶ A bluish discoloration around the lips, eyes, and nail beds
  - ▶ Wheezing
  - ▶ Weight gain
- Emphysema
  - ▶ Minimal cough
  - ▶ Scant sputum
  - ▶ Difficulty breathing
  - ▶ Often significant weight loss
  - ▶ Occasional infections
  - ▶ Barrel chest
  - ▶ Less wheezing
  - ▶ Use of accessory muscles of respiration
  - ▶ Pursed-lip breathing
  - ▶ Slight bluish discoloration around lips, eyes, and nail beds

SCOPE

- Chronic obstructive pulmonary disease affects 20–30% of the adult population in the United States and is responsible for more than 60,000 deaths annually.
- Eight million Americans have chronic bronchitis; 2 million people have emphysema.

MOST OFTEN AFFECTED

- Persons older than 40 years of age; males are affected more frequently than females.

- Although not a genetic disease, a predisposition to developing COPD may be inheritable. A rare form of emphysema is inherited.

CAUSES

- Cigarette smoking
- Air pollution
- Genetic defect (rare)
- Occupational exposure (e.g., firefighters)
- Viral infection (possibly)

RISK FACTORS

- Passive smoking (especially adults whose parents smoked)
- Severe viral pneumonia early in life
- Aging
- Alcohol consumption
- Asthma or allergies

 Diagnosis

WHAT THE DOCTOR LOOKS FOR

- The doctor will conduct a physical examination and investigate other possible respiratory diseases, such as acute bronchitis, asthma, cancer, or acute viral infection.
- The doctor will look for other conditions known to be associated with COPD, including coronary artery disease and peptic ulcer disease.

TESTS AND PROCEDURES

- Blood tests
- Arterial blood may be obtained.
- Pulmonary function may be tested to assist with diagnosis.
- Chest X-ray

 Treatment

GENERAL MEASURES

- COPD is usually managed adequately in the outpatient setting. Hospitalization may be needed for complications or diagnostic procedures.
- Respiratory failure may require intensive care and possibly mechanical breathing assistance.

- Smoking cessation
- Infections should be aggressively treated.
- Respiratory therapy
- Pulmonary rehabilitation
- Home oxygen may be required.
- Surgery may be indicated in selected cases.

ACTIVITY

As tolerated. Full activity should be encouraged.

DIET

A well-balanced, high-protein diet is suggested. Low carbohydrate intake may be helpful.

 # Medications

COMMONLY PRESCRIBED DRUGS

- Theophylline: Theo-Dur, Slo-bid, Unidur, Uniphyl
- Metaproterenol (Alupent), albuterol (Proventil, Ventolin), pirbuterol (Maxair), terbutaline (Brethaire), salmeterol (Serevent)
- Ipratropium: Atrovent
- Prednisone: Deltasone

CONTRAINDICATIONS

Read drug product information.

PRECAUTIONS

Read drug product information.

DRUG INTERACTIONS

Read drug product information.

OTHER DRUGS

Home oxygen

 # Followup

PATIENT MONITORING

- Individuals with severe disease or who are unstable should see the doctor monthly.
- When condition is stable, the doctor may be seen twice a year.
- Theophylline level may be checked every 6–12 months.
- If home oxygen is required, blood gasses should be checked annually or with any change in condition.

- Avoid travel at high altitude. Air travel with oxygen requires pre-arrangement.

PREVENTION

Smoking avoidance is the most important way to prevent COPD. Passive smoke also has been shown to be harmful.

COMPLICATIONS

- Infection is common.
- Other complications include circulatory and respiratory disease, respiratory failure, pulmonary hypertension, and malnutrition.

WHAT TO EXPECT

- Younger patients with mild disease have a fairly good prognosis. Older patients with more severe lung disease do worse.
- Supplemental oxygen, when indicated, has been shown to increase survival.
- Smoking cessation is also important for an improved prognosis.

 # Miscellaneous

OTHER FACTORS

N/A

PEDIATRIC

Repeated childhood respiratory illnesses increase the risk of COPD later in life.

GERIATRIC

The elderly have up to twice the risk as younger persons.

OTHERS

COPD is unusual among individuals younger than age 25 unless a genetic defect is present. The incidence of COPD increases as age approaches 60.

PREGNANCY

N/A

FURTHER INFORMATION

N/A

Cirrhosis of the Liver

 Basics

DESCRIPTION

Cirrhosis is a degenerative disease of the liver.

SIGNS AND SYMPTOMS

- Fatigue
- Loss of appetite
- Nausea
- Discomfort or a feeling of fullness in the abdomen
- Weakness and malaise
- Vomiting of blood
- Encephalopathy
- Yellowish discoloration of the skin and eyes (jaundice)
- Enlarged liver
- Enlargement of the breasts in men
- Testicular atrophy
- "Spider veins"

CAUSES

- Alcohol abuse
- Viral infection
- Genetic defect
- Other medical conditions

SCOPE

Cirrhosis of the liver accounts for over 30,000 deaths annually in the United States.

MOST OFTEN AFFECTED

Depends on cause

RISK FACTORS

See Causes

 Diagnosis

WHAT THE DOCTOR LOOKS FOR

- The doctor will perform a physical examination to evaluate liver function.
- The doctor will investigate conditions known to be associated with cirrhosis of the liver, such as hepatitis, gallbladder disease, cystic fibrosis, and heart failure.
- Possible sources of gastrointestinal bleeding will be investigated.

TESTS AND PROCEDURES

- A number of blood tests may be performed.
- The liver may be visually examined by laparoscopy.
- A sample of liver tissue may be obtained by biopsy for laboratory analysis.
- An imaging procedure called cholangiography may be done to evaluate the liver and gallbladder.
- Utrasound, computed tomography (CT scan), or other specialized procedures may be performed to assist in diagnosis.
- The upper digestive system may be evaluated by endoscopy.

GENERAL MEASURES

- Cirrhosis of the liver is usually managed on an outpatient basis, except for complicating emergencies such as gastrointestinal bleeding or kidney failure.
- Treatment is aimed at the underlying cause of cirrhosis, preventing further liver damage, and preventing complications.
- Therapies involve drug treatment, dietary restrictions, rest, and other supportive measures. Adequate protein intake is necessary for liver healing.
- Surgery or transplantation may be necessary.

ACTIVITY

Patients should be as active as possible. Leg elevation may be necessary for swelling of the feet and ankles.

DIET

- Adequate protein and generous calories to help the liver heal
- In some cases, protein restriction is necessary.
- In some cases, salt restriction is necessary.
- In some cases, fluid restriction is necessary.
- No alcohol

Medications

COMMONLY PRESCRIBED DRUGS

- Propranolol
- Spironolactone, furosemide
- Lactulose (Cholac)
- Ampicillin plus aminoglycoside, cefotaxime, norfloxacin, penicillamine
- Corticosteroids, azathioprine
- Interferon
- Ursodeoxycholic acid (Ursodiol)

CONTRAINDICATIONS

Read drug product information.

PRECAUTIONS

Read drug product information.

SIGNIFICANT POSSIBLE INTERACTIONS

Read drug product information.

OTHER DRUGS

N/A

 Followup

PATIENT MONITORING

- Stable patients need a yearly battery of liver tests.
- Unstable patients may need weekly tests.
- Patients should monitor weight and maintain a daily diary.

PREVENTION

- Limit use of alcohol and other substances that are toxic to the liver.
- Do not share syringes.
- Practice safe sex.

COMPLICATIONS

- Jaundice
- Bleeding disorders
- Brain damage
- Gastrointestinal bleeding
- Liver failure
- Liver cancer (uncommon)
- Infection
- Kidney failure

WHAT TO EXPECT

The course of cirrhosis depends on liver function. If a cause is identified and treated, the outcome may be good.

OTHER FACTORS

N/A

PEDIATRIC

N/A

GERIATRIC

Cirrhosis is one of the leading causes of death in people over age 65.

OTHERS

N/A

PREGNANCY

Cirrhosis may become worse during pregnancy. Higher rates of miscarriage, premature birth, and infant death occur in women with cirrhosis.

FURTHER INFORMATION

- American Liver Foundation, (800) 223-0179
- National Digestive Diseases Information Clearinghouse, Box NDDIC, Bethesda, MD 20892, (301) 468-6344

Claudication

 ## Basics

DESCRIPTION

Claudication is a feeling of muscle fatigue that occurs after a period of minimal exercise. The feeling may progress to a cramp-like pain, usually in the calf muscles. The pain is relieved by rest. Claudication may occur in the arms but is more common in the legs; calf more frequently than the thigh.

SIGNS AND SYMPTOMS

- May start gradually or suddenly
- Unable to walk distances
- Pain varies from muscle tiredness to a cramp
- May be a loss of hair on toes

CAUSES

Blockage of artery, usually due to arteriosclerosis

SCOPE

Claudication is common in the United States.

MOST OFTEN AFFECTED

Claudication is common in males over 55 years of age, females over 60 years of age. Males are affected four times as often as females.

RISK FACTORS

- Smoking
- Diabetes
- High blood pressure
- High levels of lipids and fats in the blood
- Obesity
- Heart disease

 ## Diagnosis

WHAT THE DOCTOR LOOKS FOR

- The doctor will perform a thorough assessment of the circulatory system.
- The doctor will look for other possible causes of symptoms, such as arthritis or nerve disorders.
- The doctor should diagnose and treat other cardiovascular disease.

TESTS AND PROCEDURES

- Blood tests
- Noninvasive blood pressure measurements in numerous locations on the extremities
- Specialized imaging of the circulatory system (arteriography) may be done to assist in diagnosis.
- Ultrasound may be done to assess blood vessels.

 ## Treatment

GENERAL MEASURES

- Claudication is managed in the outpatient setting, except for severe cases or advanced disease.
- Conservative measures: stop smoking, initiate walking and exercise program, control of high blood fats and cholesterol
- Reduce risk factors.
- Surgical treatment may be required.

ACTIVITY

As tolerated

DIET

N/A

Medications

COMMONLY PRESCRIBED DRUGS

- Aspirin
- Pentoxifylline (Trental)

CONTRAINDICATIONS

Read drug product information.

PRECAUTIONS

Try to reduce risk factors first before taking medications.

SIGNIFICANT POSSIBLE INTERACTIONS

Read drug product information.

OTHER DRUGS

- Ticlopidine
- Vasodilators
- Calcium channel blockers
- Blood thinners (anticoagulants)

Followup

PATIENT MONITORING

- The doctor should be seen as often as necessary.
- Imaging of blood vessels should be repeated twice a year.

PREVENTION

- Start walking program of 4 to 5 miles per day.
- Avoid smoking

COMPLICATIONS

A small number of people with claudication may ultimately require amputation of the affected leg.

WHAT TO EXPECT

The condition may gradually improve or get progressively worse.

Miscellaneous

OTHER FACTORS

N/A

PEDIATRIC

N/A

GERIATRIC

Claudication is more common with advancing age.

OTHERS

N/A

PREGNANCY

N/A

Common Cold

Basics

DESCRIPTION

The common cold is an inflammation of the
nasal passages due to any number of respiratory
viruses. The common cold is usually not serious;
the vast majority of sufferers treat themselves.

SIGNS AND SYMPTOMS

- Nasal stuffiness
- Sneezing
- Scratchy throat
- Cough
- Hoarseness
- Malaise
- Headache
- Fever

CAUSES

- Usually due to one of 200 strains of virus
- In 40% cases, no cause can be identified.

SCOPE

Preschool children average 6–10 colds annually;
children in kindergarten average 12 colds
annually; school children average 7 colds
annually; adolescents and adults average 2–4
colds annually. There are about 31 episodes of
cold per 100 persons annually.

MOST OFTEN AFFECTED

Children get colds more frequently than adults.
Males and females are affected in equal
proportions. American Indians and Eskimos are
at higher risk than other ethnic groups and have
more frequent complications, such as ear
infection. Certain genetic traits may make a
person unusually susceptible to the common
cold.

RISK FACTORS

- Exposure to infected individuals
- Touching the nose or eyes with contaminated
  fingers

Diagnosis

WHAT THE DOCTOR LOOKS FOR

The doctor will look for other conditions that
can cause similar signs and symptoms, such as
allergies or other viral infections.

TESTS AND PROCEDURES

- Blood tests
- Fluid from the nose or throat may be analyzed
  in the laboratory.
- In rare cases, virus may be cultured.

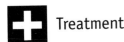 ## Treatment

GENERAL MEASURES

- Colds are usually managed by self-care
- Rest, fluids, and relief of symptoms
- The usual course of the common cold is 6–10 days.
- Use a vaporizer or humidifier.
- Stop smoking and drinking alcohol, if not already done.
- In infants, nasal passages may be cleared with a bulb syringe; incline mattress at 45°; use saline nasal drops.

ACTIVITY

Resume activity as tolerated, but rest more frequently the first few days after resuming activity.

DIET

Increase fluid intake.

 ## Medications

COMMONLY PRESCRIBED DRUGS

No cure or practical preventive measure exists for the common cold. Avoid "shotgun" medications (those that claim to treat all the symptoms of the common cold). Instead, target specific symptoms. This approach may reduce the risk of adverse effects from medications.

- Topical sprays: oxymetazoline (for stuffy nose), ipratropium (for runny nose)
- Oral decongestants: pseudoephedrine (for stuffy nose)
- Oral Antihistamines: chlorpheniramine (for sneezing, runny nose)
- Cough suppressants: codeine, dextromethorphan
- Expectorants: guaifenesin (effectiveness has not been proven)

Common Cold

CONTRAINDICATIONS

Oral decongestants are contraindicated in patients taking monoamine oxidase (MAO) inhibitors and selegiline.

PRECAUTIONS

- Oral decongestants
  - ▶ May increase blood pressure; may cause irregular heart rhythm; may interfere with diabetes management
  - ▶ Other adverse effects include headache, nervousness, sleeplessness, and dizziness.
  - ▶ Should be used with caution in patients taking guanethidine
- Antihistamines: may worsen nasal blockage and sinus congestion
- Cough suppressants: Codeine and dextromethorphan can be abused.
- Expectorants
  - ▶ Liquid preparations may contain high concentrations of alcohol.
  - ▶ Nausea, vomiting, or abdominal pain are common adverse effects.
- Vitamin C: Use is generally safe, but can cause kidney stones and interfere with urine glucose monitoring in people with diabetes.

DRUG INTERACTIONS

Read drug product information.

OTHER DRUGS

- Many mouthwashes, gargles, and lozenges are promoted to relieve the pain of sore throat. Hard candy, gargling with warm saline, and the use of products containing anesthetics such as benzocaine or phenol may all provide relief of pain. Antibacterial gargles or lozenges are of no value in treating a viral illness.
- Aromatic oils such as menthol, camphor, and eucalyptus, when applied topically or taken in a lozenge, produce a sensation of increased airflow.
- Antivirals: interferon, zinc chloride

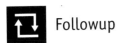

Followup

PATIENT MONITORING

Contact the physician for fever over 102°F (38.9°C), difficulty breathing, productive cough, or shaking chills.

PREVENTION

Frequent hand washing and avoiding touching the face may help prevent colds.

COMPLICATIONS

- Lower respiratory tract infection
- Asthma
- Severe worsening of asthma or chronic lung disease
- Ear infection (otitis media)
- Acute sinus infection
- Pneumonia

WHAT TO EXPECT

Complete recovery can be expected within 3–10 days.

Miscellaneous

OTHER FACTORS

N/A

PEDIATRIC

- Medications may produce toxic or adverse effects in young children.
- Do not give aspirin to children due to the risk of Reye's syndrome.
- Incidence of colds is highest among children.

GERIATRIC

Medications commonly produce adverse effects in the elderly.

OTHERS

N/A

PREGNANCY

Take medications only if clearly needed. No clear association exists between the use of decongestants or antihistamines and birth defects. Indiscriminate use of codeine during pregnancy may pose a risk to the fetus.

FURTHER INFORMATION

N/A

Congestive Heart Failure

 Basics

DESCRIPTION

Congestive heart failure (CHF) is the principal complication of heart disease. It is caused by abnormal cardiac pump function. CHF occurs at some time in all cases of severe heart disease.

SIGNS AND SYMPTOMS

- Early and mild heart failure:
  - ▶ Need to urinate during sleep hours
  - ▶ Shortness of breath on exertion
  - ▶ Diminished exercise capacity
  - ▶ Fatigue
  - ▶ Difficulty breathing
  - ▶ Weakness
  - ▶ Rapid heart rate with mild exertion
- Moderate heart failure:
  - ▶ Cough during sleep
  - ▶ Easier to breathe sitting up
  - ▶ Acute episodes of breathing difficulty during sleep
  - ▶ Wheezing, especially at night
  - ▶ Loss of appetite
  - ▶ Sensation of fullness or dull pain in abdomen
  - ▶ Rapid heart rate at rest
  - ▶ Anxiety
  - ▶ Coolness of the arms and legs
  - ▶ Swelling of the feet and ankles
- Severe heart failure:
  - ▶ Mental impairment
  - ▶ Abdominal bloating
  - ▶ A bluish discoloration around the mouth, eyes, or ears (cyanosis)
  - ▶ Low blood pressure
  - ▶ Frothy and/or pink sputum

CAUSES

- Heart attack
- Pulmonary embolism
- Metabolic disorders (hyperthyroidism, fever, stress)
- Other heart disease

SCOPE

Heart failure is the most common diagnosis in hospitalized persons over 65 years of age.

MOST OFTEN AFFECTED

Varies depending on cause. More common in males between the ages of 40 and 70; equal frequency with females 75 years of age or older.

RISK FACTORS

- Noncompliance with therapy
- Irregular heart rhythm
- Drug side effects
- Inappropriate physical, emotional, or environmental stress
- Other medical conditions

 Diagnosis

WHAT THE DOCTOR LOOKS FOR

- The doctor will perform a physical examination, in particular assessing heart function.
- The doctor should identify and treat correctable conditions, such as heart attack.

TESTS AND PROCEDURES

- A number of blood tests may be performed to assist in diagnosis.
- Urinalysis
- Chest X-ray
- The function of the heart may be studied with echocardiograhy.
- The heart may be assessed by cardiac catheterization.

 Treatment

GENERAL MEASURES

- Severe heart failure may require hospitalization.
- Underlying correctable conditions should be identified and treated.
- Surgery or transplantation may be required.

ACTIVITY

- During severe stage, bed rest with elevation of head of bed and anti-embolism stockings to help control leg swelling
- Gradual increase in activity with walking will help increase strength.

DIET

- Sodium restriction
- Weight reduction diet if overweight
- Low-fat diet to slow coronary artery disease

Medications

COMMONLY PRESCRIBED DRUGS

- Digoxin
- Diuretics: furosemide (Lasix), metolazone (Zaroxolyn), spironolactone
- Angiotensin-converting enzyme (ACE) inhibitors
- Vasodilators: nitroglycerin, hydralazine, prazosin, isosorbide dinitrate

CONTRAINDICATIONS

Read drug product information.

PRECAUTIONS

ACE inhibitors may cause low blood pressure (rare).

SIGNIFICANT POSSIBLE INTERACTIONS

Read drug product information.

OTHER DRUGS

Dopamine, dobutamine

Followup

PATIENT MONITORING

- The doctor should be seen as often as necessary depending on health status.
- Initially, the doctor may be seen every 2-3 weeks after stabilization.

PREVENTION

Treatment of underlying disorders, when possible

COMPLICATIONS

- Electrolyte disturbance
- Irregular heart rhythms
- Circulatory problems
- Digitalis toxicity

WHAT TO EXPECT

- Result of initial treatment is usually good, whatever the cause.
- The long-term outcome is variable. Death rates range from 10% with mild symptoms to 50% with advanced, progressive symptoms.

Miscellaneous

OTHER FACTORS

N/A

PEDIATRIC

Heart failure in children is usually associated with congenital heart disease.

GERIATRIC

N/A

OTHERS

N/A

PREGNANCY

Heart failure during pregnancy requires special care.

FURTHER INFORMATION

- American Heart Association, 7320 Greenville Avenue, Dallas, TX 75231, (214) 373-6300
- American College of Cardiology, 911 Old Georgetown Road, Bethesda, MD 20814, (301) 897-5400

Constipation

 Basics

DESCRIPTION

Constipation is a combination of changes in the frequency, size, consistency, and ease of stool passage, which leads to an overall decrease in volume of bowel movements. "Normal" toilet habits vary over a wide range; occasional episodes of constipation are to be expected.

SIGNS AND SYMPTOMS

- Less frequency of defecation than usual
- Harder stool than usual
- Smaller stools than usual
- Impaction of stool
- Thickening of stool
- Lack of consistent urgency to stool
- Difficulty expelling feces
- Painful evacuation of feces
- Sensation of incomplete emptying of the bowel
- Abdominal fullness
- Painful spasm of the rectum

CAUSES

- Electrolyte disturbance
- Hormonal disturbance (hypothyroidism, diabetes)
- Congenital conditions
- Other illness, injury, or debility
- Other bowel conditions
- Inadequate fluid intake
- Side effect of drugs (e.g., anticholinergic agents, opiates)
- Chronic abuse of laxatives or cathartics
- Psychiatric, cultural, emotional, environmental factors

SCOPE

- Constipation is common, affecting most persons at some point.
- More frequent among the very young and the very old

MOST OFTEN AFFECTED

- All ages can be affected by constipation, but it is more frequent in infancy and old age.
- May affect more than one member of a family
- More frequent in females than males

RISK FACTORS

- Age (very young or very old)
- Neurosis
- Drug use
- Sedentary life style or condition

 Diagnosis

WHAT THE DOCTOR LOOKS FOR

- The doctor will evalute the patient and identify and treat the cause of constipation.
- The doctor should evaluate for other signs of debility or aging (e.g, arthritis).

TESTS AND PROCEDURES

- Blood tests may be done to assist in diagnosis.
- Abdominal x-ray
- Specialized tests may be done to assess digestion, such as timing the passage of material through the tract.
- Digital rectal exam to rule out cancer and check for blood in the stool
- The lower intestinal tract may be visually examined by sigmoidoscopy or colonoscopy.

 Treatment

GENERAL MEASURES

- Constipation is usually managed in the outpatient setting, except when an underlying lesion or obstruction requires hospitalization.
- Attempt to eliminate medications that may cause or worsen constipation.
- Increase fluid intake.
- Modify diet.
- Use enemas if other remedies fail.
- Allow adequate time for bowel evacuation in a quiet, unhurried environment.
- Use commode with thighs drawn toward abdomen.

ACTIVITY

Exercise is encouraged.

DIET

- Increase fiber to approximately 15 grams per day (bran, fruit, green vegetables, and whole grain cereals and breads).
- Liberal intake of fluids is encouraged.

Constipation

 ## Medications

COMMONLY PRESCRIBED DRUGS

- Bulk-forming agents: psyllium (Konsyl, Metamucil, Perdiem), methylcellulose (Citrucel), polycarbophil (Mitrolan, Fibercon)
- Laxatives: milk of magnesia, magnesium citrate, phosphate of soda, lactulose (Chronulac), sorbitol, alumina-magnesia (Maalox, Mylanta); appropriate for short-term use
- Stool softeners: docusate sodium (Colace)

CONTRAINDICATIONS

- Any obstruction or impediment to transit in the bowel; laxatives may result in distension or perforation
- Acute abdominal inflammation
- Kidney and heart failure are relative contraindications.

PRECAUTIONS

Chronic use of laxatives can cause serious problems.

DRUG INTERACTIONS

Magnesium-containing laxatives interact with tetracycline, digitalis, and phenothiazines.

OTHER DRUGS

- Lubricants (e.g., mineral oil)
- Emollient suppositories: may relieve soreness
- Cathartics (stimulants): ricinoleic acid, castor oil (Neoloid), phenolphthalein (Ex-Lax, Modane), bisacodyl (Dulcolax)
- Anthraquinones: senna (Senokot)
- Enemas: Phospho soda (Fleets); avoid soap suds (may lead to colitis)
- Suppositories: sodium phosphate, glycerin, bisacodyl

 ## Followup

PATIENT MONITORING

See doctor if constipation persists.

PREVENTION

Some people have a tendency toward constipation. Proper diet, bowel training, and use of bulk-forming supplements are important.

COMPLICATIONS

- Serious bowel disorders
- Conditions caused by repeated laxative abuse
- Fluid and electrolyte depletion

WHAT TO EXPECT

Constipation that is occasional, brief, and responsive to simple measures is harmless. Habitual constipation can be a lifelong nuisance.

 ## Miscellaneous

OTHER FACTORS

N/A

PEDIATRIC

N/A

GERIATRIC

- Elderly persons who have had regular bowel action throughout their lives seldom develop constipation due to age alone.
- Persons with a lifelong tendency to constipation often encounter increasing difficulty with advancing age.
- An increased risk of colorectal cancer may be associated with constipation.

OTHERS

N/A

PREGNANCY

Women with a tendency toward constipation may find the condition more troublesome in the third trimester and require dietary adjustment and fiber supplements.

FURTHER INFORMATION

N/A

Contraception

 Basics

DESCRIPTION

Contraception is defined as practices designed to prevent pregnancy. Contraceptive practices either (1) prevent ovulation, (2) prevent implantation, (3) are spermicidal, or (4) prevent sperm from reaching the egg. Natural family planning aims to avoid intercourse at the time of expected ovulation. Failure rates vary among methods. The most effective form of contraception is permanent sterilization, either tubal sterilization in the female or vasectomy in the male. Neither are to be considered reversible, but it may be reversed under certain circumstances. Surgical attempts at reversal are often unsuccessful.

SIGNS AND SYMPTOMS

N/A

CAUSES

N/A

SCOPE

About two-thirds of women at risk for unwanted pregnancies use contraception.

MOST OFTEN AFFECTED

• Females: 11–52 years of age
• Males: any age after puberty

RISK FACTORS

• Pregnancy can occur in any woman who is ovulating and having intercourse with a fertile male.
• Young adolescents are at increased risk for unplanned pregnancy.
• Socioeconomic factors (e.g., less access to medical care, limited knowledge about repro-duction) can increase the risk for unplanned pregnancy.

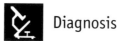 Diagnosis

WHAT THE DOCTOR LOOKS FOR

N/A

TESTS AND PROCEDURES

• Cells from the cervix may be examined by microscope (Pap smear).
• Cultures for sexually transmitted disease (gonorrhea and Chlamydia)
• Blood tests
• Female may be given a pregnancy test.
• Males may have a semen analysis after vasectomy.

Treatment

GENERAL MEASURES

- Latex condom: Use water-based lubricants; check for holes before using; leave space at tip to act as reservoir for the semen; withdraw from vagina before penis becomes flaccid; use a spermicide in addition to a condom to increase effectiveness.
- IUD: Check for the presence of the string frequently.
- Diaphragm: A diaphragm must be fitted by a physician. Before inserting, place one tablespoon of spermicidal gel or cream into the dome of diaphragm and line entire rim of the diaphragm with it; insert the diaphragm and check for proper placement; leave in for at least 8 hours after intercourse. Then remove and clean according to directions; check for holes. If another act of intercourse occurs before 8 hours, insert additional spermicidal gel or cream into vagina with an applicator device without displacing the diaphragm.

- Female condom (Reality): The female condom is available over-the-counter. Use new condom for each sex act; insert properly so that inner ring is well into vagina and outer ring lies against vulva; make sure that penis enters inside the sheath; remove condom after intercourse being careful not to spill semen.
- Periodic abstinence
  - ▶ Need accurate record of menstrual cycles for at least 12 months before use
  - ▶ Problem for women with variable cycle length
  - ▶ Added effectiveness from observing cervical mucus for disappearance of abundant clear mucus and by observing basal temperature rise of about 1 for 3 days. Both signs usually indicate ovulation.
- Permanent sterilization
  - ▶ Tubal sterilization in the female
  - ▶ Vasectomy in the male

ACTIVITY

N/A

DIET

N/A

Contraception

 Medications

COMMONLY PRESCRIBED DRUGS

- Oral contraceptives: Take pill daily at approximately same time; if a pill is missed, take two the following day but use an additional method of protection, such as a barrier method, until next menstrual period; if two menstrual periods are missed, seek medical care to rule out pregnancy. Do not stop pills if a period is missed.
- Spermicides: All contain nonoxynol-9. Choice depends on personal preference; foams and creams disperse well; suppositories or tablets must first dissolve.
- Implantable contraceptive: Levonorgestrel (Norplant) consists of six tubes implanted into the upper arm by physician; effective for up to 5 years.
- Injectable contraceptive: Medroxyprogesterone acetate (Depo-Provera); effective for up to 4 months

CONTRAINDICATIONS

- Implantable or injectable contraceptives
  - ▶ Active liver disease
  - ▶ Thrombophlebitis
  - ▶ Pregnancy
  - ▶ Unexplained, abnormal, uterine bleeding
  - ▶ High blood levels of fats and lipids
- Oral contraceptives
  - ▶ Same as implantable contraception plus noncompliance and estrogen-dependent cancer
  - ▶ May be inadvisable for women with high blood pressure, insulin-dependent diabetes mellitus, and migraine headaches
  - ▶ Not reccommended for women 35 years of age or older who smoke, due to increased risk of heart attack.

PRECAUTIONS

Read drug product information.

DRUG INTERACTIONS

Add a barrier method if taking phenytoin (Dilantin) or antibiotics.

OTHER DRUGS

N/A

Followup

PATIENT MONITORING

- The doctor should be seen annually for pelvic exam and Pap smear.
- Report side effects or problems to doctor.
- The doctor should check for presence of IUD 1 month after insertion.

PREVENTION

N/A

COMPLICATIONS

- Oral contraceptives
  - ▶ Clotting disorders
  - ▶ High blood pressure
  - ▶ Heart attack: main risk is in smoker, particularly after age 35
  - ▶ Nausea and vomiting: take pill on full stomach
  - ▶ Breakthrough bleeding : usually self-limiting after 3 months
  - ▶ Absence of menstrual period
  - ▶ Cyclic weight gain
  - ▶ Breast tenderness: rare with low-dose pill
  - ▶ Depression: rare with low-dose pill
  - ▶ Brown patches on skin
  - ▶ Acne or excessive hair growth
  - ▶ Jaundice
  - ▶ Weight gain throughout cycle

- Implantable contraceptive (Norplant)
  - ▶ Amenorrhea (absence of menstrual period): about 33%
  - ▶ Irregular bleeding: about 33%
  - ▶ Both are self limited after about 1 year.
- Injectable contraceptive (Depo-Provera)
  - ▶ Irregular bleeding during first few months
  - ▶ Not readily reversible
  - ▶ Absense of menstrual periods common after 1 year of use
- IUD
  - ▶ Pelvic inflammatory disease
  - ▶ Heavy bleeding and cramps
- Pregnancy may occur with any method.

WHAT TO EXPECT

N/A

 ## Miscellaneous

OTHER FACTORS

N/A

PEDIATRIC

N/A

GERIATRIC

N/A

OTHERS

Healthy nonsmokers may use oral contraceptives until age 50.

PREGNANCY

See above

FURTHER INFORMATION

Printed materials available from American College of Obstetrics and Gynecology (800) 673-8444

Crohn's Disease

 ## Basics

DESCRIPTION

Crohn's disease is a slowly progressive inflammatory disease of unknown cause affecting the small or large intestine.

SCOPE

Crohn's disease affects 20-100 out of 100,000 persons in the United States. It is more common in whites and Jews than African-Americans or Asians.

MOST OFTEN AFFECTED

- Most initial cases of Crohn's disease occur in people 15–25 years of age. It is also relatively common among individuals 55–65 years of age. Females are affected slightly more often than males.
- About 15% of affected persons have a member of the immediate family with the disease, with a similar pattern of symptoms and age of onset.

SIGNS AND SYMPTOMS

- Diarrhea
- Weight loss
- Pain, tenderness, or feeling of fullness in the abdomen
- Lesion of the rectum, bladder, skin, or vagina
- Disease elsewhere in the body (e.g., skin disease, arthritis)
- Bleeding

CAUSES

Unknown; condition is aggravated by infection or inflammation and by smoking cessation.

RISK FACTORS

N/A

 ## Diagnosis

WHAT THE DOCTOR LOOKS FOR

- The doctor will perform a physical examination to rule out other possible conditions, such as ulcerative colitis, intestinal infection, or cancer.
- The doctor identifies and treats other conditions known to be associated with Crohn's disease, such as arthritis and skin lesions.

TESTS AND PROCEDURES

- Blood tests
- Barium x-rays may be done to visualize the intestinal tract.
- The intestinal tract may be visually examined by colonoscopy.
- A sample of tissue may be obtained by biopsy for analysis.
- Plain x-rays or computed tomography (CT scan) of the abdomen

 ## Treatment

GENERAL MEASURES

- Crohn's disease is customarily treated in an outpatient setting.
- Hospitalization may be required for complications or special treatments.
- The disease is progressive and often requires surgery.
- Attention to maintaining weight and nutrition is important.
- Use a sitz bath at the direction of the doctor.
- Clean anal area with soap and water after bowel movements.

ACTIVITY

Full activity as tolerated

DIET

- Usually no restrictions
- If fat malabsorption is a problem, reduce dietary fat.
- Avoid highly fibrous substances if scarring or recurring obstructions develop.
- Increase dietary fiber if diarrhea is prominent; reducing dietary fat is also sometimes recommended.

Medications

COMMONLY PRESCRIBED DRUGS

- Mesalamine (5-aminosalicylic acid), methotrexate, azathioprine (Imuran), prednisone, sulfasalazine
- Prednisone, hydrocortisone (Cortenema), or mesalamine enemas
- Metronidazole (Flagyl), olsalazine (Dipentum)

CONTRAINDICATIONS

Drug allergy

PRECAUTIONS

- Sulfasalazine may not be tolerated because it frequently causes nausea, vomiting, and other gastrointestinal distress.
- Drug allergies are common.
- Male sterility is a problem with chronic use.

SIGNIFICANT POSSIBLE INTERACTIONS

Read drug product information.

OTHER DRUGS

- Antibiotics
- Mercaptopurine (6-mercaptopurine)

Followup

PATIENT MONITORING

- The doctor should be seen every 3–6 months if symptoms are stable or as often as necessary based on health status.
- Contact the doctor about changes in condition.
- The digestive tract may be periodically examined by endoscopy.

PREVENTION

- An individual with Crohn's disease should receive good medical care, including ongoing care with regular physician and use of consulting physicians when necessary.

COMPLICATIONS

- Progression of Crohn's disease is nearly certain, even after surgery.
- About 15% of patients develop an ulcer or lesion.
- About 10% have disease elsewhere in the body, such as skin disease or arthritis.
- Extensive colon disease is associated with an increased risk of cancer.
- Colon may become severely diseased or perforated, which may lead to massive bleeding.

WHAT TO EXPECT

- The average patient has surgery every 7 years.
- Short-bowel syndrome may develop after four surgeries.
- Expect the disease to recur.
- Most people have a normal life with work, children, and full activities, but overall lifespan is shortened.

Miscellaneous

OTHER FACTORS

N/A

PEDIATRIC

Crohn's disease is rare in children.

GERIATRIC

N/A

OTHERS

Occurs at any age

PREGNANCY

- Long-time use of sulfasalazine can cause sterility in males that resolves when person stops taking medication.
- Crohn's disease is not a contraindication to pregnancy.

FURTHER INFORMATION

Crohn's and Colitis Foundation of America Inc, 11th floor, Park Ave South, NY 10016, Phone (800) 343-3637

Croup

 ## Basics

DESCRIPTION

Croup is a viral illness characterized by barking cough, high-pitched breathing, and fever, that often causes upper airway obstruction in children.

SIGNS AND SYMPTOMS

- Barking, spasmodic cough
- Noisy, high-pitched breathing
- Low-grade to moderate fever
- Bluish discoloration around eyes, mouth, and nail beds (cyanosis)
- Fatigue

CAUSES

Viral infection

SCOPE

There are 15,000–40,000 cases of croup per 100,000 persons in the United States.

MOST OFTEN AFFECTED

Children, males and females in equal proportion

RISK FACTORS

- History of croup
- Recurring upper respiratory infections

 ## Diagnosis

WHAT THE DOCTOR LOOKS FOR

- The doctor will perform a physical examination to assess for the presence of croup.
- Conditions that can cause similar signs and symptoms include epiglottitis, foreign body aspiration, and other types of infection.

TESTS AND PROCEDURES

- Blood tests
- Fluid from the throat may be sampled for laboratory analysis.
- X-rays of the neck
- The airway may be examined by laryngoscopy or bronchoscopy.

 ## Treatment

GENERAL MEASURES

- Mild cases of croup may be managed in the outpatient setting.
- Severe cases may require intensive care.
- Humidification ("croup tent")
- Intravenous (IV) fluids
- Intubation may be required.
- Tracheotomy (rarely)

ACTIVITY

Must keep patient quiet; crying may worsen symptoms.

DIET

- Nothing by mouth for severe cases
- Frequent small feedings with increased fluids for mild cases

Medications

COMMONLY PRESCRIBED DRUGS

- Dexamethasone
- Racemic epinephrine (Vaponefrin)
- Antibiotics
- Oxygen as needed

PRECAUTIONS

Read drug product information.

CONTRAINDICATIONS

Read drug product information.

DRUG INTERACTIONS

Read drug product information.

OTHER DRUGS

- Budesonide
- Ribavirin
- Amantadine

 ## Followup

PATIENT MONITORING

- Patients in the hospital will be seen often by the doctor and other health care professionals.
- The doctor should be seen as often as necessary.
- Contact doctor immediately for any severe worsening of condition, or call 9-1-1.

PREVENTION

N/A

COMPLICATIONS

- Bacterial infection
- Cardiopulmonary arrest
- Pneumonia

WHAT TO EXPECT

- If required, intubation is maintained for 3–5 days.
- If required, tracheotomy is maintained for 3–7 days.
- Recovery is usually complete, without lasting effects.

 ## Miscellaneous

OTHER FACTORS

N/A

PEDIATRIC

Croup is common in children under 3 years of age.

GERIATRIC

N/A

OTHERS

N/A

PREGNANCY

N/A

FURTHER INFORMATION

N/A

Cutaneous (Skin) Drug Reactions

 Basics

DESCRIPTION

Cutaneous (skin) rashes or eruptions are the most common adverse reactions to drug therapy. The majority of reactions develop within 1 week of initiation of drug therapy but may occur up to 4 weeks later.

SCOPE

• There are about 144 cases of drug reaction among 100,000 hospitalized persons.
• Overall prevalence is unknown among the 125 million nonhospitalized Americans who regularly use prescription drugs as outpatients.

MOST OFTEN AFFECTED

All ages affected, females more often than males

SIGNS AND SYMPTOMS

• Eruptions of skin: most frequent skin reaction; reddened pimples or bumps that often itch; onset typically 7–10 days after initiation of drug; may last 1–2 weeks
• Rash: itchy red spots; may fade within 24 hours, but new rash may develop
• Acne-like eruptions
• Eczema-like reactions: itchy, scaling skin on inner surfaces of arms or legs
• Patches of dry skin or hair loss
• Sensitivity to light

CAUSES

Exposure to medication

RISK FACTORS

Drug therapy, especially with antibiotics

 Diagnosis

WHAT THE DOCTOR LOOKS FOR

• The doctor performs an examination and looks for other diseases that cause similar signs.
• The doctor will look for other conditions known to be associated with drug reactions, such as severe allergies, swelling, or bone marrow disorders.

TESTS AND PROCEDURES

• Routine blood tests are usually not helpful.
• A sample of tissue may be obtained by biopsy for laboratory analysis.
• Skin testing for allergies may be performed.

 Treatment

GENERAL MEASURES

• A person with rash or swelling should be evaluated by a doctor as soon as possible.
• Hospitalization may be required for severe allergies or other acute reactions.
• Stop taking the drug that causes reactions.
• Avoid use of the drug that caused the reaction.

ACTIVITY

• No specific restrictions in general
• For acute dry, scaly skin or rash, bathe with tepid water and avoid activities that cause sweating.

DIET

No dietary restrictions

Cutaneous (Skin) Drug Reactions

 Medications

COMMONLY PRESCRIBED DRUGS

- Most cases require no specific therapy.
- Antihistamines may relieve symptoms of rash, swelling, and inflammation.
- Skin creams or lotions may be used for dry skin.
- Topical corticosteroids

CONTRAINDICATIONS

Read drug product information.

PRECAUTIONS

Read drug product information.

DRUG INTERACTIONS

Read drug product information.

OTHER DRUGS

N/A

 Followup

PATIENT MONITORING

- The doctor should be seen often to ensure that the reaction is not progressing.
- Patients with severe reactions may require hospitalization.

PREVENTION

Avoid drugs that cause reaction.

WHAT TO EXPECT

- Eruptions generally fade within days after stopping drug therapy.
- Rash, swelling, and other severe reactions are potentially more serious and can even be life-threatening.

 Miscellaneous

OTHER FACTORS

N/A

PEDIATRIC

N/A

GERIATRIC

- Reactions may be more likely among elderly who take a greater number of medications.
- Severe reactions are less tolerated in the elderly.

OTHERS

N/A

PREGNANCY

N/A

FURTHER INFORMATION

American Academy of Dermatology, 930 N. Meacham Rd., P.O. Box 4014, Schaumberg, IL 60168-4014; (708) 330-0230

Cystic Fibrosis

 Basics

DESCRIPTION

Cystic fibrosis, or CF, is a generalized disorder of infants, children and young adults. Characteristics include chronic pulmonary disease, pancreatic disease, and abnormally high levels of salts in the sweat.

SIGNS AND SYMPTOMS

- Sweat glands
  - ▶ Increased concentrations of salt
  - ▶ Dehydration with heat and infections
- Respiratory system:
  - ▶ Wheezing
  - ▶ Chronic cough
  - ▶ Difficulty
  - ▶ Rapid breathing
  - ▶ Barrel chest
  - ▶ Repeated bouts of bronchitis or pneumonia
- Gastrointestinal system:
  - ▶ Failure to thrive
  - ▶ Chronic, recurrent abdominal pain
  - ▶ Gastroesophageal reflux
  - ▶ Voracious appetite before treatment
  - ▶ A sensation of fullness in the abdomen
  - ▶ Frequent, bulky, foul-smelling, pale stool
- Others:
  - ▶ Delayed weight gain during growth and development
  - ▶ Retarded bone growth
  - ▶ Delayed sexual development
  - ▶ Infertility in males

CAUSES

Genetic defect

SCOPE

CF is the most common lethal genetic disease. It affects about 1 in 2,000 Caucasians. It is less common in African-Americans, Native Americans, and Asians.

MOST OFTEN AFFECTED

Infants, children, and young adults are most often affected, as the average age of survival is age 29. Males and females are affected equally. CF tends to run in families.

RISK FACTORS

Family history of CF

Diagnosis

WHAT THE DOCTOR LOOKS FOR

- The doctor will perform a thorough physical examination to look for specific signs and symptoms of CF.
- Other possible causes of signs and symptoms will be investigated, such as immune system disorders, recurring pneumonia, or asthma.
- The doctor will look for known complications of CF, such as collapsed lung, heart failure, or other serious conditions.

TESTS AND PROCEDURES

- Blood tests
- Sweat tests
- Genetic screening
- Stool studies
- Fluid from airway may be cultured for laboratory analysis.
- Pulmonary function tests
- Exercise testing may be performed.
- The structures and function of the heart may be evaluated by ultrasound.
- Chest x-ray

 ## Treatment

GENERAL MEASURES

- CF is usually managed in the outpatient setting.
- Infections or other crisis may require hospitalization.
- Intravenous (IV) antibiotics to prevent infection may be provided at home.
- Care by experienced physician and team (respiratory therapist, nurse, nutritionist, physical therapist, counsellor, social worker) is crucial.
- Goals are to prevent and treat respiratory failure and pulmonary complications.
- Respiratory therapy
- Regular exercises for fitness
- Emphasis on good nutrition; supplements may be needed
- Medication for treatment of symptoms
- Insulin, if diabetes develops
- Surgery may be needed for some complications
- Organ transplants possible for lung, liver, and endocrine pancreas

ACTIVITY

Physical conditioning to the extent possible for cardiorespiratory fitness

DIET

- Allow liberal salting of foods, if desired
- High dietary protein, calories, fat
- Vitamin supplements (double the Recommended Daily Allowance)

Cystic Fibrosis

 ## Medications

COMMONLY PRESCRIBED DRUGS

- Antibiotics: may be oral, IV, or aerosolized
- Other therapies: pancreatic enzyme replacement, bronchodilators, dornase alfa (DNase), ibuprofen, oxygen therapy, annual flu vaccine

CONTRAINDICATIONS

Read drug product information.

PRECAUTIONS

Read drug product information.

SIGNIFICANT POSSIBLE INTERACTIONS

Read drug product information.

OTHER DRUGS

Other antibiotics

 ## Followup

PATIENT MONITORING

The doctor should be seen at least 3 times a year; management at a cystic fibrosis center is recommended.

PREVENTION

- Genetic counseling
- Prenatal diagnosis for future pregnancies
- For respiratory infections: vaccines, avoidance of general anesthesia, management by a good medical team

Cystic Fibrosis

COMPLICATIONS

- Collapsed lung
- Heart failure
- Pulmonary hypertension
- Emphysema
- Other circulatory and respiratory problems
- Diabetes
- Metabolic disorders
- Bleeding esophageal varices
- Liver and intestinal disorders
- Sterility in females
- Numerous psychosocial aspects
- Malnutrition
- Retarded growth

WHAT TO EXPECT

- The outcome largely depends on the involvement of the lungs.
- The prognosis is improving due to early detection and aggressive treatment.
- Average survival is to age 29.

 Miscellaneous

OTHER FACTORS

N/A

PEDIATRIC

Diagnosis is usually confirmed in infancy or early childhood but some cases go undetected until adolescence.

GERIATRIC

N/A

OTHERS

N/A

PREGNANCY

If physical condition is good at the start of pregnancy, the mother usually returns to that level following birth. If health is poor before pregnancy, health status may get worse following birth.

PATIENT EDUCATION

Cystic Fibrosis Foundation, 6931 Arlington Road, Ste. 2000, Bethesda, MD 20814, (800) 344-4823.

Section D

Dehydration

 Basics

DESCRIPTION

Dehydration is a depletion of body fluids that occurs when fluids are lost from the gastrointestinal tract, urinary tract, and skin.

SIGNS AND SYMPTOMS

- Skin that "tents" when pinched
- Dry, shrunken tongue
- Dizziness when standing
- Rapid heart rate
- Disorientation
- Shock

CAUSES

Excessive loss of fluid from the gastrointestinal tract, urinary tract and skin. May result from vomiting, diarrhea, excessive sweating, dialysis, chronic kidney disease, diuretic ("water pill") therapy, diabetes mellitus, and other disorders.

SCOPE

N/A

MOST OFTEN AFFECTED

N/A

RISK FACTORS

N/A

 Diagnosis

WHAT THE DOCTOR LOOKS FOR

N/A

TESTS AND PROCEDURES

N/A

 Treatment

GENERAL MEASURES

- Replacement of fluids and salts
- Discontinue diuretics

ACTIVITY

N/A

DIET

N/A

Dehydration

 Medications

COMMONLY PRESCRIBED DRUGS
N/A

CONTRAINDICATIONS
N/A

PRECAUTIONS
N/A

DRUG INTERACTIONS
N/A

OTHER DRUGS
N/A

 Followup

PATIENT MONITORING
N/A

PREVENTION
N/A

COMPLICATIONS
N/A

WHAT TO EXPECT
N/A

 Miscellaneous

OTHER FACTORS
N/A

PEDIATRIC
N/A

GERIATRIC
N/A

OTHERS
N/A

PREGNANCY
N/A

FURTHER INFORMATION
N/A

Dementia

 Basics

DESCRIPTION

Dementia, also called senility, is the persistent impairment of intellectual functioning.
- Alzheimer's disease is the most common form of dementia, characterized by a relentless deterioration of higher brain functioning. The rate of deterioration varies.
- Multi-infarct dementia (MID) results from strokes or "mini-strokes."
- Some forms of dementia can be reversed.

SIGNS AND SYMPTOMS

- Impaired memory, abstract thinking, and judgment
- Difficulty with language or speaking
- Personality change, emotional outbursts, wandering, restlessness, hyperactivity
- Sleep disturbances
- Mood disturbances
- Urinary incontinence
- Fecal incontinence (late)
- Tremor
- Hallucinations, delusions
- Paranoia
- Weight loss
- Seizures

CAUSES

- Alzheimer's disease
- Stroke or "mini-strokes" caused by atherosclerosis (hardening) of brain arteries
- Other brain disorders

SCOPE

- About 1.2 million people in the United States have severe dementia, and another 2.5 million have moderate illness.
- Ten percent of all persons over the age of 65 have clinically important dementia.
- At least 15% of those with Alzheimer's have a family history of the disease.

MOST OFTEN AFFECTED

The incidence of dementia increases with age. Males and females are affected in equal proportion. Some forms can occur in younger persons.

RISK FACTORS

- Increasing age
- Atherosclerotic disease
- Trisomy 21 (Down syndrome)
- History of head trauma
- History of central nervous system infection

 Diagnosis

WHAT THE DOCTOR LOOKS FOR

- The doctor will perform a physical examination to identify any medical problems.
- Psychologic functioning will be evaluated.
- Possible causes of dementia will be identified and treated.

TESTS AND PROCEDURES

- Blood tests
- Syphilis test
- Mental status testing
- Electroencephalogram (EEG) may be performed to assist in diagnosis.
- Computed tomography (CT scan), magnetic resonance imaging (MRI), or positron emission tomography (PET) may be performed to evaluate brain structures and function.

 Treatment

GENERAL MEASURES

- Dementia is managed in the outpatient setting except when complications require hospitalization.
- Nursing home care or adult day care may be necessary.
- Daily schedules and written directions can be helpful.

- Emphasis on nutrition, personal hygiene, personal safety (accident-proofing the home), and supervision
- Provide sensory stimulation (prominent displays of clocks and calendars).

ACTIVITY

Fully active with direction and supervision

DIET

No special diet

Medications

COMMONLY PRESCRIBED DRUGS

- Antipsychotics: haloperidol (Haldol), thioridazine (Mellaril)
- Depression: nortriptyline (Pamelor), desipramine (Norpramin), sertraline (Zoloft), fluoxetine (Prozac), paroxetine (Paxil), fluvoxamine (Luvox)
- Sleep disturbance: temazepam (Restoril), zolpidem (Ambien), trazodone (Desyrel), chloral hydrate
- Tacrine (Cognex)
- Donepezil (Aricept).

CONTRAINDICATIONS

- Antipsychotics (haloperidol, thioridazine): severe depression, Parkinson's disease, hypo- or hypertension
- Tricyclic antidepressants (nortriptyline, desipramine): heart attack, acute narrow-angle glaucoma
- Acute active liver disease; active, untreated peptic ulcers

PRECAUTIONS

Drugs have numerous precautions; read drug product information.

DRUG INTERACTIONS

Drugs have numerous interactions; read drug product information.

OTHER DRUGS

- Lithium carbonate
- Carbamazepine (Tegretol)

Followup

PATIENT MONITORING

The doctor should be seen as often as needed to evaluate health and mental function and monitor drug therapy.

PREVENTION

N/A

COMPLICATIONS

- Drug side effects
- Falls
- Pressure sores
- Malnutrition
- Constipation
- Infections

WHAT TO EXPECT

- Alzheimer's disease: the progression of this disease varies, but it inevitably leads to profound impairment.
- Some forms of dementia can be treated, but the course of most dementia varies.

Miscellaneous

OTHER FACTORS

N/A

PEDIATRIC

N/A

GERIATRIC

N/A

OTHERS

N/A

PREGNANCY

N/A

FURTHER INFORMATION

Alzheimer's Association, (800) 621-0379

Depression

 Basics

DESCRIPTION

Depression results when a person experiences more frustration and anger than he or she can handle. Each person is capable of handling a different amount of frustration or anger.

SIGNS AND SYMPTOMS

- Depressed mood
- Poor appetite: either weight gain or loss (may eat or drink out of boredom or reasons other than appetite)
- Sleep disorder: either insomnia or excessive sleepiness
- Fatigue: tiredness out of proportion to the amount of energy expended
- Agitation, restlessness, irritability, or withdrawal
- Lack of interest in pleasure, decreased sexual appetite, lack of pleasure in activities or things the person used to enjoy
- Poor self image: self-reproach, excessive guilt
- Difficulty concentrating, poor memory, inability to make decisions
- Suicidal thoughts

CAUSES

Neurotransmitter imbalance

SCOPE

It is estimated that 5–20% of population will experience a significant depression at some time.

MOST OFTEN AFFECTED

Average age is 30–40 years; females more often than males. A tendency to depression may be inheritable.

RISK FACTORS

- Female gender
- Family history (depression, suicide, alcoholism, other substance abuse)
- Chronic disease, especially multiple diseases
- Migraine headaches
- Chronic pain
- Recent heart attack
- Peptic ulcer disease

- Insomnia
- Stressful situations
- Adolescence
- Advancing age
- Retirement
- Children with behavioral disorders, especially hyperactivity

 Diagnosis

WHAT THE DOCTOR LOOKS FOR

The doctor will evaluate the patient to identify causes of depression, such as brain disease, hormone disorders, or other conditions.

TESTS AND PROCEDURES

- Blood tests
- Urinalysis
- Electrocardiogram (EKG)
- Measurement of brain activity may be performed, called electroencephalography (EEG).
- Computed tomography (CAT scan) or magnetic resonance imaging (MRI) may be performed to assist in diagnosis.
- Psychologic testing may be given.

 Treatment

GENERAL MEASURES

- Depression is managed in the outpatient setting.
- Psychotherapy is helpful in solving the problems caused by depression.
- Consider support groups.

ACTIVITY

No restrictions

DIET

No special diet

Medications

COMMONLY PRESCRIBED DRUGS

- Anxiety, restlessness, irritability or sleeplessness: amitriptyline (Elavil, Endep), nortriptyline (Pamelor, Aventyl), doxepin (Adapin, Sinequan), trazodone (Desyrel), trimipramine (Surmontil)
- Fatigue, excessive sleepiness, indecisiveness, or difficulty in concentration: imipramine (Tofranil, Tipramine), desipramine (Norpramin, Pertofrane), fluoxetine (Prozac), sertraline (Zoloft), paroxetine (Paxil), protriptyline (Vivactil), bupropion (Wellbutrin)
- Venlafaxine (Effexor)

CONTRAINDICATIONS

Read drug product information.

PRECAUTIONS

- Medications have sedating side effects.
- Most common side effects are dry mouth, constipation, profuse sweating, and sleepiness. Most side effects decrease or disappear in 2 to 3 weeks.

DRUG INTERACTIONS

- Read drug product information.
- Avoid nonprescription drugs containing pseudoephedrine, phenylephrine, or phenylpropanolamine (cold medicines).

OTHER DRUGS

- Clomipramine (Anafranil)
- MAO inhibitors

Followup

PATIENT MONITORING

- The doctor should be seen within 2 weeks after starting medication. Don't expect to feel greatly improved at this visit.
- Office visits about every 2 weeks until improvement begins

- If treatment is adequate, depression should improve within 4 weeks.
- The doctor should be seen 3 months thereafter.
- Treatment must continue even after improvement.

PREVENTION

See Causes and Risk factors

COMPLICATIONS

- Suicide
- Failure to improve

WHAT TO EXPECT

Properly treated, depression almost always improves.

Miscellaneous

OTHER FACTORS

N/A

PEDIATRIC

Depression occurs in children.

GERIATRIC

Depression is more common among the elderly.

OTHERS

N/A

PREGNANCY

Medications should be used with caution during pregnancy. Rely on psychotherapy and support groups until pregnancy is completed.

FURTHER INFORMATION

National Depression Manic Depression Association (DMDA) (800) 82-MDMDA

Dermatitis, Contact

 Basics

DESCRIPTION

Contact dermatitis is an inflammatory reaction of the skin in response to an external substance.
- Primary dermatitis is due to injury of the skin by specific irritants, generally producing discomfort immediately after exposure.
- Allergic contact dermatitis affects individuals previously sensitized to the substance. It is a delayed reaction, developing over several hours.

SIGNS AND SYMPTOMS

- Bumps, blisters, or rash surrounded by reddened skin
- Crusting or oozing
- Itching
- Thickening of skin
- Flaking, scaling
- Fissuring
- May occur in areas where skin is thinner (eyelids, genitalia)
- Usually occurs in areas that have been in contact with offending agent (e.g., nails and nail polish)
- Linear lesions or welts
- Lesions with sharp borders and sharp angles

CAUSES

- Plants (poison ivy, oak, sumac)
- Chemicals (jewelry, zippers, hair dyes, industrial chemicals, detergents)
- Topical medicines (antibiotics, anesthetics)

SCOPE

N/A

MOST OFTEN AFFECTED

Contact dermititis occurs in people of all ages, males and females in equal proportion. Allergic dermatitis is more common in families with a history of allergies.

RISK FACTORS

- Occupation
- Hobbies
- Travel
- Cosmetics
- Jewelry

 Diagnosis

WHAT THE DOCTOR LOOKS FOR

The doctor will look for signs and symptoms of contact dermatitis.

TESTS AND PROCEDURES

Patch tests for allergies

GENERAL MEASURES

- Contact dermatitis is managed in the outpatient setting.
- Remove the offending agent.
- Avoid irritating substances.
- Topical soaks
- Lukewarm water baths for itching
- Aveeno (oatmeal) baths
- Emollients (white petrolatum, Eucerin)

ACTIVITY

Stay active, but avoid overheating.

DIET

No special diet

Medications

COMMONLY PRESCRIBED DRUGS

- Topical
  - ▶ Lotion of zinc oxide, talc, menthol 0.25%, phenol 0.5%
  - ▶ Corticosteroids: fluocinonide (Lidex)
  - ▶ Calamine lotion
  - ▶ Topical antibiotics for secondary infection: bacitracin, gentamicin, erythromycin
- Systemic
  - ▶ Antihistamine: hydroxyzine, diphenhydramine
  - ▶ Corticosteroids: prednisone
  - ▶ Antibiotics: erythromycin

CONTRAINDICATIONS

N/A

PRECAUTIONS

- Drowsiness from antihistamines
- Local skin effects from prolonged use of potent topical steroids

DRUG INTERACTIONS

N/A

OTHER DRUGS

Other topical antibiotics

 ## Followup

PATIENT MONITORING

- The doctor should be seen as often as necessary.

PREVENTION

Avoid causative agents. Use of protective gloves (with cotton lining) when handling agents may be helpful.

COMPLICATIONS

- Severe eruption
- Secondary bacterial infection

WHAT TO EXPECT

Contact dermatitis is harmless and usually goes away by itself.

 ## Miscellaneous

OTHER FACTORS

N/A

PEDIATRIC

N/A

GERIATRIC

The elderly have an increased incidence of dermatitis due to dry skin.

OTHERS

N/A

PREGNANCY

Usual cautions with medications.

FURTHER INFORMATION

N/A

Diabetes Mellitus, Insulin-Dependent (IDDM of Type I)

 Basics

DESCRIPTION

Insulin-dependent diabetes mellitus (IDDM) is a chronic disease caused by the insufficient production of insulin. It requires the regular administration of insulin. Individuals with poorly controlled IDDM are at risk for several complications, including eye, nerve, kidney, and cardiovascular problems.

SIGNS AND SYMPTOMS

- Frequent urination
- Severe thirst, frequent drinking
- Excessive eating
- Loss of appetite
- Weight loss
- Fatigue, lethargy
- Muscle cramps
- Irritability and mood swings
- Vision changes, such as blurriness
- Altered school or work performance
- Headaches
- Anxiety attacks
- Chest pain and occasional difficult breathing
- Abdominal discomfort and pain
- Nausea
- Diarrhea or constipation

CAUSES

- Inherited genetic defect
- Environmental factors may be involved, such as viruses, diet, toxins, and stress.

SCOPE

Insulin-dependent diabetes mellitus affects 15 out of 100,000 persons annually.

MOST OFTEN AFFECTED

The average age of onset is 8–12 years. Males and females are affected in equal numbers. IDDM is more common in Caucasians, less common in African-Americans. It may be inherited.

RISK FACTORS

Genetic factors

Diabetes Mellitus, Insulin-Dependent (IDDM of Type I)

 ## Diagnosis

WHAT THE DOCTOR LOOKS FOR

- The doctor will obtain a history and perform a physical examination to identify the signs and symptoms of diabetes.
- A cause of diabetes will be identified if possible.

TESTS AND PROCEDURES

- A number of blood tests may be performed to assist in diagnosis.
- Electrolytes
- Urinalysis
- A procedure called an oral glucose tolerance test may be done to assess how the body metabolizes sugar.

 ## Treatment

GENERAL MEASURES

- Initial care may require hospitalization.
- Diabetes is usually managed on an outpatient basis, preferably in a diabetes clinic where a team approach is used.
- Routine care is done by the family at home. The child is encouraged to do as much self-care as possible.
- For the very young child, treatment is aimed at maintaining blood sugar levels within a normal range. "Tight control" of blood glucose levels, in which the individual strives to maintain normal blood glucose levels at all times, may be dangerous for the very young child. For adults, tight control may prevent or reduce the severity of diabetes complications. However, it can increase the frequency of hypoglycemia (low blood sugar levels).
- Prevention of complications is a goal of treatment.

ACTIVITY

- All normal activities, including full participation in sports activities
- Regular, rather than periodic, aerobic exercise is preferable.

DIET

A well-balanced diet is important in the management of diabetes. Meals and snacks must be coordinated with insulin injections. The advice of a nutritionist is helpful in the management of IDDM.

Diabetes Mellitus, Insulin-Dependent (IDDM or Type I)

 Medications

COMMONLY PRESCRIBED DRUGS

Insulin

CONTRAINDICATIONS

None

PRECAUTIONS

Patients will receive extensive education about how to avoid hypoglycemia and rebound hyperglycemia (high blood sugar levels).

DRUG INTERACTIONS

N/A

OTHER DRUGS

- Immunosuppressants: cyclosporine
- Other experimental drugs: azathioprine, steroids, nicotinamide

 Followup

PATIENT MONITORING

- Initially, the doctor should be seen frequently until stable; then every 2–3 months thereafter.
- Daily home blood glucose monitoring with home blood glucose meter (e.g., One-Touch, Accuchek, Glucometer, Exactech, Answer) 3–4 times daily, with adjustment/supplementation of insulin dose based on blood glucose levels
- Periodic (about every 3 months) blood tests to assess overall glycemic control
- Dietary management should be regularly reviewed and updated.

PREVENTION

None known

Diabetes Mellitus, Insulin-Dependent (IDDM or Type 1)

COMPLICATIONS

- Vascular disease
- High levels of fats in the bloodstream
- Foot problems
- Low blood sugar
- Diabetic ketoacidosis
- Excessive weight gain
- Psychologic problems related to chronic disease

WHAT TO EXPECT

- Initial remission or "honeymoon" phase with decreased insulin needs and easier overall control; usually lasts 3–6 months and rarely beyond a year
- Progression to "total diabetes" is usually gradual, but a major stress or illness may bring it on more acutely.
- Longevity and quality of life are increasing with careful blood glucose monitoring and improvements in insulin delivery
- At this time, people with IDDM probably have a reduced life expectancy, but it has improved dramatically over the past 20 years.
- Advances in understanding diabetes may prevent or minimize complications.

 Miscellaneous

OTHER FACTORS

N/A

PEDIATRIC

IDDM is more prevalent among children. For this reason, it is sometimes called "juvenile onset diabetes."

GERIATRIC

N/A

OTHERS

N/A

PREGNANCY

- Planning the pregnancy and tightly controlling blood sugar levels before conception is important.
- It is now possible to have a safe pregnancy, with vaginal delivery of a term baby (with care by a physician skilled in managing pregnant diabetic patients).

FURTHER INFORMATION

American Academy of Family Physicians Foundation, P.O. Box 8418, Kansas City, MO 64114, (800) 274-2237, ext. 4400

Diabetes Mellitus, Non-Insulin-Dependent (NIDDM)

 ## Basics

DESCRIPTION

Non-insulin-dependent diabetes mellitus (NIDDM) is a defect of insulin secretion and action, accounting for 80% of diabetic cases. People with poorly controlled NIDDM are at risk for a variety of complications, including eye, nerve, kidney, and cardiovascular problems. Despite its name, NIDDM is sometimes managed with insulin. However, many people with NIDDM manage their disease with oral medications, diet, and exercise.

SIGNS AND SYMPTOMS

- Kidney disease, nerve disease, retinal disease
- Frequent urination
- Excessive thirst, frequent drinking
- Excessive eating
- Weight loss
- Weakness
- Fatigue
- Frequent infections

CAUSES

Genetic factors and obesity are important.

SCOPE

NIDDM affects about 5,000 out of 100,000 persons in the United States.

MOST OFTEN AFFECTED

Typically occurs after age 40. Females are affected more frequently than males in white populations. May be inherited.

RISK FACTORS

- Family history
- Gestational diabetes

 ## Diagnosis

WHAT THE DOCTOR LOOKS FOR

The doctor will perform a physical examination to identify the signs and symptoms of NIDDM.

TESTS AND PROCEDURES

Blood tests, including several measurements of blood sugar levels

 ## Treatment

GENERAL MEASURES

- NIDDM is managed in the outpatient setting except for complicating emergencies requiring hospitalization.
- Home monitoring of blood or urine glucose
- Regular examination for complications

ACTIVITY

Regular aerobic exercise can improve glucose tolerance and decrease medication requirements.

DIET

- American Diabetes Association (ADA) provides dietary recommendations for NIDDM. The most important part of this diet is weight loss in obese patients. The diet is similar to that recommended by the American Heart Association and includes increased complex carbohydrate, decreased fat, and moderation in salt and alcohol.
- Dietary treatment alone can often result in adequate metabolic control in NIDDM.

Diabetes Mellitus, Non-Insulin-Dependent (NIDDM)

 Medications

COMMONLY PRESCRIBED DRUGS

- Oral medications to lower blood sugar levels (hypoglycemic drugs): tolbutamide, tolazamide, chlorpropamide, glyburide (Diabeta, Micronase), glipizide (Glucotrol)
- Insulin

CONTRAINDICATIONS

- Oral medications: IDDM, pregnancy, history of allergy; use caution in liver or renal disease and acute infection or stress.

PRECAUTIONS

Home glucose monitoring (1–4 times per day) is recommended for most patients taking insulin.

DRUG INTERACTIONS

- Drugs that enhance the effect of oral hypoglycemic drugs: salicylates, clofibrate, warfarin (Coumadin), chloramphenicol, ethanol
- Beta-blockers may mask symptoms of hypoglycemia and delay return to normal blood sugar levels.

OTHER DRUGS

- Metformin
- Phenformin
- Acarbose

 Followup

PATIENT MONITORING

- The doctor should be seen as often as necessary for control of blood sugar levels. Visits every 2–4 months are typical.
- Annual physicals

PREVENTION

Avoid weight gain and obesity. Maintenance of regular physical activity may prevent or delay NIDDM.

COMPLICATIONS

- Nerve disease
- Eye disease
- Kidney disease
- Cardiovascular disease
- Coma
- Gangrene of extremities
- Blindness
- Skin ulcers

WHAT TO EXPECT

- Maintenance of normal blood sugar levels may delay or prevent complications of diabetes.
- In susceptible individuals, complications begin to appear 10–15 years after onset, but they can also be present at time of diagnosis.

 Miscellaneous

OTHER FACTORS

N/A

PEDIATRIC

Occasional cases of NIDDM have been seen in children.

GERIATRIC

NIDDM is common in the elderly and is a significant contributing factor to blindness, renal failure, and lower limb amputations.

OTHERS

NIDDM is generally a disease of adults, appearing after age 40.

PREGNANCY

Diabetes can cause significant maternal complications and fetal wasting. Intensive management by those skilled in this area has improved the outcome dramatically.

FURTHER INFORMATION

American Diabetes Association, 430 North Michigan Ave. Chicago, IL 60611

Diaper Rash

 Basics

DESCRIPTION

Diaper rash, also called diaper dermatitis, is a rash occurring under the covered area of a diaper.

SIGNS AND SYMPTOMS

- Prominent rash on buttocks and pubic skin
- Folds of skin may or may not be affected.
- Genitalia may or may not be affected.
- Child scratches vigorously at night.
- Skin seems chapped.
- May be weeping or crusting
- Swelling

CAUSES

Irritation to skin from prolonged contact with urine or feces

SCOPE

Diaper rash is common.

MOST OFTEN AFFECTED

Infants, males and females in equal proportion

RISK FACTORS

- Infrequent diaper changes
- Waterproof diapers
- Improper laundering
- Family history of dermatitis
- Hot, humid weather
- Recent treatment with oral antibiotics
- Diarrhea

 Diagnosis

WHAT THE DOCTOR LOOKS FOR

- The doctor will perform a physical examination to look for signs of diaper rash.
- Other causes of rash should be identified and treated, such as contact dermatitis or infection.

TEST AND PROCEDURES

Rash may be cultured for laboratory analysis.

 Treatment

GENERAL MEASURES

- Diaper rash is managed in the outpatient setting.
- Expose the buttocks to air as much as possible.
- Don't use waterproof pants during treatment-day or night. They keep skin wet, making it susceptible to rash or infection.
- Change diapers frequently, even at night if the rash is extensive.
- Super absorbable diapers are beneficial.
- Discontinue use of baby lotion, powder, ointment, or baby oil (except zinc oxide).
- Apply zinc oxide ointment to the rash at the earliest sign of diaper rash, and 2 or 3 times a day thereafter (apply to clean, thoroughly dry skin).
- Use mild soap and pat dry.

ACTIVITY

Protect from overheating

DIET

No special diet

Medications

COMMONLY PRESCRIBED DRUGS

- Antifungal medications: miconazole nitrate 2% cream, miconazole powder, econazole (Spectazole), clotrimazole (Lotrimin), ketoconazole (Nizoral)
- Steroid creams: hydrocortisone 0.5–1%, clioquinol-hydrocortisone (Vioform-Hydrocortisone)
- Antibiotics

CONTRAINDICATIONS

N/A

PRECAUTIONS

N/A

DRUG INTERACTIONS

N/A

OTHER DRUGS

N/A

 ## Followup

PATIENT MONITORING

The doctor should be seen weekly until diaper rash is cleared, then at times of recurrence.

PREVENTION

See General measures

COMPLICATIONS

Infection

WHAT TO EXPECT

Quick, complete recovery with appropriate treatment

 ## Miscellaneous

OTHER FACTORS

N/A

PEDIATRIC

Diaper rash is most common among children.

GERIATRIC

Diaper rash can affect incontinent elderly persons.

OTHERS

N/A

PREGNANCY

N/A

FURTHER INFORMATION

N/A

Diarrhea, Acute

 Basics

DESCRIPTION

Acute (of short duration) diarrhea of abrupt onset in a healthy individual is most often caused by an infectious process. A variety of symptoms are often observed, including frequent passage of loose or watery stools, fever, chills, anorexia, vomiting, and malaise.

- Acute viral diarrhea: most common form, usually occurs for 1 to 3 days, is self-limited
- Bacterial diarrhea: develops within 12 hours of eating bacteria-contaminated food
- Protozoal infections: prolonged, watery diarrhea that often afflicts travelers returning from areas where the water supply has been contaminated
- Traveler's diarrhea: typically begins 3–7 days after arrival in a foreign location and is generally acute

SIGNS AND SYMPTOMS

- Loose, liquid stools
- Blood or mucus
- Fever
- Abdominal pain and distension
- Headache
- Loss of appetite
- Malaise, fatigue
- Vomiting
- Muscle ache
- Cramping, pale-greasy stools, fatigue, weight loss

CAUSES

Infection with bacteria, virus, or parasite

INCIDENCE/PREVALENCE

N/A

MOST OFTEN AFFECTED

All ages

RISK FACTORS

- Visiting a developing country
- Immune system disorders

 Diagnosis

WHAT THE DOCTOR LOOKS FOR

- The doctor will perform a thorough physical examination.
- Causes of diarrhea should be identified and treated, such as ulcerative colitis.

TESTS AND PROCEDURES

- Blood tests
- A sample of stool may be obtained for culture and laboratory analysis.
- Abdominal x-rays
- The intestinal tract may be visually examined by sigmoidoscopy.

 Treatment

GENERAL MEASURES

- Diarrhea is managed in the outpatient setting except for dehydration or other complicating emergencies requiring hospitalization.
- Replacement of lost fluid and salts
- Clear liquids such as tea, broth, carbonated beverages (without caffeine), and rehydration fluids (e.g., Gatorade) to replace lost fluid

ACTIVITY

Bed rest

DIET

- During periods of active diarrhea, avoid coffee, alcohol, dairy products, most fruits, vegetables, red meats, and heavily seasoned foods.
- After 12 hours with no diarrhea, begin eating clear soup, salted crackers, dry toast or bread, and sherbet.
- As stooling rate decreases, slowly add rice, baked potato, and chicken soup with rice or noodles to diet.
- As stool begins to retain shape, add to diet baked fish, poultry, applesauce, and bananas.

Medications

COMMONLY PRESCRIBED DRUGS

- Loperamide, bismuth subsalicylate
- Antibiotics: metronidazole, trimethoprim-sulfamethoxazole, ciprofloxacin (Cipro)

CONTRAINDICATIONS

Avoid alcoholic beverages when taking metronidazole.

PRECAUTIONS

- Antidiarrhea medications should be used with caution in cases of infectious diarrhea or antibiotic-associated colitis.
- Doxycycline, sulfamethoxazole-trimethoprim, ciprofloxacin may cause photosensitivity. Use sunscreen.

DRUG INTERACTIONS

- Bismuth subsalicylate can cause toxicity in patients taking aspirin and may alter anticoagulation control in patients taking coumadin.
- Ciprofloxacin and erythromycin increase theophylline levels.

OTHER DRUGS

- Doxycycline
- Diphenoxylate-atropine
- Tinidazole, secnidazole
- Vancomycin

 ## Followup

PATIENT MONITORING

Contact physician should diarrhea continue for 3 to 5 days with or without blood or mucus.

PREVENTION

- Avoid brushing teeth with contaminated water, ingesting ice cubes, or eating cold salads or meats when traveling.
- Avoid uncooked or undercooked seafood or meat, buffet meals left out for several hours, or food served by street vendors.

COMPLICATIONS

- Dehydration
- Sepsis
- Shock
- Anemia

WHAT TO EXPECT

Diarrhea is a common problem that is rarely life-threatening if attention is given to maintaining adequate hydration.

 ## Miscellaneous

OTHER FACTORS

N/A

PEDIATRIC

May be caused by overfeeding, medications, cystic fibrosis, and malabsorption disorders

GERIATRIC

Watery diarrhea in elderly patient with chronic constipation may be caused by fecal impaction or cancer.

OTHERS

N/A

PREGNANCY

Dehydration may lead to premature labor.

FURTHER INFORMATION

N/A

Dissociative Disorders

Basics

DESCRIPTION

Dissociative disorders are characterized by a sudden change in state of consciousness, identity, behavior, thoughts, feelings, and perception of external reality. These disorders include amnesia, identity disorder, fugue states, sleep-walking, conversion reactions, and other disorders.

SIGNS AND SYMPTOMS

- Symptoms cause significant distress or impairment in social, occupational, or other important areas of functioning.
- Dissociative amnesia:
  - ▶ Episodes of inability to recall important personal information that is too extensive to be explained by ordinary forgetfulness
  - ▶ Not due to other illness or substance abuse
- Dissociative fugue:
  - ▶ Sudden unexpected travel away from home or one's customary place of work with an inability to recall one's past
  - ▶ Confusion about personal identity or assumption of a new identity (partial or complete)
- Dissociative identity disorder:
  - ▶ The presence of two or more distinct personality states
  - ▶ Inability to recall important personal information
  - ▶ Reports of time distortion
  - ▶ Hearing voices
  - ▶ Chronic headaches
  - ▶ History of severe emotional or physical abuse as a child
  - ▶ Referring to self as "he/she," "we," "us"
  - ▶ Eating disorders
  - ▶ Flashbacks
  - ▶ Unreal feelings
  - ▶ Amnesia about important childhood events
  - ▶ Personal objects and belongings that cannot be accounted for
  - ▶ Denying unremembered behavior
  - ▶ Different handwriting styles
  - ▶ Sudden mood changes
  - ▶ Sudden behavioral changes, e.g., from adult to young child
  - ▶ Feeling controlled by "another person" from within
  - ▶ Self-inflicted violence such as wrist cutting
- Depersonalization disorder: Persistent or recurrent experiences of feeling detached from one's mental processes or body (e.g., feeling like one is in a dream)

CAUSES

- Physical, emotional, verbal, or sexual abuse in childhood
- Sudden and severe trauma or threat to one's psychological or physical integrity
- Witnessing a traumatic event, such as an industrial or car accident
- Other psychological factors

SCOPE

Dissociative disorder affects 8–10% of the general psychiatric population. As many as 70% of young adults report short periods of dissociative experiences that are self-limiting and resolve spontaneously.

MOST OFTEN AFFECTED

Adolescents and young to middle-age adults; rare as a new illness in elderly. If untreated, may linger from childhood into adult and old age. Females affected twice as frequently as males.

RISK FACTORS

- Exposure to neglect, abuse, and trauma in one's childhood
- Tendency to cope with life stresses by excessively using an escape mechanism of day dreaming and/or dissociation

Diagnosis

WHAT THE DOCTOR LOOKS FOR

- The doctor will obtain a history and perform a thorough physical examination.
- Other mental, nervous system, or medical disorders should be identified and treated.

TESTS AND PROCEDURES

- Toxicology screening
- An electroencephalogram (EEG) may be done to rule out epilepsy and sleep disorders.
- Sleep study, called polysomnogram, may be done to rule out sleep apnea.

- Computed tomography (CT scan) and magnetic resonance imaging (MRI) may be performed to assist in diagnosis.
- Psychologic testing may be done.

 ## Treatment

GENERAL MEASURES

- Dissociative disorders are usually managed in an outpatient setting.
- Hospitalization may be required during a crisis.
- Individual psychotherapy plus behavior modification and other therapy
- Support groups, group therapy, expressive art therapy, occupational and recreational therapy, reading therapy, and writing therapy
- Self-hypnosis, relaxation exercises, and guided imagery

ACTIVITY

Based on patient's condition

DIET

N/A

 ## Medications

COMMONLY PRESCRIBED DRUGS

- No specific cures
- Antidepressants
- Benzodiazepines
- Propranolol
- Neuroleptics: thioridazine, haloperidol, chlorprothixene, perphenazine, risperidone
- Droperidol

CONTRAINDICATIONS

Read drug product information.

PRECAUTIONS

Read drug product information.

DRUG INTERACTIONS

Read drug product information.

OTHER DRUGS

- Buspirone
- Clomipramine, fluvoxamine

 ## Followup

PATIENT MONITORING

- The doctor should be seen for at least an hour of psychotherapy up to 3 to 4 sessions per week to avoid hospitalizations.
- Hospitalized patients require more intensive treatment.

PREVENTION

- Child abuse prevention
- Crisis intervention following individual trauma and natural or man-made disasters is crucial for prevention of chronic illness or disability.

COMPLICATIONS

Self-inflicted violence; suicide attempts; substance abuse and chemical dependency

WHAT TO EXPECT

- Without treatment, the outcome ranges from spontaneous improvement or recovery to acute and chronic disease.
- Effective treatment produces partial or full recovery for many patients.

Miscellaneous

OTHER FACTORS

N/A

PEDIATRIC

Suspect abuse or neglect.

GERIATRIC

Dissociative disorders are less common among the elderly; drug side effects are a more likely cause of symptoms.

OTHERS

N/A

PREGNANCY

N/A

FURTHER INFORMATION

N/A

Diverticular Disease

 Basics

DESCRIPTION

Diverticular disease is caused by an abscess in or inflammation of abnormal outpouchings of the intestine.

SIGNS AND SYMPTOMS

- Symptoms may be mild or absent
- Pain
- Diarrhea or constipation
- Bloated abdomen
- Dark, tarry stool
- Fever with chills as severity increases
- Loss of appetite, nausea, vomiting
- Difficult urination

SCOPE

Diverticular disease affects up to 20% of the general population. However, incidence increases to 40–50% among individuals 50–70 years of age.

MOST OFTEN AFFECTED

Diverticular disease is rare in people younger than 40 years of age; most common in those 50–70 years of age. Males and females affected in equal proportions.

CAUSES

- Causes are not clearly proven
- Low-fiber diet

RISK FACTORS

- Age over 40
- Low-fiber diet
- Previous diverticular disease

 Diagnosis

WHAT THE DOCTOR LOOKS FOR

The doctor will perform a physical examination to identify causes of similar symptoms, such as irritable bowel syndrome, lactose intolerance, or cancer.

TESTS AND PROCEDURES

- Blood tests
- Urinalysis and culture
- Abdominal x-rays, barium enema
- Computed tomography (CT scan) may be done to assist in diagnosis.
- Blood vessels may be assessed by a radiologic procedure called angiography.
- Other special imaging procedures may be done.
- The digestive tract or urinary system may be examined by endoscopy.

 Treatment

GENERAL MEASURES

- Diverticular disease is usually managed in the outpatient setting.
- A small number of people with diverticular disease require hospitalization.
- Surgery may be necessary.

ACTIVITY

Depends on condition; activity may be restricted

DIET

- Nothing by mouth during acute episode, progress to fluids, then to high-fiber diet as normal bowel function returns.
- Increase dietary fiber with high-fiber foods and/or fiber supplement if appropriate.

Medications

COMMONLY PRESCRIBED DRUGS

- Antispasmodics: hyoscyamine (Levsin), buspirone (BuSpar), meperidine (Demerol), high-fiber diet
- Antibiotics: metronidazole (Flagyl), amoxicillin, ciprofloxacin, gentamicin, clindamycin
- Pain reliever
- Bleeding: vasopressin

CONTRAINDICATIONS

Allergic reaction

PRECAUTIONS

Morphine and other opiates should be avoided.

DRUG INTERACTIONS

Read drug product information.

OTHER DRUGS

Tobramycin, metronidazole, cephalosporins

 ## Followup

PATIENT MONITORING

The doctor should be seen as often as necessary based on symptoms and health status.

PREVENTION

High-fiber diet and use of soluble fiber suppplements, such as psyllium, agar, and methylcellulose

COMPLICATIONS

- Bleeding
- Perforation
- Inflammation of the abdominal lining
- Bowel obstruction
- Abscess
- Fistula

WHAT TO EXPECT

- Outcome is good with early detection and treatment of complications.
- After successful treatment of initial episode, up to 67% of patients have no repeat attacks that require hospitalization.
- Of those with bleeding, up to 20% will rebleed in a period of months to years.

 ## Miscellaneous

OTHER FACTORS

N/A

PEDIATRIC

Very rare among children

GERIATRIC

More common among the elderly

OTHERS

N/A

PREGNANCY

Could be confused with ectopic pregnancy

FURTHER INFORMATION

National Digestive Diseases Information Clearinghouse, Box NDDIC, Bethesda, MD 20892, (301) 468-6344

Dysfunctional Uterine Bleeding

 Basics

DESCRIPTION

Dysfunctional uterine bleeding is abnormal uterine bleeding in the absence of a detected disease. It is also called "breakthrough bleeding" or "estrogen withdrawal bleeding."

SIGNS AND SYMPTOMS

- Uterine bleeding:
  - ▶ Unrelated to menstrual cycle
  - ▶ Heavier than normal menstrual flow
  - ▶ Occurs in an irregular pattern
  - ▶ Rarely painful
- Absence of other systemic symptoms or bleeding elsewhere

CAUSES

- Hormonal disturbance
- Other: uterine lesions, cancer, vaginal infection, foreign body, ectopic pregnancy, other medical conditions
- Tends to run in families

SCOPE

Widespread, but exact prevalence is unknown

MOST OFTEN AFFECTED

Females 12–45 years of age

RISK FACTORS

See Causes

 Diagnosis

WHAT THE DOCTOR LOOKS FOR

The doctor will perform a physical examination to identify and treat causes of uterine bleeding.

TESTS AND PROCEDURES

- Blood tests
- Pregnancy test
- Basal body temperature may be charted.
- Ultrasound may be done to assist with diagnosis.
- Pap smear
- Cells from the uterus may be obtained by biopsy for laboratory analysis.

 Treatment

GENERAL MEASURES

- Dysfunctional uterine bleeding is almost always managed as an outpatient.
- Hospitalization may be required.
- Surgery (e.g., hysterectomy, dilatation and curretage) may be required.

ACTIVITY

As tolerated

DIET

Normal; include adequate iron

Medications

COMMONLY PRESCRIBED DRUGS

- Conjugated estrogens
- Medroxyprogesterone, ethinyl estradiol
- Supplemental iron therapy
- Naproxen sodium, mefenamic acid
- Leuprolide acetate, nafarelin, goserelin

CONTRAINDICATIONS

N/A

PRECAUTIONS

Read drug product information.

DRUG INTERACTIONS

Read drug product information.

OTHER DRUGS

- Progesterone
- Danazol

 Followup

PATIENT MONITORING

- The doctor should be seen as often as necessary.
- Maintain a menstrual calendar to document the pattern of bleeding and its relation to therapy.

PREVENTION

Avoid prolonged stress or emotional turmoil.

COMPLICATIONS

- Anemia
- Cancer
- Drug side effects

WHAT TO EXPECT

- The outcome varies.
- In young women, most cases can be treated successfully without surgery.

 Miscellaneous

OTHER FACTORS

N/A

PEDIATRIC

N/A

GERIATRIC

Cancer should be ruled out.

OTHERS

Young females and those in their later reproductive years are most often affected.

PREGNANCY

N/A

FURTHER INFORMATION

American College of Obstetricians & Gynecologists (ACOG), 409 12th St., SW, Washington, DC 20024-2188, (800) 762-ACOG

Dysmenorrhea

 Basics

DESCRIPTION

Dysmenorrhea is pelvic pain that occurs around the time of menstruation. It is a leading cause of absenteeism for women under age 30.

SIGNS AND SYMPTOMS

- Mild: pelvic discomfort, cramping, or feeling of heaviness on first day of menstrual bleeding with no associated symptoms
- Moderate: discomfort occurring on first 2–3 days of menses and accompanied by mild malaise, diarrhea, and headache
- Severe:intense, cramp-like pain lasting 2–7 days and often with gastrointestinal upset, back pain, thigh pain, and headache

CAUSES

- Hormone disturbance
- Anatomical abnormalities
- Other physical conditions

SCOPE

About 40% of adult females have menstrual pain; 10% are incapacitated for 1 to 3 days each month.

MOST OFTEN AFFECTED

Females 20–30 years of age

RISK FACTORS

- Never given birth
- Positive family history
- Pelvic infection
- Sexually transmitted diseases
- Endometriosis

 Diagnosis

WHAT THE DOCTOR LOOKS FOR

- The doctor will obtain a history and perform a physical examination.
- Causes of dysmenorrhea should be identified and treated, such as infection, complications of pregnancy, or endometriosis.

TESTS AND PROCEDURES

- Ultrasound may be done to assist in diagnosis.
- The reproductive system may be examined by laparoscopy.

 Treatment

GENERAL MEASURES

- Dysmenorrhea is usually managed in the out-patient setting.
- Treatment is directed at general physical conditioning.
- Infections must be treated if present.
- Transcutaneous electrical nerve stimulator (TENS) may relieve symptoms.
- Surgery may be required.

ACTIVITY

Normal

DIET

Normal

Medications

COMMONLY PRESCRIBED DRUGS

- Nonsteroidal anti-inflammatory drugs (NSAIDs): ibuprofen (Motrin, Advil, Nuprin), naproxen sodium (Anaprox, Aleve), aspirin
- Other nonsteroidal anti-inflammatory drugs
- Oral contraceptives

CONTRAINDICATIONS

- Platelet disorders
- Gastric ulcers or gastritis
- Blood clotting disorders
- Vascular disease
- Contraindications to oral contraceptives

PRECAUTIONS

- May irritate gastrointestinal tract
- May cause blood clotting disorders
- May impair kidney function
- May contribute to heart failure
- May lead to liver disorder

DRUG INTERACTIONS

- Blood thinners (anticoagulants)
- Aspirin with other NSAIDs
- Methotrexate
- Furosemide
- Lithium

OTHER DRUGS

- Nafarelin acetate
- Calcium channel blockers (e.g., nifedipine)
- Hydrocodone or tramadol (Ultram)
- Other NSAIDs

 ## Followup

PATIENT MONITORING

N/A

PREVENTION

- None known
- Reduce risk of sexually transmitted diseases

COMPLICATIONS

- Anxiety and/or depression
- Infertility from underlying pathology

WHAT TO EXPECT

Dysmenorrhea often improves with age and childbirth. Some forms require therapy based on underlying cause.

 ## Miscellaneous

OTHER FACTORS

N/A

PEDIATRIC

N/A

GERIATRIC

N/A

OTHERS

N/A

PREGNANCY

N/A

FURTHER INFORMATION

N/A

Section E

Eclampsia

 ## Basics

DESCRIPTION

Eclampsia, or toxemia of pregnancy, is the presence of seizures in a pregnant female without underlying neurological disease who also has pre-eclampsia. Pre-eclampsia is hypertension (high blood pressure), swelling, and protein in the urine, during pregnancy. Eclampsia can also occur after birth, almost always within 24 hours.

SIGNS AND SYMPTOMS

- Seizures
- Headache, visual disturbances, and stomach pain often precede seizure.
- Seizures may occur once or repeatedly.
- After-seizure coma and bluish discoloration around mouth, eyes, and nail beds (cyanosis)
- Swelling, fluid in lungs

CAUSES

Exact cause of seizures remains unclear.

SCOPE

- Preeclampsia affects 5% of all pregnancies; incidence of eclampsia is unclear.
- Up to 2% of women with pre-eclampsia progress to eclampsia, a number that is decreasing with improved monitoring and care.

MOST OFTEN AFFECTED

Preeclampsia and eclampsia are more common in younger women, but the incidence of seizures is much greater among older women. Predisposition may be genetic.

RISK FACTORS

- First pregnancy
- Obstetric conditions (e.g., multiple fetuses)
- Preexisting high blood pressure or kidney disease
- Strong family history of preeclampsia-eclampsia
- Poor prenatal care

 ## Diagnosis

WHAT THE DOCTOR LOOKS FOR

- The doctor will perform a physical examination to identify the signs and symptoms of eclampsia.
- Other possible causes of seizures will be considered, such as epilepsy.
- Until other causes are proven, all pregnant women with seizures should be considered to have eclampsia.

TESTS AND PROCEDURES

- A variety of blood tests may be ordered to assist in diagnosis.
- Urinalysis, 24-hour urine collection

 ## Treatment

GENERAL MEASURES

- The management of eclampsia requires hospitalization. Intravenous (IV) medications are given, and the patient is monitored if necessary.
- Needs of the newborn should be considered; transfer to a specialized neonatal care facility may be required.
- Treatment consists of controlling seizures, giving oxygen, lowering blood pressure, and delivery of newborn as soon as possible.

ACTIVITY

Bed rest

DIET

Nothing by mouth until stable, then usual seizure precautions; low-salt diet is commonly recommended.

Medications

COMMONLY PRESCRIBED DRUGS

- Magnesium sulfate
- IV fluids

CONTRAINDICATIONS

Drug allergies

PRECAUTIONS

N/A

DRUG INTERACTIONS

N/A

OTHER DRUGS

Diazepam, lorazepam, phenytoin, phenobarbital

Followup

PATIENT MONITORING

The doctor will be seen often to monitor the health status of mother and baby.

PREVENTION

- Adequate prenatal care
- Good control of preexisting hypertension
- Recognition and treatment of preeclampsia

COMPLICATIONS

- Temporary deficits, such as blindness, affect 56% of women with eclampsia.
- Most women do not suffer long-term effects.
- Death from toxemia or its complications
- Death of fetus

WHAT TO EXPECT

- One fourth of women with eclampsia have hypertension in subsequent pregnancies, but only 5% of these will have severe hypertension, and only 2% will be eclamptic again.
- Women who have been eclamptic and have many children may be at higher risk for essential hypertension later in life
- Women who have been eclamptic and have many children are at greater risk of death in subsequent pregnancies than women who are pregnant for the first time.

Miscellaneous

OTHER FACTORS

N/A

PEDIATRIC

Adequate neonatal care and facilities are essential.

GERIATRIC

N/A

OTHERS

N/A

PREGNANCY

A complication of pregnancy

FURTHER INFORMATION

Additional materials from: American College of Obstetricians & Gynecologists, 409 12th St., SW, Washington, DC 20024-2188, (800) 762-ACOG

Endometriosis

 Basics

DESCRIPTION

Endometriosis is a disorder of the uterus that leads to painful menstruation, infertility, and other conditions. It is caused by the misplacement of uterine lining tissue outside the uterus, such as on the ovaries or in the fallopian tubes. Endometriosis can also affect distant sites throughout the abdomen and chest.

SIGNS AND SYMPTOMS

- Infertility
- Painful intercourse
- Menstrual cramps
- Difficulty with defecation
- Chronic pelvic pain
- Premenstrual spotting
- Miscarriage

CAUSES

- Unknown

SCOPE

Endometriosis affects 8–30% of women of childbearing age.

MOST OFTEN AFFECTED

Women of reproductive age

RISK FACTORS

- Hereditary/genetic predisposition
- Personality traits (achieving, egocentric, over-anxious, perfectionist, intelligent, underweight; however, the validity of these observations lacking)
- Delayed childbearing
- Hormonal disturbance (luteinized unruptured follicle syndrome)

 Diagnosis

WHAT THE DOCTOR LOOKS FOR

- The doctor will perform a thorough physical examination to identify and rule out other potential causes of pelvic pain including complications of pregnancy, urinary tract infection, irritable bowel syndrome, ulcerative colitis, Crohn's disease, ruptured ovarian cyst, and other conditions.
- The doctor will look for other conditions known to be associated with endometriosis.

TESTS AND PROCEDURES

- Blood tests, urinalysis
- Ultrasound or magnetic resonance imaging (MRI) may be done to assess the pelvic structures.
- The reproductive tract may be visually examined by laparoscopy.
- A sample of uterine tissue may be obtained by biopsy for laboratory analysis.

 Treatment

GENERAL MEASURES

- Endometriosis should be diagnosed and treated early to prevent infertility and pelvic pain.
- Prevention of disease is difficult; however, disease may be managed with oral contraceptive agents.
- Treatment of endometriosis may require hospitalization.
- Surgery may be required.

ACTIVITY

Activity may be limited depending upon severity of pelvic pain.

DIET

No special diet

Medications

COMMONLY PRESCRIBED DRUGS

- Nafarelin (Synarel), leuprolide acetate (Lupron, Depo-Lupron), goserelin (Zoladex)
- Maintenance: oral contraceptives, calcium supplements

CONTRAINDICATIONS

Any contraindication to the drug itself or low estrogen levels.

PRECAUTIONS

- Drugs may cause calcium loss, hot flashes, tingling sensation of face and arms.
- Contraception should be used by sexually active women.

SIGNIFICANT POSSIBLE INTERACTIONS

Refer to manufacturer's literature.

OTHER DRUGS

- Danazol (Danocrine)
- Medroxyprogesterone (Provera)
- Megestrol (Megace)
- "Continuous" oral contraceptives, e.g., norgestrel-ethinyl estradiol (Lo/Ovral, Ovral) until childbearing is desired

Followup

PATIENT MONITORING

- The doctor should be seen every 8–12 weeks.
- Ultrasound should be done every 8–12 weeks.
- Additional surgery may be needed.

PREVENTION

- Pregnancy seems to temporarily improve the disease.
- Endometriosis is generally a recurring disorder that may persist even into early menopause.

COMPLICATIONS

- Fertility problems
- Chronic pelvic pain
- Hysterectomy

WHAT TO EXPECT

- Pregnancy can occur, but depends upon the severity of the disease.
- Disease gradually improves with the onset of menopause, but can usually be controlled during the reproductive years.

Miscellaneous

OTHER FACTORS

N/A

PEDIATRIC

N/A

GERIATRIC

Endometriosis can persist during early menopause and may be worsened with estrogen replacement therapy (ERT).

OTHERS

N/A

PREGNANCY

See a board certified reproductive endocrinologist or gynecologist with expertise in infertility.

FURTHER INFORMATION

The American Fertility Society, 2140 11th Ave South, Suite 200, Birmingham, AL 35205-2800, (205) 933-8494

Epididymitis

 Basics

DESCRIPTION

Epididymitis is an inflammation of the epididymis, an elongated structure attached to the testicle. This condition causes pain of the scrotum, swelling and hardening of the epididymis, and eventually the formation of a fluid-filled cavity.

SIGNS AND SYMPTOMS

- Scrotal pain, sometimes extending to the groin region
- Urethral discharge
- Symptoms of urinary tract infection: frequent urination, painful urination, cloudy urine, or blood in the urine
- A swollen, firm mass within the scrotum
- Swelling of the scrotum
- Fever and chills occur with severe infection and abscess formation.

CAUSES

- Infection (e.g., chlamydia, gonorrhea, other bacteria)
- Urinary tract obstruction
- Inflammation
- Birth defect

SCOPE

Epididymitis is common in the United States.

MOST OFTEN AFFECTED

Epididymitis primarily affects younger, sexually active men or older men with urinary infection, but it may also rarely occur in prepubertal boys.

RISK FACTORS

- Urinary tract infection
- Use of urinary catheter
- Urethral instrumentation or surgery
- Urethral scarring

 Diagnosis

WHAT THE DOCTOR LOOKS FOR

The doctor will perform a physical examination to identify causes of scrotal pain, such as testicular torsion, mumps, or trauma.

TESTS AND PROCEDURES

- Urinalysis and culture
- Ultrasound may be used to evaluate the scrotum.

 Treatment

GENERAL MEASURES

- Epididymitis is usually managed on an outpatient basis.
- Hospitalization may be required for severe infection or surgery.
- Elevate the scrotum.
- Apply a cold pack to the affected area.
- Local anesthetic may be used in severe cases.
- Surgery may be required.

ACTIVITY

Bed rest for minimum of 1 to 2 days

DIET

No restrictions, but drink large amounts of fluids.

Medications

COMMONLY PRESCRIBED DRUGS

- Antibiotics: doxycycline, tetracycline, trimethoprim-sulfamethoxazole (Bactrim, Septra), ciprofloxacin (Cipro), ofloxacin (Floxin), norfloxacin (Noroxin), ceftriaxone, gentamicin
- Pain relievers: nonsteroidal anti-inflammatory drugs (e.g., naproxen or ibuprofen), aceta-minophen-codeine, oxycodone-acetaminophen

CONTRAINDICATIONS

None

PRECAUTIONS

Read drug product information.

DRUG INTERACTIONS

Read drug product information.

OTHER DRUGS

N/A

 ## Followup

PATIENT MONITORING

The doctor should be seen often until all signs of infection have cleared.

PREVENTION

- Vasectomy
- Antibiotics
- Early treatment
- Avoid vigorous rectal examination

COMPLICATIONS

- Recurrent epididymitis
- Infertility
- Gangrene

WHAT TO EXPECT

- Pain improves within 1 to 3 days, but it may take several weeks or months to completely resolve.
- Sterility may result.

Miscellaneous

OTHER FACTORS

N/A

PEDIATRIC

N/A

GERIATRIC

Diabetic patients with nerve disease may have little pain despite severe infection.

OTHERS

N/A

PREGNANCY

N/A

FURTHER INFORMATION

N/A

Epiglottitis

 ## Basics

DESCRIPTION

Epiglottitis is an acute inflammation of the epiglottis, a flap of tissue above the larynx, and related structures. It can cause severe airway obstruction. Epiglottitis is a medical emergency that requires prompt emergency care.

SIGNS AND SYMPTOMS

- Develops rapidly
- Fever
- Difficulty swallowing, drooling
- Sore throat
- Swollen glands in neck
- Difficulty breathing
- Muffled voice/cry
- Minimal cough
- Shock

CAUSES

Infection with *Haemophilus influenzae* (in children and adults) or Group A Streptococcus in adults.

SCOPE

The incidence of epiglottitis has dropped dramatically since the introduction of the Haemophilus b vaccine.

MOST OFTEN AFFECTED

- Epiglottitis most commonly affects children 3–7 years old, although any age can be affected.
- Infrequent in adults
- Occurs with equal frequency in males and females

RISK FACTORS

N/A

 ## Diagnosis

WHAT THE DOCTOR LOOKS FOR

- The doctor will perform a complete physical examination to assess the degree of symptoms.
- Other airway conditions will be identified, such as croup, infection, or foreign body.

TESTS AND PROCEDURES

- Blood tests
- A sample of blood may be cultured for laboratory analysis.
- Fluid from the throat may be cultured.
- X-rays of the neck and chest may be taken to assist in diagnosis.
- The airway may be visually examined by intubation.
- A sample of spinal fluid may be obtained for laboratory analysis.

 ## Treatment

GENERAL MEASURES

- Acute epiglottitis requires emergency care and hospitalization.
- Mechanical breathing may be required.
- A surgical opening may be made in the neck.
- Other surgery may be required.

ACTIVITY

N/A

DIET

N/A

Medications

COMMONLY PRESCRIBED DRUGS

Antibiotics: cefotaxime, ceftriaxone

CONTRAINDICATIONS

Read drug product information.

PRECAUTIONS

Read drug product information.

DRUG INTERACTIONS

Read drug product information.

OTHER DRUGS

- Ampicillin, chloramphenicol
- Antifever medication

 ## Followup

PATIENT MONITORING

The doctor will be seen often during hospitalization.

PREVENTION

- *H. influenzae* vaccine (not 100% protective)
- Prevention with rifampin

COMPLICATIONS

- Pneumonia, meningitis, other inflammatory conditions
- Septic shock
- Air in the chest cavity
- Death from asphyxia

WHAT TO EXPECT

The risk of death or serious illness is low with appropriate intervention.

 ## Miscellaneous

OTHER FACTORS

N/A

PEDIATRIC

N/A

GERIATRIC

N/A

OTHERS

N/A

PREGNANCY

N/A

FURTHER INFORMATION

N/A

Section F

Fatigue

 Basics

DESCRIPTION

Fatigue is a state of discomfort and decreased level of energy resulting from prolonged or excessive exertion or loss of ability to respond appropriately to stimulation. Fatigue is also called lassitude, tiredness, lethargy, malaise, and ennui.

SIGNS AND SYMPTOMS

N/A

CAUSES

Drug or alcohol use, overexertion, anemia, chronic fatigue syndrome, diabetes mellitus or other medical conditions, emotional problems (depression, etc.), inadequate nutrition, inadequate rest, obesity, poor physical conditioning, and others.

SCOPE

N/A

MOST OFTEN AFFECTED

N/A

RISK FACTORS

N/A

 Diagnosis

WHAT THE DOCTOR LOOKS FOR

N/A

TESTS AND PROCEDURES

N/A

 Treatment

GENERAL MEASURES

Treatment is directed at the underlying cause of fatigue.

ACTIVITY

N/A

DIET

N/A

Medication

COMMONLY PRESCRIBED DRUGS

N/A

CONTRAINDICATIONS

N/A

PRECAUTIONS

N/A

DRUG INTERACTIONS

N/A

OTHER DRUGS

N/A

 Followup

PATIENT MONITORING

N/A

PREVENTION

N/A

COMPLICATIONS

N/A

WHAT TO EXPECT

N/A

 Miscellaneous

OTHER FACTORS

N/A

PEDIATRIC

N/A

GERIATRIC

N/A

OTHERS

N/A

PREGNANCY

N/A

FURTHER INFORMATION

N/A

Fecal Incontinence

 Basics

DESCRIPTION

Fecal incontinence (encopresis) is the regular passage of feces into clothes or other inappropriate places by a child older than 4 years of age.

SIGNS AND SYMPTOMS

- Constipation, usually
- Pasty stool found on underclothes
- Fecal or foul odor surrounds the child
- Pain around the navel
- Occasional passage of a large volume of stool
- History of painful bowel movements
- Shyness and withdrawal, acting out, or aggressive behavior
- Some have had psychotherapy.
- Some have had recurrent urinary tract infections.

CAUSES

- Psychologic (toilet training issues)
- Rectal disorders (e.g. painful defecation, poor muscle tone)
- Dietary or metabolic (lack of fiber, excessive protein or milk intake, inadequate water intake, hypothyroidism)

SCOPE

Encopresis affects 1.3% of all children over 4 years of age.

MOST OFTEN AFFECTED

Seventy percent have onset before 5 years of age; males are affected more frequently than females.

RISK FACTORS

- Boys are more often affected.
- Difficulty with bowel training
- Unresolved defecation problems

 Diagnosis

WHAT THE DOCTOR LOOKS FOR

- Fecal incontinence is often noticed by the doctor during the physical examination; many parents and children do not mention the problem to their doctors.
- Underlying causes of constipation should be identified and treated.

TESTS AND PROCEDURES

- Urinalysis and urine culture
- Blood tests
- X-ray of the abdomen
- A barium enema may be done to assess the digestive tract.
- A sample of colon tissue may be obtained by biopsy for laboratory analysis.

 Treatment

GENERAL MEASURES

- Hospital admission may be necessary.
- If impaction is present, it must be treated.
- Avoid development of impaction.
- Avoid frequent and repeated digital examinations, enemas, and suppositories.
- Biofeedback training can be used as alternative therapy or when conventional therapy has been unsuccessful.
- Child should sit on toilet twice a day at the same times each day for 10 to 15 minutes and 10 to 15 minutes after a meal.

ACTIVITY

Unrestricted

DIET

- Avoid excessive milk, bananas, apples, gelatin.
- Increase fiber.

Medications

COMMONLY PRESCRIBED DRUGS

- Stool impaction: mineral oil, enemas, polyethylene glycol (Colyte, Nulytely)
- Maintenance: mineral oil, lactulose, methylcellulose (Citrucel), psyllium (Metamucil, Perdiem), polycarbophil (Mitrolan), malt soup extract (Maltsupex), fiber wafers, multivitamins

CONTRAINDICATIONS

Read drug product information.

PRECAUTIONS

Avoid mineral oil at bedtime. Read drug product information.

DRUG INTERACTIONS

Read drug product information.

OTHER DRUGS

N/A

Followup

PATIENT MONITORING

- Maintenance treatment program should be followed for at least 6 months and maybe for as long as 1 to 2 years.
- The doctor should be seen every 4–10 weeks.
- Contact doctor as needed by telephone.

PREVENTION

- Improve feeding practices.
- Bowel training
- Early detection
- Use dark Karo syrup and fiber for hard stools.
- Prompt treatment of skin problems to avoid painful defecation
- Look for signs of relapse, which include large caliber stools, decrease in frequency of defecation, soiling.

COMPLICATIONS

- Excessive enemas or suppositories may cause colitis.
- Dermatitis around the anal area
- Anal fissure

WHAT TO EXPECT

- The outcome is usually good, although relapses may occur.
- Children with psychosocial or emotional problems preceding the fecal incontinence are more resistant to treatment.

Miscellaneous

OTHER FACTORS

N/A

PEDIATRIC

N/A

GERIATRIC

N/A

OTHERS

N/A

PREGNANCY

N/A

FURTHER INFORMATION

N/A

Fertility Problems

 Basics

DESCRIPTION

Fertility problems are usually suspected if a couple fails to conceive after 1 year of unprotected intercourse.

SIGNS AND SYMPTOMS

- Hormone disorder (e.g., hypothyroidism, abnormal puberty)
- Sexual dysfunction (e.g., premature ejaculation)
- Irregular ovulation
- Excessive body hair (hirsutism)
- Endometriosis

CAUSES

- Most couples have more than 1 factor.
- Male factors are responsible for 30 to 40% of fertility problems.
- Ovulation factors are responsible for 15% of fertility problems.
- Cervical and uterine factors are responsible for 10% of fertility problems; fallopian tube and other anatomical problems are responsible for 25 to 30%.
- Immune factors are responsible for 5% of fertility problems.
- Psychological/nutritional/metabolic factors are responsible for 5% of fertility problems.

SCOPE

Fertility problems affect 10–15% of all couples.

MOST OFTEN AFFECTED

Fertility problems increase with age. They affect 14% of individuals ages 30–34, 20% of those ages 35–39, and 25% of those ages 40–45.

RISK FACTORS

Genital/pelvic infections (VD or STD)

 Diagnosis

WHAT THE DOCTOR LOOKS FOR

A thorough history and physical examination should be performed on each partner.

TESTS AND PROCEDURES

- Blood tests
- Semen analysis, post-coital test
- The basal body temperature may be charted.
- Tissue from the uterus may be obtained by biopsy for laboratory analysis.
- The reproductive tract may be evaluated with a special radiology procedure called a hysterosalpingogram (HSG).
- The reproductive tract may be visually examined by laparoscopy.
- Many specialized tests are available, but only from fertility specialists in specialized facilities.

 Treatment

GENERAL MEASURES

- Infertility is managed in the outpatient setting.
- The cause of infertility should be identified and treated.
- Information about adoption may be provided when appropriate.
- Donor insemination may be considered.
- Surgery may be required.

ACTIVITY

- Males with low sperm counts should avoid hot tubs/saunas.
- If the male has a low sperm count, intercourse should be timed to occur approximately every 36 hours during the fertile period. Delay of intercourse beyond 7 days also adversely affects semen quality.

DIET

N/A

Fertility Problems

 Medications

COMMONLY PRESCRIBED DRUGS

- Clomiphene citrate
- Bromocriptin

CONTRAINDICATIONS

N/A

PRECAUTIONS

Drugs have many precautions; read drug product information.

DRUG INTERACTIONS

Bromocriptine: alcohol, antihypertensives, tricyclic antidepressants, phenothiazines

OTHER DRUGS

- Human chorionic gonadotropin
- Menotropins; human menopausal go- nadotropin (hMG)
- Gonadotropin releasing hormone (GnRH) analogs

 Followup

PATIENT MONITORING

See Diagnosis

PREVENTION

Prevention of sexually transmitted disease (STD) and pelvic inflammatory disease

COMPLICATIONS

Complications of pregnancy

WHAT TO EXPECT

- About half of couples conceive during the second year of unprotected intercourse.
- If the couple has been infertile for 4 or more years, the prognosis tends to be poor.

 Miscellaneous

OTHER FACTORS

N/A

PEDIATRIC

N/A

GERIATRIC

N/A

OTHERS

With aging, the effects of diseases such as endometriosis increase; cumulative exposure from environmental or occupational hazards may also play a role in fertility problems.

PREGNANCY

N/A

FURTHER INFORMATION

- RESOLVE, 5 Water St, Arlington, MA 02174
- Fertility Research Foundation, 1430 Second Avenue, Suite 103, New York, NY 10021, (212) 744-5500
- American College of Obstetricians & Gynecologists, 409 12th St, SW, Washington, DC 20024-2188, (800) 762-ACOG

Fibrocystic Breast Disease

 Basics

DESCRIPTION

Fibrocystic breast disease, also called benign breast disease, includes benign disorders such as lumps and pain. The disease does not have a well-defined set of symptoms and has no clear cause. Benign lumps are usually smooth, regular, and somewhat mobile beneath the skin. Benign breast disease may also include nipple discharge, pain, inflammatory conditions, and growth disorders.

SIGNS AND SYMPTOMS

- May have no symptoms
- Breast pain
- Breast tenderness
- Pain subsides after menstrual cycle
- Smooth masses
- Tense masses
- Masses that change
- Masses in both breasts
- Breast engorgement
- Breast thickening
- Nipple discharge

CAUSES

- The cause of benign breast disease is unknown.
- Possible causes include hormone disorders, dietary fat intake.

SCOPE

It is estimated that at least 50% of women have benign breast symptoms during their lifetime.

MOST OFTEN AFFECTED

Symptoms tend to occur in menstruating women.

RISK FACTORS

- Unknown
- The effect of methylxanthine-containing substances, e.g., coffee, tea, cola, and chocolate, is uncertain.

 Diagnosis

WHAT THE DOCTOR LOOKS FOR

The doctor will do a complete physical examination and identify the cause of symptoms.

TESTS AND PROCEDURES

- Blood tests
- Mammography
- Ultrasound may be used to assist in diagnosis.
- A sample of breast tissue may be obtained by biopsy for laboratory analysis.

 Treatment

GENERAL MEASURES

- Benign breast disease is managed in the outpatient setting.
- Biopsy or surgery may require hospitalization.
- Symptoms frequently resolve spontaneously.
- Cold compresses may be helpful.
- Use a well-fitting, supportive brassiere (worn night and day).
- Surgery may be required.

ACTIVITY

No restrictions. Avoid activities that may cause trauma to the breasts.

DIET

Avoid methylxanthines (coffee, tea, chocolate).

Medications

COMMONLY PRESCRIBED DRUGS

- Spironolactone (Aldactone), vitamin A, vitamin E, oral contraceptives
- Danazol (Danocrine), bromocriptine

CONTRAINDICATIONS

Read drug product information.

PRECAUTIONS

Read drug product information.

DRUG INTERACTIONS

Read drug product information.

OTHER DRUGS

N/A

 ## Followup

PATIENT MONITORING

- Patients may have an increased risk of cancer.
- The doctor should be seen as often as necessary.
- Women should have a mammogram at age 35, at least every 1 to 2 years after age 40, and yearly after age 50.
- When physical examination, mammography, and needle aspiration are used in combination, detection rates for breast cancer range from 93 to 100%.

PREVENTION

Avoiding caffeine may reduce breast pain.

COMPLICATIONS

- Physical examinations and mammograms may be difficult to interpret.
- Cancer

WHAT TO EXPECT

Benign breast disease is chronic, recurring, and intermittent.

 ## Miscellaneous

OTHER FACTORS

N/A

PEDIATRIC

Biopsy in children should be avoided.

GERIATRIC

Not as common among the elderly.

OTHERS

N/A

PREGNANCY

N/A

FURTHER INFORMATION

- American College of Obstetricians & Gynecologists, 409 12th St., SW, Washington, DC 20024-2188, (800) 762-ACOG
- Booklet on Breast Self Examination from Primary care and Care and Cancer, 17 Prospect St., Huntington, NY 11743, (516) 424-8900
- National Cancer Institute, (800) 4-CANCER

Food Allergy

 Basics

DESCRIPTION

Food allergy is a hypersensitivity reaction caused by certain foods.

SIGNS AND SYMPTOMS

- Gastrointestinal: nausea, vomiting, diarrhea, abdominal pain, flatulence, bloating
- Dermatologic: hives, rash, swelling, dermatitis, pallor, flushing
- Respiratory: runny nose, asthma, cough, earache
- Neurologic: fatigue, fainting, headache
- Other symptoms: systemic reaction, growth retardation, bed-wetting

CAUSES

- Any food or ingested substance can cause allergic reactions. Most commonly implicated foods include cow's milk, egg whites, wheat, soy, peanut, fish, tree nuts (walnut and pecan), shellfish, melons, sesame seeds, sunflower seeds, and chocolate.
- Several food dyes and additives can cause allergic-like reactions.

SCOPE

- The incidence of food allergy ranges from 1 to 7% of the population.
- In children up to 4 years of age, the incidence is between 8 to 16%.
- Only about 3–4% of children over 4 years of age have persisting food allergy.

MOST OFTEN AFFECTED

- Food allergy can affect all ages but is more common in infants and children.
- Males are affected twice as often as females.
- A family history may increase the risk of food allergy by 50%.

RISK FACTORS

- Allergies
- Family members with a history of food allergies

 Diagnosis

WHAT THE DOCTOR LOOKS FOR

- The doctor will take a careful history and perform a thorough physical examination to rule out other causes of symptoms.
- The gastrointestinal, dermatologic, respiratory, neurologic, or other signs and symptoms can mimic a variety of diseases.

TESTS AND PROCEDURES

- Blood tests
- Allergy tests: prick test, challenge test
- A stool sample may be obtained for laboratory analysis.
- The digestive tract may be evaluated with X-rays.

 Treatment

GENERAL MEASURES

- Food allergies are usually managed in the outpatient setting.
- Avoiding the offending food is the most effective way to manage food allergy.
- Individuals with severe allergy should carry epinephrine for self-administration in the event that the offending food is ingested unknowingly and a severe reaction develops immediately.
- The success of immunotherapy and hyposensitization has not been proven.

ACTIVITY

No restrictions

DIET

As determined by tests

Medications

COMMONLY PRESCRIBED DRUGS

- Treatment of symptoms: antihistamine
- Cromolyn
- Ketotifen (not available in the United States)

CONTRAINDICATIONS

Read drug product information.

PRECAUTIONS

Read drug product information.

DRUG INTERACTIONS

Read drug product information.

OTHER DRUGS

N/A

 ## Followup

PATIENT MONITORING

The doctor should be seen as often as needed.

PREVENTION

Avoid the offending food(s).

COMPLICATIONS

- Severe allergic reaction (anaphylaxis)
- Swelling
- Asthma
- Intestinal distress
- Patches of rash or dry skin

WHAT TO EXPECT

- Most infants will outgrow their food hypersensitivity by 2 to 4 years of age. It may be possible to reintroduce the offending food cautiously into the diet (particularly helpful when the food is one that is difficult to avoid).
- Adults with food hypersensitivity (particularly to milk, fish, shellfish, or nuts) tend to maintain their allergy for many years.

 ## Miscellaneous

OTHER FACTORS

N/A

PEDIATRIC

N/A

GERIATRIC

N/A

OTHERS

N/A

PREGNANCY

N/A

FURTHER INFORMATION

Patient support—Food Allergy Network, 4744 Holly Ave., Fairfax, VA 22030-5647, (703) 691-3179

Food Poisoning, Bacterial

 Basics

DESCRIPTION

Bacterial food poisoning includes a variety of illnesses resulting from ingestion of food contaminated with disease-causing bacteria.

SCOPE

Although the true extent of food poisoning is unknown, an estimated 6.3 million cases occur per year in the United States. About 1 in 10 Americans suffer food-borne diarrhea annually.

MOST OFTEN AFFECTED

Food poisoning affects all ages, males and females with equal frequency.

SIGNS AND SYMPTOMS

- Food poisoning is suspected when multiple persons become ill after eating the same meal.
- Nausea, vomiting, cramps, diarrhea, fever 1–72 hours after meal
- Bloody diarrhea without fever 3–5 days after meal

CAUSES

Bacterial contamination

RISK FACTORS

Ingestion of
- Egg salad, cream-filled pastries, gravies
- Cereals, fried rice, dried foods, herbs
- Raw or under-cooked pork, poultry beef, seafood, eggs, dairy products
- Raw vegetables, contaminated water

 Diagnosis

WHAT THE DOCTOR LOOKS FOR

- The doctor conducts a history and physical examination to identify the cause of signs and symptoms.
- Identifying the source of contamination may involve epidemiological study.

TESTS AND PROCEDURES

- A stool sample may be obtained for laboratory analysis.
- Suspected food sources may be cultured.
- The intestinal tract may be examined by sigmoidoscopy.

 Treatment

GENERAL MEASURES

- Most cases of food poisoning are self-limiting and do not require therapy.
- Food poisoning is usually managed in the outpatient setting.
- Individuals with severe food poisoning may require hospitalization.
- Oral solutions for rehydration; intravenous (IV) fluids may be necessary for severe dehydration (particularly among the elderly).
- For infants, rehydration products (e.g., Pedialyte) provide adequate fluid and salt replacement. Do not use for more than 1 to 2 days without seeing the doctor again.

ACTIVITY

Bed rest for comfort if needed during the acute phase

DIET

- Eliminate contaminated food.
- Bland diet during recovery
- Nothing by mouth if there is excessive vomiting or diarrhea

Medications

COMMONLY PRESCRIBED DRUGS

Antibiotics

CONTRAINDICATIONS

Read drug product information.

PRECAUTIONS

Read drug product information.

DRUG INTERACTIONS

Read drug product information.

OTHER DRUGS

N/A

 Followup

PATIENT MONITORING

The doctor should be seen as often as necessary based on symptoms and health status. Serious cases require hospitalization.

PREVENTION

- Do not eat raw seafood, meats, or poultry.
- Avoid unpasteurized dairy products.
- Thoroughly clean food preparation areas.
- Cool any prepared foods not immediately consumed.

COMPLICATIONS

- Cardiovascular collapse
- Irregular heart rhythm
- Severe infection
- Seizures or coma

WHAT TO EXPECT

In most cases, signs and symptoms resolve over a few days.

 Miscellaneous

OTHER FACTORS

N/A

PEDIATRIC

- Outbreaks of food poisoning may occur at day-care centers.
- Newborns and infants are a high risk for complications and death.

GERIATRIC

- Outbreaks of food poisoning can occur in nursing homes.
- Significant cause of death

OTHERS

N/A

PREGNANCY

Some infections can affect the newborn, with severe consequences.

FURTHER INFORMATION

N/A

Frostbite

Basics

DESCRIPTION

Frostbite is a complication of exposure to cold, resulting in diminished blood flow to the affected part (especially hands, face, or feet). Dehydration, tissue destruction, and ultimately cell death occurs. In severe cases, deep tissue freezing may damage underlying blood vessels, muscles, and nerve tissue.

SIGNS AND SYMPTOMS

- Injured area first appears cold, hard, and white and has no sensation.
- After rewarming, the area is blotchy-red, swollen, and painful
- Loss of skin sensation
- Numbness
- Throbbing pain
- Tingling sensation
- Excessive sweating
- Joint pain
- Pallor
- Swelling
- Sensation of heat
- Blistering
- Blue discoloration
- Skin death
- Gangrene

CAUSES

- Prolonged exposure to cold
- Refreezing thawed extremities

SCOPE

There are about 4,800 cases of frostbite annually in the United States.

MOST OFTEN AFFECTED

Frostbite affects all ages, males and females with equal frequency.

RISK FACTORS

- Impaired mental function
- Alcohol or drug abuse
- Mental illness
- Ambient temperature less than 0°F (-17.8°C)
- Smoking
- Elderly
- Circulatory disorders

Diagnosis

WHAT THE DOCTOR LOOKS FOR

The doctor will perform a physical examination to determine the extent and severity of frostbite.

TESTS AND PROCEDURES

- Blood tests
- Decreased hepatic function
- Electrocardiogram (EKG)
- Ultrasound may be used to assist in diagnosis.

Treatment

GENERAL MEASURES

- Frostbite may be managed in the outpatient setting or require hospitalization, depending on severity.
- Provide emergency first aid as needed, including rescue breathing and cardiopul-monary resuscitation (CPR).
- Prevent refreezing. It may be necessary to keep frostbitten part frozen until patient can be transported to a care facility.
- Rewarming must be done carefully and cautiously.
- Keep victim dry. If conscious, give warm fluids with high sugar content.
- Prevent damage to other body parts.

ACTIVITY

- As tolerated; protect injured body parts.
- Physical therapy should begin once healing progresses sufficiently.

DIET

- As tolerated
- Warm oral fluids

 # Medications

COMMONLY PRESCRIBED DRUGS

- Warm intravenous (IV) fluids
- Heated oxygen
- Levothyroxine, hydrocortisone
- Tetanus toxoid
- Pain relievers
- Antibiotics

CONTRAINDICATIONS

Read drug product information.

PRECAUTIONS

Read drug product information.

DRUG INTERACTIONS

Read drug product information.

OTHER DRUGS

Nifedipine, pentoxifylline

 # Followup

PATIENT MONITORING

- The doctor will be seen often during hospitalization.
- The doctor should be seen as often as necessary during followup.

PREVENTION

- Dress in layers with appropriate cold weather gear.
- Cover exposed areas and extremities appropriately.
- Prepare properly for trips to cold climates.

- Avoid alcohol when out in the cold; alcohol interferes with the body's heat conservation mechanism.
- Recognize the early signs of cold exposure and take appropriate action.

COMPLICATIONS

- Metabolic disturbance
- Irregular heart rhythm
- Tissue loss, gangrene
- Death

WHAT TO EXPECT

- Loss of sensation and the formation of blisters may occur.
- The affected areas will heal or mummify without surgery. The process may take 6–12 months. Person may be sensitive to cold and experience burning and tingling.

 # Miscellaneous

OTHER FACTORS

N/A

PEDIATRIC

N/A

GERIATRIC

- Increased risk of death
- More sensitive to temperature extremes

OTHERS

N/A

PREGNANCY

N/A

FURTHER INFORMATION

N/A

Section G

Gallstones

 ## Basics

DESCRIPTION

Gallstones, or cholelithiasis, is the formation of cholesterol- or pigment-containing stones in the gallbladder.

SIGNS AND SYMPTOMS

- Most people have no symptoms.
- About 5–10% of people with gallstones develop symptoms annually.
- Fewer than half of those with gallstones develop symptoms over their lifetime.
- Episodes of stomach pain, radiating to the back
- Nausea
- Vomiting
- Intolerance for fatty food (not proven)
- Indigestion

CAUSES

- Production of cholesterol-rich bile
- Changes in bile composition or flow
- Blood disorders
- Gallbladder infection

SCOPE

Gallstones affect 8–10% of the U.S. population.

MOST OFTEN AFFECTED

The incidence of gallstones increases with age, peaking in the 50s. Gallstones occur more frequently in American Indians and Hispanics and are twice as frequent in females as males.

RISK FACTORS

- Digestive disorders (short gut syndrome, inflammatory bowel disease)
- Multiple births
- Long-term total parenteral nutrition (TNP)
- Cirrhosis of the liver
- Blood disorders
- Prosthetic cardiac valves
- Rapid weight loss
- Childhood cancer
- Native-American descent
- Female gender

 ## Diagnosis

WHAT THE DOCTOR LOOKS FOR

- The doctor will perform a physical examination to identify the cause of symptoms.
- Causes of similar symptoms include hepatitis, pancreatitis, coronary artery disease, appendicitis, pneumonia, cancer, kidney stones, and numerous other conditions.

TESTS AND PROCEDURES

- A specialized imaging procedure, hepatobiliary radionuclide scan, may be done to assist in diagnosis.
- The gallbladder may be evaluated by a radiology procedure called oral cholecystogram.
- Ultrasound or computed tomography (CT scan) may be used.

Treatment

GENERAL MEASURES

- Gallstones may be medically managed in the outpatient setting.
- Surgical procedures for the treatment of gallstones require hospitalization.
- Only gallstones that cause symptoms are treated.
- Stones that do not cause symptoms are observed.
- Surgery may be open or minimally invasive.
- Direct contact dissolution may be an option.
- Extracorporeal shock wave lithotripsy, i.e., "stone busting" (under study—not FDA approved)

ACTIVITY

N/A

DIET

Low-fat diet may be helpful.

Medications

N/A

DIET

ACTIVITY

Rest with legs elevated

DIET

- Cool or cold clear liquids only (noncarbonated)
- Avoid caffeine.
- Unrestricted salt

 ## Medications

COMMONLY PRESCRIBED DRUGS

IV saline (salt water) fluids

CONTRAINDICATIONS

N/A

PRECAUTIONS

N/A

DRUG INTERACTIONS

N/A

OTHER DRUGS

N/A

 ## Followup

PATIENT MONITORING

- The doctor will be seen often if hospitalization is required.
- For minor cases of heat injury, no followup may be needed.
- The doctor should be seen as often as necessary.

PREVENTION

- Avoid dehydration with proper fluids during activity or exercise—8 ounces of fluid for every 15 minutes of moderate exercise.
- Allow acclimatization to hot weather through proper conditioning and activity modification.
- Dress appropriately with loose-fitting, open weave, light-colored clothing.

- Maintain as much skin exposure as possible in hot, humid conditions, while using proper sun block protection.
- Recognize the signs and symptoms of heat stress and act accordingly.

COMPLICATIONS

- Major organ system failure
- Irregular heart rhythms or heart attack
- Pulmonary conditions
- Coma, seizures
- Acute kidney failure
- Bleeding disorders
- Liver disease

WHAT TO EXPECT

- Recovery is good when mental function is not altered. Recovery occurs within 24 to 48 hours in most cases.
- The death rate for heat stroke (10–80%) is directly related to the duration and intensity of injury, as well as to the speed and effectiveness of treatment.

 ## Miscellaneous

OTHER FACTORS

N/A

PEDIATRIC

Children are more susceptible to heat injury.

GERIATRIC

The elderly are more susceptible to heat injury.

OTHERS

N/A

PREGNANCY

Pregnant women may be more prone to dehydration.

FURTHER INFORMATION

N/A

Hemorrhoids

 Basics

DESCRIPTION

Hemorrhoids, or piles, are varicose or enlarged veins of the rectum. They may be internal or external. Hemorrhoids may be acute (of short duration), chronic (long-lasting), or relapsing.

SIGNS AND SYMPTOMS

- Rectal bleeding
- Anal protrusion
- Anal pain
- Itching
- Constipation
- Straining with defecation
- Bowel incontinence
- Blood or mucus in stool
- Sensation of incomplete emptying of the bowel
- Anal fissure
- Anal infection
- Anal ulceration

CAUSES

Dilated veins of rectum

SCOPE

Common

MOST OFTEN AFFECTED

Hemorrhoids primarily affect adults, although they may occur at any age. Males and females are affected with equal frequency.

RISK FACTORS

- Pregnancy
- Colon cancer
- Liver disease
- Constipation
- Occupations that require prolonged sitting
- Loss of muscle tone in old age, rectal surgery, episiotomy, anal intercourse
- Obesity

 Diagnosis

WHAT THE DOCTOR LOOKS FOR

The doctor will perform a physical examination to identify the presence of hemorrhoids.

TESTS AND PROCEDURES

The colon may be examined by anoscopy or sigmoidoscopy.

 Treatment

GENERAL MEASURES

- Hemorrhoids are managed in the outpatient setting except when surgery is required.
- Mild symptoms or prevention:
  - ▶ Avoid prolonged sitting on toilet
  - ▶ Avoid straining
  - ▶ Avoid constipation by using stool softeners
  - ▶ Use soap and water for clean-up after stool
- For pain: sitz baths with soapy water or Epson salts
- Surgery may be needed for persistent and severe disease.
- Other treatments include incision of hemorrhoid, rubber band ligation, injection therapy, cryosurgery, and laser surgery.

ACTIVITY

- No restrictions
- Physical fitness is encouraged.
- Avoid prolonged sitting and straining on the toilet.

DIET

High-fiber diet

 Medications

COMMONLY PRESCRIBED DRUGS

- Prevention:
  - ▶ Fiber supplements
  - ▶ Stool softeners

- Pain:
  ▶ Analgesic sprays or ointments: benzocaine (Hurricaine), dibucaine (Nupercainal)
- Itching
  ▶ Hydrocortisone ointment (Anusol-HC; Cortifoam)
- Bleeding:
  ▶ Astringent suppositories (Preparation H)
  ▶ Hydrocortisone ointment (Anusol; Cortifoam)

CONTRAINDICATIONS

Read drug product information.

PRECAUTIONS

Read drug product information.

DRUG INTERACTIONS

Read drug product information.

OTHER DRUGS

N/A

 ## Followup

PATIENT MONITORING

The doctor should be seen as often as needed, depending on treatment.

PREVENTION

- Avoid constipation
- Lose weight, if overweight
- Avoid prolonged sitting on the toilet.
- Avoid prolonged sitting at work. Get up and move around periodically.

COMPLICATIONS

- Thrombosis
- Infection
- Ulcers
- Anemia (rare)
- Incontinence

WHAT TO EXPECT

- Spontaneous improvement
- Recurrence

 ## Miscellaneous

OTHER FACTORS

N/A

PEDIATRIC

Hemorrhoids are uncommon in infants and children. Occasionally, hemorrhoids may result from chronic constipation, fecal impaction, and straining at stool. Surgery is rarely required.

GERIATRIC

Hemorrhoids are common in the elderly along with rectal prolapse.

OTHERS

N/A

PREGNANCY

Hemorrhoids are common in pregnancy, and they usually resolve after pregnancy. No treatment is required unless they are extremely painful.

FURTHER INFORMATION

N/A

Hepatitis, Viral

 Basics

DESCRIPTION

Viral hepatitis is a group of viral infections involving the liver.

SCOPE

- Hepatitis A virus (HAV): 50% of people over age 49 have been exposed; HAV is found in 25% of cases of acute hepatitis.
- Hepatitis B virus (HBV): About 200,000 persons are infected annually. There are more than 500,000 carriers of HBV.
- Hepatitis C virus (HCV): HCV is becoming the most common cause of acute and chronic viral hepatitis; 150,000 persons are infected annually.

MOST OFTEN AFFECTED

Hepatitis occurs in all ages. It is rare in infants, and susceptibility increases with age. Males are affected more often than females.

SIGNS AND SYMPTOMS

- Fever
- Malaise, fatigue
- Nausea
- Loss of appetite
- Jaundice
- Dark urine
- Abdominal pains
- Headache
- Vomiting

CAUSES

- Viral infection
- Infection may be caused by multiple, different viruses.
- Maximum infectivity occurs 2 weeks before the appearance of jaundice.
- Transmitted sexually, by blood or its products, or during pregnancy.

RISK FACTORS

- Health care workers/other occupational risks
- Dialysis
- Recipients of blood and/or blood products
- Intravenous (IV) drug users; individuals with tattoos
- Sexually active homosexual males
- Household exposure
- Unprotected sex
- Needle stick
- Organ transplantation

 Diagnosis

WHAT THE DOCTOR LOOKS FOR

- The doctor will perform a physical examination to identify the signs and symptoms of viral hepatitis.
- Other causes of similar symptoms include Infectious mononucleosis, drug or alcohol abuse, and other liver disorders.

TESTS AND PROCEDURES

- Blood tests
- Tests may be done to identify virus.
- A sample of liver tissue may be obtained for laboratory analysis.
- Ultrasound may be used to assist with diagnosis.

 Treatment

GENERAL MEASURES

- Viral hepatitis is usually managed on an outpatient basis.
- Hospitalization may be required.
- Segregation advisable for food handlers or health care workers.
- Acute cases must be reported to public health department.
- Liver transplantation may be necessary.

ACTIVITY

As tolerated

DIET

Adequate calories; balanced nutrition

Medications

COMMONLY PRESCRIBED DRUGS

- Interferon, ribavirin (Virazole)
- Amantadine (Symmetrel)
- Steroids

CONTRAINDICATIONS

Read drug product information.

PRECAUTIONS

Bleeding disorders, immune system disorders, seizures, pregnancy, fertile age group, lactation. Read drug product information.

DRUG INTERACTIONS

Read drug product information.

OTHER DRUGS

N/A

 Followup

PATIENT MONITORING

- The doctor should be seen as often as necessary.
- Blood tests will be periodically repeated.
- Biopsy of liver may need to be repeated in chronic cases.
- Monitoring for metabolic complications

PREVENTION

- Use safe sex practices.
- Don't share needles.
- Practice good sanitation habits.
- It is currently recommended that all individuals receive vaccination against HBV.
- Vaccination against HAV is recommended for some individuals, including travelers, sewage workers, military personnel, day-care staff and children, homosexual men, and food handlers.

COMPLICATIONS

Severe liver disease, cancer, or failure

WHAT TO EXPECT

- The outcome varies depending on the virus causing hepatitis.
- Severity of liver disease is a good indicator of outcome.
- May progress to chronic disease

 Miscellaneous

OTHER FACTORS

N/A

PEDIATRIC

N/A

GERIATRIC

N/A

OTHERS

Alcohol abuse is a major factor for chronic liver disease.

PREGNANCY

Hepatitis virus may be transmitted to babies. Pregnant women should be screened for HBV.

FURTHER INFORMATION

N/A

Herpes Simplex

 Basics

DESCRIPTION

Herpes simplex is a viral disease that usually causes painful blisters in clusters on the skin, cornea, or mucous membranes. Herpes simplex may occur in other, more serious forms. Newborns or individuals with immune system disorders are at greater risk of complications or death.

SIGNS AND SYMPTOMS

- Blisters: usually cluster and open as painful ulcerated lesions, often with a reddened base
- Variations include:
  - ▶ Infection on a finger: intense itching and pain, followed by blisters that may merge; accompanied by swelling, reddening, and pain; heals over 2 to 3 weeks
  - ▶ Fever; sore, swollen, and reddened throat; small blisters on throat and mouth, rapidly increasing to involve roof of mouth, cheek, tongue, and often lips and cheeks; resolves in 10 to 14 days
  - ▶ Genital herpes: see Herpes, genital
  - ▶ Infection of eye or lid; lasts 2–3 weeks
  - ▶ Diffuse rash-like eruption
  - ▶ Newborn infection; life-threatening and usually acquired by vaginal birth of infected mother
- Recurring diseases include:
  - ▶ Recurrent lesions on lips; usually less than 1 recurrence per 6 months, but 5–25% may have more than 1 attack per month; may be precipitated by sunlight, fever, trauma, menstruation, stress; pain, burning, itching may last 6–48 hours before blisters appear, often at edge of lip; will ulcerate and crust within 48 hours; heals within 8 to 10 days
  - ▶ Eye infection: may affect cornea, eye lid, or whites of eye; ulcers, vision loss; may cause permanent visual loss
  - ▶ Genital herpes: see Herpes, genital

CAUSES

Infection with herpes simplex virus

SCOPE

- Herpes infection is widespread; up to 20% of adults may be contagious.
- From 30% to 100% of population subgroups have been exposed to herpes simplex virus.

MOST OFTEN AFFECTED

Herpes affects all ages, males and females in equal proportion.

RISK FACTORS

- Immune system disorders
- Newborns: if exposed to infected mother during birth canal or if exposed in nursery
- Prior herpes infection
- Sexual intercourse with infected person
- Occupational exposure (health care worker)

 Diagnosis

WHAT THE DOCTOR LOOKS FOR

- The doctor will complete a physical examination to look for the signs of herpes infection.
- Other conditions that may appear similar include impetigo and numerous other skin diseases.

TESTS AND PROCEDURES

- Fluid from a blister may be sampled for laboratory analysis.
- A sample of skin may be obtained by biopsy.
- Tests for other sexually transmitted diseases may be performed.

Treatment

GENERAL MEASURES

- Herpes is managed on an outpatient basis.
- Intermittent, cool, moist dressings
- Genital herpes: Painful urination may be helped by pouring a cup of warm water over genitals while urinating or sitting in a warm bath to urinate.

ACTIVITY

No restrictions

DIET

Avoid acidic foods if mouth is involved.

 ## Medications

COMMONLY PRESCRIBED DRUGS

- Acyclovir (Zovirax)
- Valacyclovir (Valtrex)
- Famciclovir (Famvir)

CONTRAINDICATIONS

Allergy to or intolerance of drug

PRECAUTIONS

Numerous precautions; read drug product information.

DRUG INTERACTIONS

Read drug product information.

OTHER DRUGS

- Foscarnet
- Other topical medications: Acyclovir, vidarabine (Vira-A), idoxuridine and trifluorothymidine, n-docosanol

 ## Followup

PATIENT MONITORING

The doctor should be seen as often as necessary.

PREVENTION

- Avoid contact with newborns or individuals with immune system disorders.
- Wash hands often.
- For genital herpes: Avoid sexual contact while disease is active; condoms can reduce the risk of transmission but are not perfect; maintain mutually monogamous sexual relations.

COMPLICATIONS

- Brain infection or inflammation
- Pneumonia
- Blood poisoning

WHAT TO EXPECT

- Good for treatment of recurrent episodes
- Expect frequent recurrences.

 ## Miscellaneous

OTHER FACTORS

N/A

PEDIATRIC

N/A

GERIATRIC

Decreased immune response of old age may increase risk of herpes.

OTHERS

N/A

PREGNANCY

N/A

FURTHER INFORMATION

N/A

Herpes, Genital

 Basics

DESCRIPTION

Genital herpes is caused by herpes simplex virus infection of the genital organs.

SIGNS AND SYMPTOMS

- 60–70% of individuals infected with herpes simplex show no symptoms.
- Fever
- Headache
- Malaise
- Muscle ache and pain
- Burning genital pain
- Painful urination
- Pain during intercourse
- Numbness or tingling of the lower back
- Swollen glands in groin
- Urinary retention
- Blisters: Blisters appear on a swollen, reddened base; they ulcerate, crust over, and heal within 21 days. Blisters persist longer on dry skin.
- Recurrent genital herpes: Symptoms (burning, numbness, tingling of skin) may occur at site of old lesion about 24 hours before the eruption of new blisters.

SCOPE

Up to one-third of the U.S. population is infected with herpes. There are 300,000–700,000 new cases annually.

MOST OFTEN AFFECTED

Individuals 18–40 years of age, females more frequently than males

CAUSES

Herpes simplex virus

RISK FACTORS

- Sexual activity
- Clothing, wet towels (rare)
- Triggers (recurrent)
  - ▶ Genital trauma
  - ▶ Menstrual period
  - ▶ Infection
  - ▶ Emotional stress
  - ▶ Sunlight

 Diagnosis

WHAT THE DOCTOR LOOKS FOR

- The doctor will perform a physical examination to identify the presence of genital herpes.
- The doctor will also look for conditions known to be associated with genital herpes, including other sexually transmitted diseases.

TESTS AND PROCEDURES

- Blood tests
- A sample of blister fluid may be obtained for laboratory analysis.
- Pap smear

 Treatment

GENERAL MEASURES

- Genital herpes is managed in the outpatient setting.
- Most care of genital herpes is self-care.
- Cool compresses, ice packs to perineum, sitz baths
- Local perineal hygiene
- Analgesics: nonsteroidal anti-inflammatory drugs (NSAIDs)
- Topical anesthetics: lidocaine

ACTIVITY

- Avoid intercourse in the presence of genital lesions.
- Appropriate rest if systemic symptoms are present

DIET

No special diet

Medications

COMMONLY PRESCRIBED DRUGS

Acyclovir (Zovirax)

CONTRAINDICATIONS

Allergy to acyclovir

PRECAUTIONS

Acyclovir is not approved for routine use in pregnancy; drug is excreted in breast milk.

DRUG INTERACTIONS

Drugs have many interactions; read drug product information.

OTHER DRUGS

- Acyclovir topical ointment: less effective
- Foscarnet
- Vidarabine
- Famciclovir (Famvir)
- Valacyclovir (Valtrex)

 ## Followup

PATIENT MONITORING

- Acute episode: See the doctor if complications develop.
- Latent infection: annual Pap smear

PREVENTION

- Use condoms and spermicide during sexual intercourse.
- Avoid multiple sexual partners.
- Avoid stress when possible.

COMPLICATIONS

- Vaginal discharge
- Bacterial infection
- Urinary retention
- Meningitis
- Transmission to baby
- Increased risk for human immunodeficiency virus (HIV) infection

WHAT TO EXPECT

- Resolution of signs and symptoms in 14–21 days; recurring episodes heal in 7–10 days
- Blisters recur in more than 50% of infected individuals; individuals with immune system disorders average 3–4 episodes per year.

 ## Miscellaneous

OTHER FACTORS

N/A

PEDIATRIC

Genital herpes in a child may be a sign of sexual abuse.

GERIATRIC

N/A

OTHERS

N/A

PREGNANCY

- First episode of genital herpes infection during pregnancy is associated with increased rate of miscarriage and preterm labor.
- Greatest risk for neonatal infection occurs at time of delivery.
- Cesarean section may be required.
- Acyclovir therapy is not approved for routine use during pregnancy.

FURTHER INFORMATION

Herpes Resource Center ASHA/HRC, P.O. Box 13827, Research Triangle Park, North Carolina 27709-9940, HRC Hotline (919) 361-8488; web page http://sunsite.unc.edu./ASHA/

Hirsutism

 Basics

DESCRIPTION

Hirsutism is excessive hair growth due to increased male hormones.
- Often accompanied by menstrual irregularities
- Extreme masculinization effects (deep voice, enlarged clitoris, balding) is known as virilization.

SIGNS AND SYMPTOMS

- Hair thickens and darkens in "male" pattern, i.e., beard, moustache, chest hair
- Usually accompanied by irregular menstruation and absence of ovulation
- Usually accompanied by acne
- May be accompanied by infertility
- Onset is usually gradual.

CAUSES

- Hormone disorder
- Ovarian disease
- Ovarian cancer

SCOPE

Hirsutism affects about 8% of adult women.

MOST OFTEN AFFECTED

Females, after puberty

RISK FACTORS

- Family history of hirsutism
- Absence of ovulation

 Diagnosis

WHAT THE DOCTOR LOOKS FOR

- The doctor will perform a thorough physical examination to evaluate hirsutism and identify the cause.
- Other conditions known to be associated with hirsutism should be identified and treated, such as acne.

TESTS AND PROCEDURES

- A number of blood tests may be performed to assist with diagnosis.
- Computed tomography (CT scan) or ultrasound may be used to assess the reproductive tract.
- A sample of uterine tissue may be obtained by biopsy for laboratory analysis.
- Other specialized diagnostic testing may be done.

GENERAL MEASURES

- Hirsutism is managed in the outpatient setting.
- Cosmetic measures include plucking, bleaching, shaving, electrolysis and cover-up cosmetics.
- Treatment is slow and often lifelong.
- Ovulation may need to be induced if pregnancy is desired.
- Use contraception as needed.
- Maintain ideal weight.
- Treat accompanying acne.

ACTIVITY

No special activity

DIET

No special diet

Medications

COMMONLY PRESCRIBED DRUGS

- Oral contraceptives: estrogen, progesterone, medroxyprogesterone (Depo-Provera)
- Dexamethasone

CONTRAINDICATIONS

Avoid medications in pregnancy.

PRECAUTIONS

N/A

DRUG INTERACTIONS

N/A

OTHER DRUGS

Anti-androgenic drugs: spironolactone, cyproterone, flutamide, ketoconazole, leuprolide (Lupron), danazol, metformin

 ## Followup

PATIENT MONITORING

The doctor should be seen as often as needed to monitor drug therapy.

PREVENTION

- Tumor must be ruled out.
- As hormone balance improves, fertility may increase; use contraception as needed.
- Avoid quackery and unlicensed electrolysis.

COMPLICATIONS

- Uterine bleeding and anemia
- Hormone excess may affect lipids, cardiac disease risk, and bone density.
- Poor self-image/shame

WHAT TO EXPECT

- Treatment takes 6–24 months and may be lifelong.
- Excellent outcome with long term therapy for halting further hair growth
- Moderate to poor outcome for reversing current hair growth

 ## Miscellaneous

OTHER FACTORS

N/A

PEDIATRIC

N/A

GERIATRIC

Can occur after menopause

OTHERS

N/A

PREGNANCY

Hirsutism may be accompanied by infertility.

FURTHER INFORMATION

N/A

HIV Infection and AIDS

 Basics

DESCRIPTION

The human immunodeficiency virus (HIV) infects immune system cells, causing cell death and a decline in immune function. As a result, a person infected with HIV eventually develops acquired immunodeficiency syndrome (AIDS), which includes opportunistic infections, cancer, and neurologic lesions. HIV appears to have direct effects on the central nervous system, the gastrointestinal tract, and other systems.

SIGNS AND SYMPTOMS

- Chronic infection with variable course (50% of persons develop AIDS within 10 years)
- Acute infection: fever, rash, muscle aches, and malaise; this self-limited syndrome occurs about 6–8 weeks after infection
- Following infection, there is a variable period of time without symptoms.
- Lymph node enlargement persisting longer than 3 months
- Other diseases:
  - ▶ Constitutional: fever lasting more than 1 month, weight loss, persistent diarrhea, skin rash, severe chronic fatigue
  - ▶ Neurologic disease: dementia, nerve disorders
  - ▶ AIDS-defining opportunistic infections: *Pneumocystis carinii* pneumonia (PCP); toxoplasmosis, candidiasis, tuberculosis, other infections
  - ▶ Cancers: Kaposi's sarcoma, non-Hodgkin's lymphoma, other cancers

HIV Infection and AIDS

CAUSES

Human immunodeficiency virus (HIV)

SCOPE

There are more than 500,000 cases of AIDS cases in the United States, and more than 300,000 deaths.

MOST OFTEN AFFECTED

Young adults 25–44 years of age. Males are affected more frequently than females.

RISK FACTORS

- Sexual activity: Homosexual men are at greatest risk, but all sexually active people are at risk, depending on the risk factors of, and number of sexual partners.
- Intravenous (IV) drug use (sharing of contaminated needles)
- Recipients of blood products
- Hemophiliacs who have received pooled plasma products are at high risk.
- Children of HIV-infected women
- Health care workers' greatest risk is needle stick.

 Diagnosis

WHAT THE DOCTOR LOOKS FOR

- The doctor will perform a physical examination to identify any of the conditions associated with HIV infection or AIDS.
- The doctor should screen for HIV infection when there is prolonged illness without ready explanation.

TESTS AND PROCEDURES

- Blood tests. CD4 cells (the cells infected and destroyed by HIV) are counted; CD4 cell count gives an indication of the severity of HIV infection.
- Any number of radiology procedures or special tests may be done to assist in diagnosis, depending on the nature of opportunistic infections or other conditions.

HIV Infection and AIDS

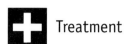 Treatment

GENERAL MEASURES

- HIV infection is managed by a primary care provider in an outpatient setting.
- Infectious disease or HIV specialist may be involved in acute episodes.
- Depending on CD4 cell counts, individuals with HIV infection may receive anti-viral therapy or preventive treatment for PCP, toxoplasmosis, or mycobacterium avium complex.

ACTIVITY

Regular exercise is encouraged. Many community HIV groups have organized "wellness" activities.

DIET

- Good nutrition is encouraged.
- Avoid raw eggs, unpasteurized milk, and other potentially contaminated foods.
- Vitamin supplements may be required.

 Medications

COMMONLY PRESCRIBED DRUGS

- Didanosine (ddI, Videx), lamivudine (3TC, Epivir), stavudine (d4T, Zerit), zalcitabine (ddC, Hivid), zidovudine (AZT, Retrovir)
- Indinavir (Crixivan), ritonavir (Norvir), saquinavir (Invirase)
- Nevirapine (Viramune)

CONTRAINDICATIONS

Significant drug interactions; read drug product information.

PRECAUTIONS

Anti-retroviral drugs have significant toxicities; read drug product information.

DRUG INTERACTIONS

Drugs have potentially life-threatening interactions; read drug product information.

OTHER DRUGS

N/A

HIV Infection and AIDS

 ## Followup

PATIENT MONITORING

- The doctor should be seen as frequently as needed based on the person's health, psychological status, and the need to monitor drug therapy.
- Blood tests every 3–6 months.

PREVENTION

- Avoid unscreened blood products.
- Avoid unprotected sexual intercourse.
- Use condoms.
- Avoid injection drug abuse.
- Avoid contact with body fluids of HIV-infected individuals.

COMPLICATIONS

- Immune system deficiency
- Opportunistic infections
- Neuropsychiatric symptoms
- HIV-associated cancers

WHAT TO EXPECT

- When HIV infection leads to AIDS, life expectancy is 2–3 years.
- AIDS-defining opportunistic infections usually do not develop until CD4 counts are less than 200.
- CD4 counts decline at a rate of 50 to 80 per year with more rapid decline as counts drop below 200.

 ## Miscellaneous

OTHER FACTORS

N/A

PEDIATRIC

Progresses more rapidly in infants

GERIATRIC

Progresses more rapidly in individuals over the age of 50

OTHERS

N/A

PREGNANCY

The risk of bacterial pneumonia may be increased during pregnancy, and the risk of premature birth is also increased in HIV-infected women. Zidovudine (AZT) has been shown to decrease the risk of HIV transmission to infants.

FURTHER INFORMATION

- National AIDS Hotline (800) 342-2437 [Spanish (800) 342-7432]
- National Institute of Health AIDS Clinical Trials Group (800) 874-2572; Information on AIDS/HIV clinical trials
- American Foundation for AIDS Research: (212) 719-0033; new treatments and research

Hodgkin's Disease

 Basics

DESCRIPTION

Hodgkin's disease is a cancer of the lymph system.

SIGNS AND SYMPTOMS

- Painless, enlarged lymph nodes
- Fever
- Night sweats
- Weight loss
- Fatigue
- Loss of appetite

CAUSES

Unknown

SCOPE

There are about 7,900 new cases of Hodgkin's disease annually.

MOST OFTEN AFFECTED

Hodgkin's disease peaks at 20 and 70 years of age. It is more common in males than females, and it may be inherited.

RISK FACTORS

Immune system disorder

 Diagnosis

WHAT THE DOCTOR LOOKS FOR

- The doctor will perform a physical examination to identify the signs and symptoms of Hodgkin's disease.
- Other similar-appearing conditions include other types of cancer, sarcoidosis, or drug reaction.

TESTS AND PROCEDURES

- Blood tests
- Chest x-ray
- Computed tomography (CT scan) of the chest, abdomen, and pelvis may be done.
- Specialized radiology procedures may be done, including lymphangiogram, gallium scan, and bone scan.
- Ultrasound may be used to assist in diagnosis.
- A sample of liver or lymph tissue may be obtained for laboratory analysis.
- A sample of bone marrow may be obtained for laboratory analysis.
- Exploratory surgery may be necessary to assess the extent of disease.

 Treatment

GENERAL MEASURES

- Hodgkin's disease may be managed in the inpatient or outpatient setting.
- Hospitalization may be required.
- The disease will be "staged" to define its nature.
- Treatment is aimed at cure with minimum toxicity.
- Treatment can be radiation, chemotherapy, or a combination.
- Bone marrow transplantation may be required.

ACTIVITY

As tolerated

DIET

No restrictions

Medications

COMMONLY PRESCRIBED DRUGS

- MOPP chemotherapy
  - ▶ Mechlorethamine (Mustargen)
  - ▶ Vincristine (Oncovin)
  - ▶ Procarbazine
  - ▶ Prednisone
- "ABVD" chemotherapy
  - ▶ Doxorubicin (Adriamycin)
  - ▶ Bleomycin
  - ▶ Vinblastine
  - ▶ Dacarbazine

CONTRAINDICATIONS

Read drug product information.

PRECAUTIONS

Read drug product information.

DRUG INTERACTIONS

Read drug product information.

OTHER DRUGS

N/A

 Followup

PATIENT MONITORING

The doctor should be seen as often as necessary to monitor health status.

PREVENTION

N/A

COMPLICATIONS

- Secondary cancers
- Sterility
- Hypothyroidism
- Bone marrow suppression
- Infections
- Anemia
- Bleeding disorders
- Heart disease
- Lung disease

WHAT TO EXPECT

Hodgkin's disease has a 75% overall survival rate.

 Miscellaneous

OTHER FACTORS

N/A

PEDIATRIC

N/A

GERIATRIC

N/A

OTHERS

N/A

PREGNANCY

- If fertility is maintained after treatment, pregnancy can be normal.
- Pregnancy is not known to have a negative impact on the course of Hodgkin's disease.
- Hodgkin's disease is not known to adversely affect the pregnancy or fetus if treatment can be postponed until delivery.
- Disease may progress during pregnancy if treatment is delayed.

FURTHER INFORMATION

Leukemia Society of America, 733 3rd Avenue, New York, NY 10017, (212) 573-8484

Huntington's Chorea

 Basics

DESCRIPTION

Huntington's chorea is an inherited disease characterized by dementia and spasmodic muscle movement. It has a gradual onset and slow progression. Symptoms usually do not develop until after 30 years of age. By the time the disease is diagnosed, the patient has usually had children and passed the disease to another generation.

SIGNS AND SYMPTOMS

- Spasmodic, involuntary movement of the limb and facial muscles
- Difficulty swallowing
- Difficulty speaking
- Impaired memory, judgment
- Intellectual decline
- Emotional disturbances, mood swings
- Depression, anxiety, mania
- Delusions
- Agitation, aggression
- Urinary incontinence
- Bowel incontinence
- Weight loss
- Difficulty walking
- Unsteadiness
- Hyperkinesia
- Abnormal eye movements
- Facial twitching
- Apathy, withdrawal
- Dementia
- Rigidity
- Mania
- Hallucinations
- Delusions
- Paranoia
- Impulsiveness

CAUSES

Hereditary genetic defect

SCOPE

There are 4–8 cases of Huntington's chorea per 100,000 people in the United States.

MOST OFTEN AFFECTED

Individuals 16–75 years of age, males and females in equal frequency

RISK FACTORS

Family history

 Diagnosis

WHAT THE DOCTOR LOOKS FOR

- The doctor will perform a physical examination to identify the signs and symptoms of Huntington's chorea.
- The doctor may take a detailed family medical history.

TESTS AND PROCEDURES

- Blood tests
- Genetic tests
- Special imaging procedures may be used to assist in diagnosis, including computed tomography (CT scan), magnetic resonance imaging (MRI), or positron emission tomography (PET).

 Treatment

GENERAL MEASURES

- Huntington's chorea is managed in the outpatient setting.
- Genetic counseling should be considered.
- Electroconvulsive therapy (ECT) for drug-resistant depression may be considered.
- Speech and occupational therapy may be of benefit.

ACTIVITY

Full activity as long as possible

DIET

No special diet, but soft diet with liquid supplements may be needed.

 ## Medications

COMMONLY PRESCRIBED DRUGS

Haloperidol (Haldol)

CONTRAINDICATIONS

Read drug product information.

PRECAUTIONS

Can cause reactions; read drug product information.

DRUG INTERACTIONS

Read drug product information.

OTHER DRUGS

- Reserpine
- Tetrabenazine
- Tricyclic antidepressants
- Antipsychotics

 ## Followup

PATIENT MONITORING

The doctor should be seen as often as necessary.

PREVENTION

Genetic counseling

COMPLICATIONS

- Choking
- Brain injury
- Spasmodic muscle movement
- Personality changes
- Dementia
- Death
- Suicide

WHAT TO EXPECT

The outcome is poor; disease leads to progressive impairment and is fatal within 20 years.

 ## Miscellaneous

OTHER FACTORS

N/A

PEDIATRIC

Usually does not occur until after puberty

GERIATRIC

Usually fatal before reaching old age

OTHERS

N/A

PREGNANCY

N/A

FURTHER INFORMATION

Newsletter and printed information available from: Huntington's Disease Society of America, 140 W. 22nd St, 6th Fl, New York, NY 10011-2420, phone (212) 242-1968; fax (212) 243-2443

Hypertension, Essential

 Basics

DESCRIPTION

Essential hypertension is the sustained elevation of blood pressure (systolic blood pressure 140 millimeters of mercury [mm Hg] or greater and/or diastolic blood pressure of 90 mm Hg or greater). Hypertension is a strong risk factor for cardiovascular disease. Essential hypertension is also known as benign, idiopathic, familial, genetic, or chronic hypertension. It is sometimes referred to simply as high blood pressure.

SIGNS AND SYMPTOMS

- Hypertension typically causes no symptoms except in extreme cases or after related cardiovascular complications.
- Hypertension can cause headaches, especially at higher blood pressures. Headaches are commonly felt in the back of the head and are present upon awakening.
- Damage to the retina of the eye caused by hypertension may be observed by the doctor.

CAUSES

- More than 90% of hypertension has no identified cause. This type of hypertension is called essential or primary hypertension.
- Secondary causes of hypertension include:
  ▶ Kidney disease
  ▶ Hormonal disorders
  ▶ Blood vessel conditions
  ▶ Chemical: drugs, industrial substances

SCOPE

Hypertension affects 50 million Americans, or about 20% of the adult population.

MOST OFTEN AFFECTED

Essential hypertension usually occurs in individuals in their 20s and 30s. It is more common in males than females. Blood pressure tends to run higher in males. Most importantly, men have a significantly higher risk of cardiovascular disease at any given blood pressure. Blood pressure levels appear to run in families, but no clear genetic pattern has been identified.

RISK FACTORS

- Family history of hypertension or cardiovascular disease
- Obesity
- Alcohol consumption
- Excess dietary sodium
- Stress
- Physical inactivity

WHAT PHYSICIAN LOOKS FOR

- The doctor will do a thorough history and examination to assess physical condition. The examination should include evaluation of the heart and pulses, examination of the abdomen, and examination of the eyes.
- A diagnosis of hypertension is made if the average of at least three properly performed blood pressure measurements exceeds 90 mm Hg diastolic or 160 mm Hg systolic.
- The doctor will look for potential cardiovascular, cerebrovascular, and renal disease as well as diabetes.

TESTS AND PROCEDURES

- Blood workup includes a complete blood count and chemistry tests.
- Complete urinalysis (sometimes reveals proteinuria)
- Chest X-ray
- Tests may be performed to assess the kidney, such as an intravenous pyelogram (IVP) or a renal arteriogram.
- Special urine tests may be ordered.
- Special imaging may be done to assess blood vessels.
- The kidney may be biopsied if disease is suspected.
- An electrocardiogram (EKG) may be done to evaluate the heart.

 Treatment

GENERAL MEASURES

- Hypertension is generally treated on an outpatient basis.
- The goal of treatment is to achieve a blood pressure diastolic less than 90 mm Hg and systolic less than 160 mm Hg.
- Treatment should be individualized based on risk factors.
- Obese persons may significantly lower blood pressure by reducing weight.
- Smoking cessation is an important part of a cardiovascular risk reduction program.
- Biofeedback and relaxation exercises may reduce blood pressures.

ACTIVITY

Normal activity with an appropriate aerobic fitness program

DIET

- A reduced-salt diet may benefit some patients.
- Alcohol consumption should be reduced to less than 1 ounce per day.
- Decrease saturated fats and increase monounsaturated fats in the diet.
- Potassium and calcium may be helpful.

Hypertension, Essential

 Medications

COMMONLY PRESCRIBED DRUGS

- First-line choices of drugs include the following categories and their representatives:
  - ▶ Diuretics (hydrochlorothiazide, chlorthalidone, indapamide)
  - ▶ Alpha adrenergic agents (prazosin, terazosin, doxazosin)
  - ▶ Angioteasin converting enzyme (ACE) inhibitors (captopril, enalapril, fosinopril, lisinopril, ramipril, quinapril, benazepril)
  - ▶ Angiotensin II receptor blocker (losartan)
  - ▶ Calcium-channel blockers (diltiazem, felodipine, isradipine, nicardipine, nifedipine, nitrendipine, verapamil, amlodipine)
  - ▶ Beta blockers (acebutolol, atenolol, metoprolol, nadolol, penbutolol, pindolol, propranolol, timolol, betaxolol, bisoprolol)

CONTRAINDICATIONS

- Diuretics may worsen gout and diabetes.
- Beta blockers may be contraindicated in reactive airway disease (asthma), heart failure, heart block, diabetes, and peripheral vascular disease.
- Diltiazem or verapamil should be used cautiously with heart failure or block.

PRECAUTIONS

See product information.

DRUG INTERACTIONS

See product information.

OTHER DRUGS

- Other drugs may be used in combination with those listed above:
  - ▶ Centrally acting adrenergic inhibitors (clonidine, guanabenz, guanfacine, methyldopa)
  - ▶ Peripherally acting adrenergic inhibitors (guanadrel, guanethidine, reserpine labetalol)
  - ▶ Vasodilators (hydralazine, minoxidil)
  - ▶ Loop diuretics (furosemide, bumetanide, ethacrynic)
  - ▶ Potassium-sparing diuretics (amiloride, spironolactone triamterene)

Followup

PATIENT MONITORING

- Patients should be seen by the doctor at least every 3-6 months.
- The effectiveness of treatment should be evaluated.
- Quality of life issues should be considered, including sexual function.

PREVENTION

- Be aware of risks of cardiovascular disease.
- Make healthful changes to diet and lifestyle.
- Maintain an appropriate level of physical activity.
- Reduce or manage stress, and stop smoking.
- Limit consumption of alcoholic beverages.
- Comply with drug regimens and other treatment.
- Hypertension usually causes no symptoms and requires a lifetime of treatment even if you're feeling well.

COMPLICATIONS

- Congestive heart failure
- Myocardial infarction (heart attack)
- Stroke
- Hypertensive heart disease
- Kidney disease
- Eye disease

WHAT TO EXPECT

The outcome of hypertension is good if adequately controlled.

 Miscellaneous

OTHER FACTORS

N/A

PEDIATRIC

- Blood pressure should be measured during routine examinations.
- Hypertension can accompany a wide variety of acute and chronic illnesses among children.

GERIATRIC

Isolated systolic hypertension is more common among the elderly. Therapy is effective, although adverse reactions to medications are more frequent.

OTHERS

N/A

PREGNANCY

Elevated blood pressure during pregnancy may be either chronic hypertension or preeclampsia. Some medications may adversely affect the fetus.

FURTHER INFORMATION

N/A

Hyperthyroidism

 Basics

DESCRIPTION

Hyperthyroidism is caused by the excess production of thyroid hormone. Types of hyperthyroidism include Grave's disease and goiter.

SIGNS AND SYMPTOMS

- In adults:
  - ▶ Nervousness
  - ▶ Increased sweating
  - ▶ Heat intolerance
  - ▶ Palpitations and rapid heart rate
  - ▶ Difficulty breathing
  - ▶ Fatigue and weakness
  - ▶ Weight loss
  - ▶ Increased appetite
  - ▶ Protruding eyes
  - ▶ Goiter
  - ▶ Tremor
  - ▶ Warm and moist skin
  - ▶ Mood swings
- In children:
  - ▶ Growth abnormalities
  - ▶ Eye abnormalities

SCOPE

Hyperthyroidism affects 1 out of 1,000 women and 1 in 3,000 men.

MOST OFTEN AFFECTED

Hyperthyroidism can affect any age. It peaks in individuals 20–30 years old. It is more common in females than males.

CAUSES

- Autoimmune disease
- Iodine disturbance
- Unknown

RISK FACTORS

- Positive family history
- Female gender
- Other autoimmune disorders
- Iodide replacement after iodide deprivation

 Diagnosis

WHAT THE DOCTOR LOOKS FOR

- The doctor will perform a thorough physical examination to identify the presence of hyper-thyroidism.
- Other conditions that can cause similar signs and symptoms include anxiety, cancer, diabetes, and other disorders.

TESTS AND PROCEDURES

- Blood tests
- A special radiology procedure called a thyroid scan may be done to assist in diagnosis.

 Treatment

GENERAL MEASURES

- Hyperthyroidism is managed in the outpatient setting except for treatment of thyroid storm, a life-threatening condition that can cause heart failure, fever, and mania.
- Treatment consists of antithyroid drugs, thera-peutic iodine.
- Surgery may be required (rare).

ACTIVITY

Modified according to severity of disease

DIET

Sufficient calories to prevent weight loss

Medications

COMMONLY PRESCRIBED DRUGS

- Propylthiouracil (PTU)
- Methimazole (Tapazole)
- Radioiodine therapy: sodium iodine131 (Iodotope I-131).
- Beta-blocker: propranolol (Inderal)

CONTRAINDICATIONS

- Radioiodine therapy: pregnancy and nursing
- Propranolol: congestive heart failure, asthma, chronic bronchitis, pregnancy, hypoglycemia

PRECAUTIONS

- May cause dermatitis or liver damage
- Radioiodine therapy often causes permanent hypothyroidism and may cause birth defects if given during pregnancy.

DRUG INTERACTIONS

Oral blood-thinners (anticoagulants)

OTHER DRUGS

Ipodate sodium (Oragrafin)

 Followup

PATIENT MONITORING

- The doctor should be seen as often as necessary.
- Repeat blood tests twice a year
- After radioiodine therapy, blood tests at 6 weeks, 12 weeks, 6 months, and annually thereafter

PREVENTION

N/A

COMPLICATIONS

- Hypoparathyroidism
- Hypothyroidism
- Visual loss or double vision
- Cardiac failure in the elderly with underlying heart disease
- Muscle wasting

PREVENTION

N/A

WHAT TO EXPECT

With precise diagnosis and adequate treatment, the outcome of treatment is good.

 Miscellaneous

OTHER FACTORS

N/A

PEDIATRIC

N/A

GERIATRIC

- Characteristic symptoms and signs may be absent in elderly.
- Harder to diagnose
- Cardiac failure more likely

OTHERS

N/A

PREGNANCY

- Symptoms may be confusing.
- Radioiodine therapy is absolutely contraindicated.

FURTHER INFORMATION

N/A

Hypothermia

 Basics

DESCRIPTION

Hypothermia occurs when the core body temperature falls below 95°F (35°C). It may take several hours or several days to develop. As the body temperature falls, all organ systems are affected. Blood flow to the brain decreases and the metabolic rate declines rapidly. Patients who have been immersed for as long as 45 minutes in very cold water and appear to be dead have still been resuscitated.

SIGNS AND SYMPTOMS

- Mild (34–35°C):
  - ▶ Lethargy
  - ▶ Mild confusion
  - ▶ Shivering
  - ▶ Loss of fine motor coordination
  - ▶ Increased pulse and blood pressure
- Moderate (30–34°C):
  - ▶ Delirium
  - ▶ Slow heart rate
  - ▶ Low blood pressure
  - ▶ Slow breathing rate
  - ▶ Bluish discoloration around lips, eyes, and nail beds
  - ▶ Irregular heart rhythm
  - ▶ Semicoma and coma
  - ▶ Muscular rigidity
  - ▶ Generalized swelling
- Severe (< 30°C):
  - ▶ Very cold skin
  - ▶ Rigidity
  - ▶ No breathing
  - ▶ No pulse
  - ▶ Unresponsive
  - ▶ Fixed pupils

CAUSES

- Decreased heat production
- Increased heat loss
- Impaired temperature regulation

SCOPE

Unknown

MOST OFTEN AFFECTED

Very young and the elderly; males and females affected with equal frequency

RISK FACTORS

- Malnutrition
- Cold water immersion
- Homelessness
- Outdoor workers
- Trauma victims
- Alcohol or drug consumption
- Mental illness
- Drug intoxication
- Hormone disorders
- Central nervous system disorders
- Severe infection
- Cardiovascular disease
- Pneumonia
- Liver failure
- Kidney failure
- Extensive skin disease
- Excessive fluid loss

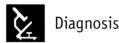

Diagnosis

WHAT THE DOCTOR LOOKS FOR

- The doctor will perform a physical examination, including the measurement of core body temperature.
- Other conditions known to be associated with hypothermia should be investigated, including trauma, stroke, and intoxication.

TESTS AND PROCEDURES

- Arterial blood may be drawn for analysis.
- A number of blood tests may be performed to assist in diagnosis.
- Blood may be cultured for microbiological analysis.
- Electrocardiogram (EKG)
- X-rays of the neck, chest, and abdomen may be done.

Treatment

GENERAL MEASURES

- Hypothermia is usually managed at a hospital emergency department or intensive care unit.
- Provide emergency first aid as needed, including rescue breathing and cardiopulmonary resuscitation (CPR).
- Remove wet garments.
- Protect against heat loss and wind chill.
- Maintain horizontal position.
- Move victim to a warm location as quickly as possible; alert 9-1-1.

ACTIVITY

Bed rest

DIET

Warm fluids only, if alert and able to swallow. Avoid fluids containing caffeine (coffee, hot chocolate).

Hypothermia

 Medications

COMMONLY PRESCRIBED DRUGS

- Antibiotics
- Resuscitation: bretylium, magnesium sulfate, sodium bicarbonate, dextrose intravenous (IV) solution
- Thiamine
- Naloxone
- Levothyroxine

CONTRAINDICATIONS

N/A

PRECAUTIONS

N/A

DRUG INTERACTIONS

N/A

OTHER DRUGS

N/A

 Followup

PATIENT MONITORING

- The doctor and other health care providers will be seen often during hospitalization.
- The doctor will be seen as often as necessary following acute episode for treatment of the underlying cause of hypothermia.

PREVENTION

- Wear appropriate clothing for cold weather, with particular attention to head, feet, and hand coverings.
- If walking or climbing in cold climate, carry survival bags lined with "space" blankets for use if stranded or injured.
- Avoid alcohol, especially if anticipating exposure to cold weather.
- Pay attention to early symptoms and take proper action, e.g., drinking warm fluids, moving indoors.
- Keep the home adequately heated.

COMPLICATIONS

- Irregular heart rhythms
- Shock
- Pneumonia
- Fluid in lungs
- Pancreatitis
- Peritonitis
- Gastrointestinal bleeding
- Kidney damage
- Bleeding disorder
- Metabolic disorder
- Gangrene of extremities

WHAT TO EXPECT

- Death from hypothermia is declining due to faster recognition and better care.
- Death rate depends on the severity of underlying cause of hypothermia.
- In previously healthy individuals, recovery is usually complete.
- Death rate in healthy patients is less 5%.
- Death rate in patients with other medical illness is more than 50%.

 Miscellaneous

OTHER FACTORS

N/A

PEDIATRIC

- Infants are at increased risk of hypothermia because of their limited ability to produce heat when placed in a cold environment.
- A child's body temperature drops faster than an adult's when immersed in cold water.

GERIATRIC

- Older adults have a lower metabolic rate and it is more difficult for them to maintain normal body temperature when environmental temperature drops below 18°C.
- Aging also impairs the ability to detect temperature changes.
- This population also has increased incidence of diseases that decrease heat production or impair temperature regulation.

OTHERS

N/A

PREGNANCY

N/A

FURTHER INFORMATION

N/A

Hypothyroidism, Adult

 Basics

DESCRIPTION

Hypothyroidism, or myxedema, is a condition resulting from the decreased action of thyroid hormone in the body.

SIGNS AND SYMPTOMS

- Onset may be insidious, subtle
- Weakness, fatigue, lethargy
- Cold intolerance
- Diminished memory
- Hearing impairment
- Constipation
- Muscle cramps
- Joint pain
- Loss of sensation, tingling feeling
- Modest weight gain
- Decreased sweating
- Heavy menstrual flow
- Depression
- Carpal tunnel syndrome
- Dry, coarse skin
- Dull facial expression
- Coarsening or huskiness of voice
- Puffiness around eyes
- Swelling of hands and feet
- Slow heart rate
- Low body temperature
- Reduced body and scalp hair
- Enlarged tongue

CAUSES

- Iodine therapy or thyroid surgery
- Thyroid disorders

SCOPE

- Hypothyroidism affects up to 5 to 10 per 1,000 persons in the United States.
- Affects 6–10% of women and 2–3% of men over 65 years of age

MOST OFTEN AFFECTED

Individuals over 40 years of age; 5–10 times more common in females than males

RISK FACTORS

- Risk increases with increasing age.
- Autoimmune diseases

 Diagnosis

WHAT THE DOCTOR LOOKS FOR

- The doctor will perform a thorough physical examination to identify the signs and symptoms of hypothyroidism.
- Conditions that can cause similar signs and symptoms include heart failure, kidney disease, depression, and other disorders.
- Other conditions known to be associated with hypothyroidism should be investigated, such as diabetes mellitus and other hormone disorders.

TESTS AND PROCEDURES

Blood tests

 Treatment

GENERAL MEASURES

- Hypothyroidism is managed in the outpatient setting except for complicating emergencies (coma, hypothermia).
- The goals of treatment are to restore and maintain a normal thyroid state.

ACTIVITY

As tolerated

DIET

- High-bulk diet may be helpful to avoid constipation.
- Low-fat diet for obese patients

Hypothyroidism, Adult

 Medications

COMMONLY PRESCRIBED DRUGS

- Levothyroxine (Synthroid, Levothroid)

CONTRAINDICATIONS

Read drug product information.

PRECAUTIONS

Read drug product information.

DRUG INTERACTIONS

- Oral anticoagulants
- Insulin
- Oral hypoglycemics
- Estrogen
- Oral contraceptives
- Cholestyramine
- Ferrous sulfate

OTHER DRUGS

N/A

 Followup

PATIENT MONITORING

- The doctor should be seen every 6 weeks until condition is stabilized, then every 6 months.
- Contact the physician to report any signs of infection or heart problems.

PREVENTION

N/A

COMPLICATIONS

- Congestive heart failure
- Coma
- Increased susceptibility to infection
- Colon disorder
- Organic psychosis with paranoia
- Adrenal crisis
- Infertility
- Hypersensitivity to opiates
- Bone softening

WHAT TO EXPECT

- With early treatment, striking transformations in approved appearance and mental function. Return to normal state is the rule.
- Relapses will occur if treatment is interrupted.
- If untreated, may progress to myxedema coma

 Miscellaneous

OTHER FACTORS

N/A

PEDIATRIC

N/A

GERIATRIC

Characteristic signs and symptoms are different or absent in the elderly. Hypothyroidism is common in elderly.

OTHERS

N/A

PREGNANCY

N/A

FURTHER INFORMATION

N/A

Section I

Immunizations

Basics

DESCRIPTION
Immunizations, also called vaccinations, are substances that prevent specific diseases.

SIGNS AND SYMPTOMS
N/A

CAUSES
N/A

SCOPE
N/A

MOST OFTEN AFFECTED
N/A

RISK FACTORS
N/A

Diagnosis

WHAT THE DOCTOR LOOKS FOR
N/A

TESTS AND PROCEDURES
N/A

Treatment

GENERAL MEASURES
- Individuals should discuss the consequences of specific diseases and risks of immunizations with their doctors.
- Minor redness, swelling, and or soreness at the site of injections can be expected; ice packs and acetaminophen may help relieve discomfort.
- Acetaminophen may relieve fever caused by immunizations.
- Adverse effects should be promptly reported to the doctor.

ACTIVITY
No restrictions after immunization

DIET
No specific restrictions after immunization

Medication

COMMONLY PRESCRIBED DRUGS
Recommendations for vaccinations are as follows:
- Hepatitis B:
  - ▶ Infants
  - ▶ Health care workers
  - ▶ Laboratory personnel who might be exposed to the virus
  - ▶ Intravenous drug users
  - ▶ Male homosexuals
  - ▶ Persons with a sexually transmitted disease
- Pneumococcal:
  - ▶ All persons over age 65
  - ▶ Individuals with chronic disease, diabetes mellitus, or infected with the human immunodeficiency virus (HIV)
- Influenza:
  - ▶ All persons over age 65
  - ▶ Health care workers
  - ▶ Individuals with chronic disease, diabetes mellitus, or infected with the human immunodeficiency virus (HIV)
- Diphtheria, tetanus, pertussis (DTP):
  - ▶ All children starting at age 2 months
  - ▶ May be given up to the 7th birthday
- Tetanus and diphtheria:
  - ▶ All persons age 7 or over, every 10 years
- Measles, mumps and rubella (MMR):
  - ▶ Children at 12 to 15 months, and again at 4 to 6 or 11 to 12 years of age
  - ▶ Adults (especially medical personnel and day-care workers) without prior immunization or uncertain immunizations born after 1957
  - ▶ International travelers
  - ▶ College students
- Varicella (Chickenpox):
  - ▶ Children at 2 to 18 months of age
  - ▶ Children 18 months to 12 years who have not already had chickenpox

- ▶ Health care workers who have not already had chickenpox
- ▶ Others who have not already had chicken-pox
- • Polio:
  - ▶ All children starting at 2 months of age
  - ▶ Adults traveling to areas where polio is prevalent
- • Haemophilus influenzae type B:
  - ▶ All children starting at 2 months of age
- • Hepatitis A:
  - ▶ Travelers to high-risk countries
  - ▶ Patients with chronic liver disease
  - ▶ Members of high-risk communities and ethnic groups
  - ▶ Homosexual males
  - ▶ Street-drug users
  - ▶ Laboratory personnel who might be exposed

CONTRAINDICATIONS

Vaccination may be contraindicated by allergies, pregnancy, active tuberculosis and immune deficiency

PRECAUTIONS

- • Precautions should be taken with DTP if an individual has suspected neurological disease or has had an adverse event (fever, seizure, spell of inconsolable crying) after a previous DPT vaccination.
- • The following are NOT contraindications and DTP may be given if present:
  - ▶ Family history of convulsions
  - ▶ Family history of sudden infant death syndrome (SIDS)
  - ▶ Family history of adverse event following DTP
  - ▶ Temperature of 105 F or less following a prior DTP

POSSIBLE DRUG INTERACTIONS

Avoid aspirin and other salicylates for 6 weeks before varicella vaccination.

OTHER DRUGS

None

 Followup

PATIENT MONITORING

None routinely needed

PREVENTION/AVOIDANCE

N/A

POSSIBLE COMPLICATIONS

- • Fever, malaise and minor local reactions (redness, pain) are the most common results of immunization.
- • Vaccines rarely cause allergic reaction, high fever, or seizures.
- • Some debatable evidence suggests that DTP may cause encephalopathy on rare occasions.

WHAT TO EXPECT

The outcome after vaccination is usually good. Most people who receive immunization develop protective antibodies.

 Miscellaneous

OTHER FACTORS

N/A

PEDIATRIC

Most vaccines are given to children before they enter school. DTP immunization of the preterm infant should not be delayed unless there are specific contraindications.

GERIATRIC

Pneumococcal, influenza, and tetanus are needed in older age groups.

OTHERS

N/A

PREGNANCY

MMR and varicella should not be routinely given to women who are pregnant or who are planning pregnancy in the next 3 months (MMR) or next 1 month (varicella).

FURTHER INFORMATION

N/A

Impetigo

 ## Basics

DESCRIPTION

Impetigo is a superficial infection of the skin that produces fluid-filled blisters. Impetigo typically begins as a reddened, tender pimple that rapidly progresses into a blister before forming a shallow ulcer covered by a yellowish crust.

SIGNS AND SYMPTOMS

- Begins as a tender red bump or pimple in the skin
- May develop slowly or spread rapidly
- Develops into fluid-filled blisters
- When blisters break, produces a weeping, shallow red ulcer that becomes covered with a honey-colored crust
- Most often occurs on the face around the mouth and nose or at site of trauma
- May form "satellite lesions" at multiple areas of the body

CAUSES

- Bacterial infection
- May be transmitted by direct contact or by insect bite
- May be the result of contamination at site of trauma

SCOPE

Unknown

MOST AFFECTED

Impetigo primarily affects children 2–5 years of age, males and females in equal proportion

RISK FACTORS

- Warm, humid environment
- Tropical or subtropical climate
- Summer or fall season
- Minor trauma, insect bites, etc.
- Poor hygiene, epidemics during war, etc.
- Person-to-person spread within families
- Poor health with anemia and malnutrition
- Complication of head lice, scabies, chicken-pox, eczema
- Contact dermatitis

 ## Diagnosis

WHAT THE DOCTOR LOOKS FOR

- The doctor will rule out other causes of similar conditions, such as chickenpox, herpes, insect bites, and burns.

TESTS AND PROCEDURES

- No blood tests are usually required.
- A small amount of the lesion contents may be sampled after removal of the crust and tested for the presence of bacteria.

 ## Treatment

GENERAL MEASURES

- Impetigo is managed on an outpatient basis.
- Remove crusts from lesions and gently wash 2–3 times a day.
- May be associated with malnutrition and anemia, crowded living conditions, poor hygiene, and neglected minor trauma; these factors should also be addressed during treatment if present.
- Good hygiene habits are important to prevent possible spread.

ACTIVITY

No restrictions

DIET

No special diet

Impetigo

Medications

COMMONLY PRESCRIBED DRUGS

- Antibiotics for 7–10 days: erythromycin base, mupirocin (Bactroban) topical ointment, dicloxacillin.

CONTRAINDICATIONS

Some antibiotics should not be given to people with known allergies.

PRECAUTIONS

Refer to product information.

POSSIBLE DRUG INTERACTIONS

- Erythromycin interacts with theophyllines, astemizole, Fexofenadine (Allegra), and other drugs.
- Refer to product information.

OTHER DRUGS

- 1st generation cephalosporins: cephalexin, cefaclor, cephradine, cefadroxil
- Amoxicillin-clavulanate acid
- Vancomycin
- Clindamycin
- Ciprofloxacin plus rifampin (rifampicin)

Followup

PATIENT MONITORING

If the lesions do not clear within 7–10 days, they should be cultured for microbiological evaluation.

PREVENTION

Close attention to good hygiene habits, particularly hand washing, is important to prevent the spread of impetigo within families.

COMPLICATIONS

- Infection may persist, or become worse.
- In rare cases, bacterial infection can affect the kidney or cause blood poisoning.

WHAT TO EXPECT

Impetigo usually completely resolves within 7–10 days with treatment.

Miscellaneous

OTHER FACTORS

N/A

PEDIATRIC

Impetigo may occur in newborns by contamination in the nursery.

GERIATRIC

N/A

OTHERS

N/A

PREGNANCY

N/A

OTHER INFORMATION

N/A

Impotence

 ## Basics

DESCRIPTION

Erectile problems (dysfunction), or impotence, is the dissatisfaction with size, rigidity, or duration of erection. Includes problems of arousal, desire, orgasm, sensation, and relationships. Temporary periods of impotence occur in about half of adult males and are not abnormal.

SIGNS AND SYMPTOMS

- Reduction of erectile size and rigidity
- Inability to maintain or achieve an erection
- Reduced body hair
- Breast growth
- Testicular atrophy or absence
- Deformed penis
- Vascular disease
- Nerve disease

CAUSES

- Endocrine
- Neurologic
- Vascular
- Medication
- Psychological
- Structural

SCOPE

About 10% of men have erectile dysfunction, but the true incidence is probably higher.

MOST OFTEN AFFECTED

Men 40 years of age and older

RISK FACTORS

- Pelvic surgery
- Medication
- Disorders listed in Causes

 ## Diagnosis

WHAT THE DOCTOR LOOKS FOR

The doctor will perform a complete physical examination to identify causes of erectile dysfunction, such as hormone, neurological, vascular, and psychological disorders or drug side effects.

TESTS AND PROCEDURES

- Blood tests
- Special nerve tests may be performed.
- Tests may be performed to assess penile blood flow.
- Ultrasound may be used to assist in diagnosis.

 ## Treatment

GENERAL MEASURES

- Erectile dysfunction is managed by a primary care provider in an outpatient setting.
- Therapy includes vacuum erectile devices, sensate focus therapy, injection therapy, and penile implants.
- Reduce performance pressure.
- Psychiatrists, psychologists, sex therapists, vascular surgeons, urologists, endocrinologists, neurologists, plastic surgeons, etc., may be consulted for cases that do not improve with therapy.

ACTIVITY

No restrictions

DIET

Control diabetes if present.

Medications

COMMONLY PRESCRIBED DRUGS

- Testosterone cypionate
- Bromocriptine
- Penile injection of phentolamine and papaverine
- Alprostadil (Caverject)

CONTRAINDICATIONS

- Injections should not be used by men with bleeding disorders, sickle cell disease or trait, or penile deformities.
- Avoid drug allergies.

PRECAUTIONS

Injection therapy may cause persistent erection, scarring, low blood pressure, or nausea.

DRUG INTERACTIONS

N/A

OTHER DRUGS

Use vacuum erection device before injections.

 Followup

PATIENT MONITORING

- The doctor should be seen as often as needed.
- Therapy may include sex partner.

PREVENTION

Sex therapist or marriage counselor may help to speed recovery and prevent future problems.

COMPLICATIONS

N/A

WHAT TO EXPECT

- Since the cause of erectile dysfunction is unspecified for most men, vacuum erection device, injection therapy, and penile implants have improved the outlook greatly.
- Vacuum erection device fails in about 20% of cases.
- Many men stop injection therapy.
- 10 to 30% of men with penile implants don't use them.
- About 15% of men improve spontaneously.

 Miscellaneous

OTHER FACTORS

N/A

PEDIATRIC

N/A

GERIATRIC

Aging alone is not a cause of erectile dysfunction.

OTHERS

N/A

PREGNANCY

N/A

FURTHER INFORMATION

N/A

Influenza

 Basics

DESCRIPTION

Influenza is an acute, usually self-limited illness caused by the influenza virus. Also called the flu or grip. It is marked by fever and inflammation of the nose, throat, eyes, and respiratory tract. Outbreaks occur almost every winter with varying degrees of severity.

SIGNS AND SYMPTOMS

Sudden onset of:
- High Fever
- Muscle aches, sometimes severe and lasting for days
- Sore throat
- Nonproductive cough
- Headache
- Swollen neck lymph nodes
- Chills
- Nasal congestion
- Malaise
- Runny nose
- Sneezing

CAUSES

Influenza virus is transmitted from person to person, usually by an airborne route

SCOPE

There are 250,000–500,000 new cases of influenza each year. Attack rates in healthy children are 10–40% each year.

MOST OFTEN AFFECTED

- Influenza most often affects school-aged children (3 months–16 years of age) and young adults (16–40 years of age).
- Males and females affected with equal frequency
- Deaths are highest among the elderly (more than 75 years of age) and those with other medical illnesses, such as lung disease.

RISK FACTORS

- People at increased risk for contracting influenza include:
  - ▶ Patients in semi-closed environments such as nursing homes
  - ▶ Students, prisoners
  - ▶ People living in crowded, close environments during times of epidemics
- Medical conditions that increase the risks of complications arising from influenza include:
  - ▶ Chronic lung diseases
  - ▶ Heart disease
  - ▶ Metabolic diseases
  - ▶ Blood disorders
  - ▶ Cancer
  - ▶ Pregnancy in the third trimester
  - ▶ Infants and the elderly
  - ▶ Suppression of the immune system

Diagnosis

WHAT THE DOCTOR LOOKS FOR

- Other causes of similar signs and symptoms, such as the common cold, bronchitis, pneumonia, tonsillitis, and other viral infections
- During the physical examination, the doctor will consider infectious illnesses that are currently spreading throughout the local community.

TESTS AND PROCEDURES

- Blood tests
- The nose or throat may be cultured for microbiological analysis.
- Chest x-ray

 ## Treatment

GENERAL MEASURES

- Influenza is managed on an outpatient basis except for treatment of severe complications or treatment of persons in high-risk groups.
- Treatment of symptoms: saline nasal spray, gargling
- Cool-mist, ultrasonic humidifier to increase moisture of breathed air.
- Hospitalized patients may require oxygen or ventilatory support.
- Smoking should be avoided.

ACTIVITY

Physical activity as tolerated

DIET

Fluid intake should be increased

Influenza

 Medications

COMMONLY PRESCRIBED DRUGS

- Amantadine and rimantadine are effective against influenza A:
  ▶ Recommended for patients with pneumonia, severe disease, or at high risk for complications. Effective if given within the first 48 hours of onset of symptoms.
  ▶ Rimantadine is not approved for influenza in children.
- Anti-fever drugs:
  ▶ Acetaminophen. This drug should be used to control fever in children.
  ▶ Aspirin should not be given to children under 16 years of age due to risk of Reye's syndrome
- Antibiotics, if there is a bacterial infection

CONTRAINDICATIONS

Nursing mothers; pregnancy unless benefits outweigh risks

PRECAUTIONS

- Amantadine and rimantadine:
  ▶ May cause mild side effects including light-headedness, insomnia, and anxiety which are related to the dose and resolve when the drug is stopped. Drugs may impair the ability to perform hazardous activities or to drive a motor vehicle. Amantadine causes more side effects than rimantadine.
  ▶ May affect underlying seizure disorders and worsen epilepsy
  ▶ Can cause psychosis in some people
  ▶ Patients with congestive heart failure who take amantadine should be observed closely for deterioration.
  ▶ Patients older than 65 years of age or with kidney impairment should receive a lower dose

SIGNIFICANT POSSIBLE INTERACTIONS

Read drug product information.

OTHER DRUGS

- Ribavirin is reported to be effective against influenza types A and B.
- Ibuprofen or other nonsteroidal anti-inflammatory drugs (NSAIDs) can be used for relief of symptoms.

Influenza

Followup

PATIENT MONITORING

- In mild cases, usually no followup is required.
- Moderate or severe cases should be followed until symptoms resolve and any complications are treated effectively.

PREVENTION

- The incubation period of influenza is 1–4 days. Infected persons are most contagious during period of peak symptoms.
- Influenza vaccine
  ▶ Recommended for all adults 65 years of age and older
  ▶ Recommended for high-risk individuals with heart, lung, metabolic or kidney diseases; diabetes; suppression of the immune system (e.g., HIV-infected individuals); alcoholism; long-term aspirin therapy
  ▶ Recommended for health care providers, home care providers, staff and residents of nursing homes and other chronic care facilities, homeless persons, public safety workers, and those in close contact with high-risk individuals
  ▶ Should be administered in the fall prior to influenza season
  ▶ Some side effects possible, e.g., fever and mild, local reaction at vaccination site.
- Amantadine and rimantadine:
  ▶ May be used for prevention in high-risk groups during epidemics of influenza A. It should not be considered a substitute for vaccination unless vaccine is contraindicated.
  ▶ Take for duration of outbreak, if no vaccine given. Discontinue after 14 days if used in addition to vaccine.

WHAT TO EXPECT

Recovery from influenza is favorable

COMPLICATIONS

- Middle-ear infection
- Pneumonia
- Reye's syndrome
- Acute sinusitis
- Croup
- Apnea in neonates
- Bronchitis
- Death

Miscellaneous

OTHER FACTORS

N/A

PEDIATRIC

Reye's syndrome is a rare and severe complication associated with aspirin use. Do not give aspirin to children with influenza; use acetaminophen.

GERIATRIC

- The elderly are more likely to have complications.
- Immunization is recommended for all individuals 65 years of age and older.

OTHERS

N/A

PREGNANCY

- Women with medical problems that place them at risk for complications of influenza should receive influenza vaccine regardless of trimester.
- Women who are in the third trimester of pregnancy during influenza season should consider being vaccinated.
- Amantadine should not be given to pregnant women.

FURTHER INFORMATION

N/A

Inner Ear Infection

 ## Basics

DESCRIPTION

Labyrinthitis is an inflammation of the vestibular system of the inner ear. There are many possible causes. The most constant and pervasive symptom is vertigo.

SIGNS AND SYMPTOMS

- Vertigo
- Dizziness
- Hearing loss
- Nausea and vomiting
- Ringing in ear (tinnitus)
- Perspiration
- Increased salivation
- Generalized malaise

CAUSES

- Physiological: mismatch of sensory systems, such as a stop after whirling turns, heights, motion sickness
- Disorder of inner ear, nerve or brain
- Infections
- Tumors
- Blood vessel disorders
- Drug side-effects
- Head injury

SCOPE

Unknown

MOST OFTEN AFFECTED

All ages beyond infancy, males and females in equal proportion

RISK FACTORS

- Trauma
- Stress
- Drug use
- Virus infection
- Cardiovascular disease

 ## Diagnosis

WHAT THE DOCTOR LOOKS FOR

- The doctor will perform a physical examination to identify the signs and symptoms of labyrinthitis.
- Other conditions that can cause similar signs and symptoms include Meniere's syndrome, head injury, bacterial infection, cancer, and multiple sclerosis.

TESTS AND PROCEDURES

- Special diagnostic tests may be performed, such as electronystagmography, caloric test, doll's eye test.
- Computed tomography (CT scan) or magnetic resonance imaging (MRI) has been used to assist in diagnosis.

 ## Treatment

GENERAL MEASURES

- Labyrinthitis is managed in the outpatient setting.
- When possible, treatment is directed at the underlying disorder causing labyrinthitis.
- Treatment of symptoms accompanies specific treatment.

ACTIVITY

Lie still with eyes closed in darkened room during acute attacks. Otherwise, activity as tolerated.

DIET

Reduced-sodium diet

Medications

COMMONLY PRESCRIBED DRUGS

- Promethazine (Phenergan)
- Diazepam
- Prochlorperazine suppositories
- Meclizine
- Scopolamine, transdermal

CONTRAINDICATIONS

Read drug product information.

PRECAUTIONS

All the listed medications have significant adverse reactions. Use with caution. Avoid scopolamine in the elderly. Read drug product information.

SIGNIFICANT POSSIBLE INTERACTIONS

Read drug product information

OTHER DRUGS

N/A

 ## Followup

PATIENT MONITORING

The doctor should be seen as often as needed

PREVENTION

No preventive measures

COMPLICATIONS

Permanent hearing loss

WHAT TO EXPECT

The outcome depends on cause. Labyrinthitis often clears completely.

 ## Miscellaneous

OTHER FACTORS

PEDIATRIC

Labyrinthitis is unusual in children.

GERIATRIC

- Labyrinthitis is common in the elderly.
- Avoid scopolamine or use with extreme caution in this age group.

OTHERS

N/A

PREGNANCY

Avoid medications.

FURTHER INFORMATION

N/A

Insect Bites and Stings

 Basics

DESCRIPTION

Insects may bite or sting and inject poison,
invade tissue, or transmit disease. This
discussion is limited to the irritative, poisonous,
and allergic effects of insects.
- Harmful insects of the United States include:
  - ▶ Bees: Bumblebees, sweat bees, honeybees
  - ▶ Wasps: Hornets, wasps
  - ▶ Ants: Fire ants, harvester ants
  - ▶ Brown recluse spider
  - ▶ Black widow spider
  - ▶ Hobo spiders
  - ▶ Scorpions
  - ▶ Mosquitoes
  - ▶ Flies: Deer, horse, black, stable, and biting
    midges
  - ▶ Lice: Body, head, pubic
  - ▶ Bugs: Kissing, bed, wheel
  - ▶ Fleas: Human, cat, dog
  - ▶ Mites: Itch mite (scabies), red bugs
    (chiggers)
  - ▶ Ticks
  - ▶ Caterpillars: Puss, browntail, buck
  - ▶ Centipedes
- Typical reactions include:
  - ▶ Local tissue irritation, inflammation, and
    destruction
  - ▶ Systemic (whole body) effects related to
    bite or sting toxin
  - ▶ Allergic reactions: immediate or delayed

SIGNS AND SYMPTOMS

- Local reactions:
  - ▶ Redness at site of bite or sting
  - ▶ Pain
  - ▶ Heat
  - ▶ Swelling
  - ▶ Itching
  - ▶ Blisters
  - ▶ Formation of ulcers
  - ▶ Weeping from site of bite or sting
- Toxic reactions:
  - ▶ Nausea
  - ▶ Vomiting
  - ▶ Headache
  - ▶ Fever
  - ▶ Diarrhea
  - ▶ Lightheadedness, fainting
  - ▶ Drowsiness
  - ▶ Muscle spasms
  - ▶ Swelling
  - ▶ Convulsions
- Systemic reactions: Allergic
  - ▶ Itching eyes
  - ▶ Facial flushing
  - ▶ Hives
  - ▶ Dry cough
  - ▶ Chest/throat constriction
  - ▶ Difficulty breathing
  - ▶ Noisy breathing
  - ▶ Bluish discoloration around eyes, mouth,
    and nail beds (cyanosis)
  - ▶ Abdominal cramps
  - ▶ Nausea, vomiting
  - ▶ Vertigo
  - ▶ Chills/fever
  - ▶ Shock
  - ▶ Loss of consciousness
  - ▶ Involuntary bowel/bladder action
  - ▶ Frothy saliva
  - ▶ Respiratory failure
  - ▶ Cardiovascular collapse
  - ▶ Death
- Delayed reaction:
  - ▶ Serum-sickness-like reactions
  - ▶ Fever
  - ▶ Malaise
  - ▶ Headache
  - ▶ Rash
  - ▶ Swollen hands
  - ▶ Aching of joints
- Unusual reactions:
  - ▶ Brain damage
  - ▶ Inflammation of nerves or blood vessels
  - ▶ Kidney failure
  - ▶ Extreme fear/anxiety

CAUSES

- Local tissue inflammation and destruction from poison
- Allergic reaction from previous sensitization
- Toxic reaction from large dose of poison

SCOPE

Insect bites and stings are widespread throughout the United States, with seasonal and regional variations.

MOST OFTEN AFFECTED

All age groups are affected, males and females in equal proportions

RISK FACTORS

- Living environment
- Climate
- Season
- Clothing
- Lack of protective measures
- Perfumes, colognes
- Previous sensitization to insect toxin
- Increased risk in young and elderly individuals

Diagnosis

WHAT THE DOCTOR LOOKS FOR

- Local reaction: Punctures, foreign bodies, infection, inflammation, lesions, or eruptions of the skin
- Toxic reaction: Chemical exposure, drug abuse, plants
- Allergic reaction: Medications, illicit drugs, foods, topical products, environmental, plants, chemicals

TESTS AND PROCEDURES

- Any number of blood tests may be ordered by the doctor
- The insect causing sting or bite may be identified if available

Insect Bites and Stings

 Treatment

GENERAL MEASURES

- The insect bite or sting victim may be treated as an outpatient or inpatient, depending on individual response to injury.
- Victims are hospitalized for severe reactions that threaten breathing or for shock, bronchospasm, severe swelling, or pain.
- First aid measures: Activate emergency medical services in severe reactions.
- If the amount of venom or toxin is large (e.g., a swarm of bees) or victim has a history of allergic reaction, seek emergency care immediately.
- If victim carries epinephrine (a drug used to manage severe allergic reactions to insect bites or stings), use it.
- If available, over-the-counter antihistamines can also help alleviate allergic reactions.
- Local effects (depending on severity)
  - ▶ Remove stinger (scrape it out with a credit card or other flat, thin object—don't squeeze with tweezer).
  - ▶ Cleanse wound.
  - ▶ Apply cold packs to bite or sting site (alternate 10 minutes on/10 minutes off).
  - ▶ Elevate and rest affected part.
- Systemic effects (depending on severity and type of reaction)
  - ▶ Oxygen, if needed for respiratory distress
  - ▶ Rescue breathing may be needed.
  - ▶ Victim may be hospitalized and observed for 24–48 hours.
- Surgical repair may be required for severe spider-bite lesions.

ACTIVITY

Rest to limit spread of poison.

DIET

No special diet; nothing by mouth if severe systemic reaction

 Medications

COMMONLY PRESCRIBED DRUGS

- Local effects (depending on severity)
  - ▶ Analgesics: acetaminophen, ibuprofen
  - ▶ Antihistamines: diphenhydramine (Benadryl) 25–50 mg four times a day
  - ▶ Steroids, topical or oral: prednisone 20–40 mg/day
  - ▶ Antibiotics
- Systemic effects (depending on severity and type of reaction)
  - ▶ Diphenhydramine for rash, wheezing, swelling
  - ▶ Aminophylline if needed for bronchospasm
  - ▶ Intravenous (IV) fluids if needed for shock
  - ▶ Hydrocortisone if needed for severe hives or spider bite
  - ▶ Tetanus prophylaxis and antibiotics if indicated
  - ▶ Diazepam (Valium)
  - ▶ Morphine or meperidine (Demerol) if needed for pain
- Anti-venoms (e.g., Black Widow spider, scorpion) may be used in certain cases based on availability and identification of organism.

CONTRAINDICATIONS

Read drug product information.

PRECAUTIONS

Treatment should not be delayed if the reaction is severe.

DRUG INTERACTIONS

Read drug product information.

OTHER DRUGS

Other antihistamines, such as loratadine and fexofenadine

Followup

PATIENT MONITORING

See primary care provider after caring for a significant wound.

PREVENTION

- Known hypersensitive persons should avoid re-exposure.
- Future exposures could cause a more severe allergic response.
- An epinephrine injection may be prescribed for emergency use.
- Individuals with known sensitivity should wear medical identification (bracelet, tag) or carry a card.
- Persons who experience severe allergic reactions may consider desensitization with immunotherapy.

COMPLICATIONS

- Infection
  - ▶ Bacterial
  - ▶ Diseases associated with tick, fly, and mosquito bites: Lyme disease, rickettsial disease (Rocky Mountain spotted fever), arborviral encephalitis, malaria, leishmaniasis, trypanosomiasis
- Scarring
- Drug reactions
- Multisystem failure
- Death

WHAT TO EXPECT

- Minor reactions: excellent recovery
- Severe reactions: excellent recovery with prompt appropriate treatment

 Miscellaneous

OTHER FACTORS

N/A

PEDIATRIC

More at risk

GERIATRIC

More at risk

OTHERS

N/A

PREGNANCY

Not a contraindication to treatment

FURTHER INFORMATION

N/A

Insomnia

 Basics

DESCRIPTION

Insomnia is difficulty falling asleep or maintaining sleep, intermittent wakefulness, early morning awakening, or a combination. May be:

- Transient, due to a life crisis, medical illness, grief or change in environment
- Chronic, associated with medical and psychiatric conditions or drug use

SIGNS AND SYMPTOMS

- Perceived reduction in sleeping time
- Initial insomnia: difficulty falling asleep at the usual time
- Middle insomnia: wakefulness during the usual sleep cycle, "tossing and turning"
- Terminal insomnia: early awakening
- Daytime fatigue, sleepiness, and napping
- Anxiety in anticipation of sleep

CAUSES

- Medical illnesses: arthritis, gastroesophageal reflux disease, duodenal ulcer, Alzheimer's disease, restless leg syndrome, sleep apnea, lung disease, painful conditions (e.g., muscle cramps)
- Psychiatric illnesses: depression, anxiety, schizophrenia, manic disorders
- Drug-induced insomnia: alcohol, caffeine, nicotine
- Nonprescription drugs: diet aids, decongestants, cough preparations
- Prescribed drugs: steroids, theophylline, phenytoin (Dilantin), levodopa (Sinemet, Dopar)
- Jet lag (transient)
- Heavy smoking

SCOPE

Insomnia affects an estimated 30% of the adult population. It is one of the most common complaints in primary care practice.

WHO MOST AFFECTED

Insomnia can affect all age groups but is more common in the elderly. Males and females are affected equally.

RISK FACTORS

- Chronic illnesses
- Age over 50
- Multiple drug use
- Obesity

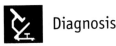 ## Diagnosis

WHAT THE DOCTOR LOOKS FOR

- The doctor will evaluate for known causes of insomnia.
- Some patients may have obstructive sleep apnea (snoring) that requires treatment.
- Patient may be evaluated for drug or alcohol dependence.
- Patient may be evaluated for depression or anxiety.

TESTS AND PROCEDURES

A sleep study (polysomnography) may be done to evaluate the patient.

 ## Treatment

GENERAL MEASURES

- Insomnia is usually managed in the outpatient setting.
- Sleep study may involve an overnight stay in a hospital.
- Transient insomnia
  - ▶ Lasts less than 3–4 weeks
  - ▶ Reassurance and supportive counseling may be helpful.
- Chronic insomnia
  - ▶ The underlying cause should be identified and addressed: pain, drugs, depression
  - ▶ Avoid alcohol after 5 PM or within 6 hours of retiring because it has a stimulant effect.
  - ▶ Person with insomnia should avoid daytime napping and should develop bedtime rituals conducive to sleep.
  - ▶ A thorough review of habits, drug intake, diet, and exercise pattern may reveal correctable causes of insomnia.
  - ▶ Drugs should be prescribed only if the above strategies fail.

ACTIVITY

- No restriction on physical activity
- A daily exercise routine is helpful. Avoid exercise close to bedtime.

DIET

- Avoid caffeine
- Avoid heavy, late-night snacks
- Sometimes a light snack before bedtime may help.
- Avoid alcohol after 5 PM or within 6 hours of retiring. In some people, alcohol acts as a stimulant.

Insomnia

 Medications

COMMONLY PRESCRIBED DRUGS

- Analgesics as indicated for pain
- Benzodiazepines for insomnia: flurazepam (Dalmane), temazepam (Restoril), triazolam (Halcion)
- Tricyclic antidepressants: amitriptyline (Elavil)
- Non-benzodiazepine agent: zolpidem (Ambien)

CONTRAINDICATIONS

- Pregnancy and lactation
- Severe mental illness
- Acute narrow-angle glaucoma
- Significant liver disease
- Depressed patient who may be suicidal

PRECAUTIONS

- Benzodiazepines may cause agitated states in some people.
- Flurazepam may impair coordination and judgement.
- Triazolam has been associated with antero-grade amnesia.
- Withdrawal psychosis and seizures may occur in some patients after abrupt cessation of insomnia drugs.
- Sedatives may cause "rebound insomnia."
- Sedatives may cause physical or psychological dependence.
- Amitriptyline can cause constipation and dizziness upon standing.
- Zolpidem should be used with the same pre-cautions as other sedative drugs. Most common reported side effects are drowsiness, dizziness, headache, and nausea.

DRUG INTERACTIONS

- Alcohol may magnify the sedative effects of the benzodiazepines.
- Blood levels of digoxin may be increased.
- Effect of levodopa may be reduced.

OTHER DRUGS

- Diphenhydramine (Benadryl) has been used to induce sleep in the elderly, but it may also cause confusion and "hangover."
- Chloral hydrate (Noctec) is favored by some physicians since it does not cause tolerance or withdrawal.
- Melatonin, a pineal hormone, is marketed as a dietary supplement. It is increasingly being used as a self-medication for insomnia. Not FDA approved. Appears useful for jet lag. Has mild hypnotic effect. No adverse effects have been reported, but controlled studies are lacking.
- L-Tryptophan, formerly widely used, is no longer available as a single ingredient in the United States.

Insomnia

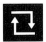 Followup

- Followup is based on the needs of the individual patient.
- The need for benzodiazepines should be reassessed periodically.
- A referral to psychosocial counseling may be made, if appropriate.

PREVENTION

Avoid all known causes of insomnia (e.g., caffeine, smoking), when possible.

COMPLICATIONS

- Transient insomnia may become chronic.
- Increased daytime sleepiness

WHAT TO EXPECT

Insomnia should resolve with time. The treatment of underlying symptoms is helpful.

 Miscellaneous

OTHER FACTORS

N/A

PEDIATRIC

N/A

GERIATRIC

- Benzodiazepines or other sedative-hypnotics should be prescribed with caution to elderly persons.
- Sleep habits normally change with age.

OTHERS

N/A

PREGNANCY

Transient insomnia may occur during pregnancy due to the discomfort of sleeping positions.

FURTHER INFORMATION

N/A

Iron Deficiency Anemia

 ## Basics

DESCRIPTION

Iron deficiency anemia is anemia due to decreased stores of iron in the body. Other forms of anemia are related to the poor absorption or utilization of iron. The onset of iron deficiency anemia may be acute with rapid blood loss, or chronic with poor diet or slow blood loss. Iron deficiency is the most common cause of anemia in the United States.

SIGNS AND SYMPTOMS

- Initially, no symptoms
- Dry, peeling lips
- Shortness of breath
- Fatigue, listlessness
- Rapid heart rate, palpitations
- Headache
- Irritability, inability to concentrate
- Pain or tingling sensation in extremities
- Pallor
- Susceptibility to infection

CAUSES

- Blood loss (e.g., menstruation, gastrointestinal bleeding)
- Poor iron intake
- Poor iron absorption
- Increased demand for iron (e.g., infancy, adolescence, pregnancy)
- Hookworms
- Stomach cancer

SCOPE

About 10–30% of the adult population have iron deficiency anemia.

MOST OFTEN AFFECTED

Iron deficiency anemia affects all ages. It is more common in females than males.

RISK FACTORS

See Causes

 ## Diagnosis

WHAT THE DOCTOR LOOKS FOR

- The doctor will rule out anemia due to poor iron metabolism or other causes.
- The doctor will evaluate for the presence of stomach cancer, especially in the elderly.
- Potential sources of bleeding will be investigated and ruled out.

TESTS AND PROCEDURES

- Blood tests to measure cells, hemoglobin, and iron compounds
- Bone marrow may be sampled for analysis to assist in diagnosis.
- Special tests may be done to identify other causes of iron loss, such as stool guaiac testing, endoscopy, and blood-clotting studies.
- Endoscopy (insertion of a tube with a small camera at its end into the esophagus) of the gastrointestinal tract may be done to identify hidden sources of bleeding.

 ## Treatment

GENERAL MEASURES

- Iron deficiency anemia is usually treated on an outpatient basis.
- The doctor should search for a cause of bleeding and treat it.

ACTIVITY

Patients with heart disease may reduce their physical activity

DIET

- Adults should limit milk to 1 pint a day.
- Consume adequate protein- and iron-containing foods, such as meat, beans, and leafy green vegetables.
- Increase dietary fiber to decrease likelihood of constipation during iron replacement therapy.
- Do not ingest milk, other dairy products, antacids, or tetracycline within 2 hours of iron dosage.

Medications

COMMONLY PRESCRIBED DRUGS

Ferrous sulfate (iron). Dose may be reduced to ease gastrointestinal effects, which affect 15% of patients on standard iron therapy.

CONTRAINDICATIONS

Do not take iron while also taking antacids or tetracycline.

PRECAUTIONS

- Iron preparations cause black bowel movements.
- Iron overdose is highly toxic. Tablets should be kept out of the reach of small children.

DRUG INTERACTIONS

- Allopurinol
- Antacids
- Penicillamine
- Tetracyclines
- Vitamin E

OTHER DRUGS

N/A

Followup

PATIENT MONITORING

The doctor should be seen regularly after blood tests return to normal, in order to detect any return of anemia.

PREVENTION

- Good nutrition with adequate iron intake
- Gynecologic or other problems causing excess blood loss should be treated.

COMPLICATIONS

Hidden sources of bleeding, such as a malignancy, may not be identified.

WHAT TO EXPECT

Iron deficiency anemia is curable with iron therapy if the underlying cause can be identified and treated.

Miscellaneous

OTHER FACTORS

N/A

PEDIATRIC

Frequent problem in infants whose major source of nutrition is cow's milk

GERIATRIC

Accounts for 60% of anemias in people over 65 years of age

OTHERS

N/A

PREGNANCY

Common during pregnancy unless iron supplements are included in the diet

FURTHER INFORMATION

National Heart, Lung & Blood Institute, Communications & Public Information Branch, National Institutes of Health, Building 31, Room 41-21, 9000 Rockville Pike, Bethesda, MD 20892, (301)251-1222

Irritable Bowel Syndrome

 Basics

DESCRIPTION

Irritable bowel syndrome, also called spastic or irritable colon, is a set of signs and symptoms of altered bowel habits, abdominal pain, and gaseousness in the absence of other disease.

SIGNS AND SYMPTOMS

- Most patients have all signs and symptoms, but not with every episode.
- Abdominal pain, usually lower quadrant, relieved by defecation
- Mucus in stools
- Constipation
- Diarrhea
- Distention
- Upper abdominal discomfort after eating
- Straining for normal consistency stools
- Urgency of defecation
- Feelings of incomplete evacuation
- Hard, round stool
- Nausea, vomiting (rarely)

CAUSES

The cause of irritable bowel syndrome is unknown.

SCOPE

- The incidence of irritable bowel syndrome in the United States is unknown, but it is second to upper respiratory infection as the cause for lost workdays.
- At least 15% of population (uncommon in children and early teens) is affected.

MOST OFTEN AFFECTED

- Irritable bowel syndrome is rare in the late teens and more commonly affects those in the late 20's.
- If a person is over age 40, symptoms are more likely to be due to another disease.
- Females are affected twice as often as males in the United States, while irritable bowel syndrome is more common in males than females in other parts of the world.

RISK FACTORS

- Other members of the family with the same or similar gastrointestinal disorder
- History of childhood sexual abuse
- Sexual or domestic abuse in women

 Diagnosis

WHAT THE DOCTOR LOOKS FOR

- Other causes of similar signs and symptoms, such as inflammatory bowel syndromes, lactose intolerance or infections.

TESTS AND PROCEDURES

- Laboratory tests may be ordered as needed to rule out other diseases and conditions.
- Imaging may be done of the gastrointestinal tract.
- Sigmoidoscopy may be done to visually inspect the large intestine.

 Treatment

GENERAL MEASURES

- Irritable bowel syndrome is managed on an outpatient basis.
- Heat to abdomen may help relieve discomfort.
- Biofeedback or other techniques may help reduce stress.
- Problem stimulants should be avoided.

ACTIVITY

As normal

DIET

- Increase fiber.
- Avoid large meals; spicy, fried, fatty foods; and milk products.

Irritable Bowel Syndrome

 Medications

COMMONLY PRESCRIBED DRUGS

- Bulk producing agents: psyllium-containing products (Metamucil)
- Constipating agents (if diarrhea is significant): loperamide (Imodium), diphenoxylate-atropine (Lomotil)
- Antispasmodics/anticholinergics: dicyclomine (Bentyl) or lactase (Lactaid)
- Anticholinergics/sedatives: chlordiazepoxide-clidinium (Librax), phenobarbital-hyoscyamine-atropine-hyoscine (Donnatal), amitriptyline HCL (Elavil)
- Antiflatulents: simethicone (Mylicon)
- For milk intolerance: lactase capsules or tablets

CONTRAINDICATIONS

Read drug product information.

PRECAUTIONS

Read drug product information.

DRUG INTERACTIONS

Read drug product information.

OTHER DRUGS

N/A

 Followup

PATIENT MONITORING

See the doctor as needed for symptoms.

PREVENTION

See Diet

COMPLICATIONS

N/A

WHAT TO EXPECT

- Irritable bowel syndrome does not progress to cancer or inflammatory disease.
- Acute episodes may recur throughout life, particularly when an individual is under stress. The frequency of episodes decreases with increasing age.

 Miscellaneous

OTHER FACTORS

N/A

PEDIATRIC

N/A

GERIATRIC

N/A

OTHERS

N/A

PREGNANCY

Some experts suggest that irritable bowel syndrome worsens during pregnancy. However, irritable bowel syndrome in the mother causes no increased risks to fetus or mother.

FURTHER INFORMATION

N/A

Section J

Jaundice

 Basics

DESCRIPTION

Jaundice is a term that describes the accumulation of bile pigment in the skin, mucous membranes, and eyes, resulting in a yellowish appearance.

CAUSES

- Jaundice is usually caused by blood disorders, heart or liver disease, viral infection, alcohol or drug use, stones in the bile ducts, or cancer of the pancreas or liver.
- A form of jaundice may be caused by pregnancy.
- Jaundice is common in newborns and usually resolves quickly with no longterm effects.

 Treatment

Because jaundice is a symptom rather than a disease in itself, treatment is directed at the underlying cause.

FURTHER INFORMATION

N/A

Jet Lag

 Basics

DESCRIPTION

Jet lag, also called circadian dysrhythmia, is a syndrome resulting from travel between different time zones. North-south travel does not cause jet lag. A person experiences jet lag when his or her body is out of synch with the local time, e.g., the clock shows that it is lunchtime, but the body says it is the middle of the night. The severity of jet lag depends on the number of time zones crossed and the direction of travel. Most people find traveling eastward and adapting to a shorter day more difficult than traveling westward and adapting to a longer day.

SIGNS AND SYMPTOMS

Extreme fatigue, sleep disturbances, loss of concentration, malaise, disorientation, sluggishness, gastrointestinal upset, and loss of appetite.

CAUSES

Jet lag is a disturbance of the body's physiological processes that control sleep and wakefulness, as well as alertness, hunger, digestion, temperature, and hormones.

 Treatment

- There is no clear evidence that elaborate preventive self-remedies to avoid jet lag are effective.
- The doctor may prescribe a short-acting sedative (e.g., lorazepam) for sleep during travel.
- Travelers should plan their destination activities to accommodate local time differences.
- The hormone melatonin shows promise as a jet lag remedy.

FURTHER INFORMATION

N/A

Section K

Kaposi's Sarcoma

 ## Basics

DESCRIPTION

Kaposi's sarcoma (KS) is a form of skin cancer characterized by vascular tumors of skin and viscera. There are several different forms of KS, including a classic indolent (slow-growing) type and a form associated with acquired immune deficiency syndrome (AIDS) and other immune system disorders.

SIGNS AND SYMPTOMS

- Multiple purplish tumors on the skin
- Lesions may be tender or itchy.
- Skin tumors may appear on the face, arms, legs or trunk.
- Lesions may also be in the mouth or other mucous membranes or on internal organs or lymph nodes.

CAUSES

It is believed that transmission of an as-yet unidentified agent leads to the formation of KS. A herpes-related virus may be the cause of KS.

SCOPE

The indolent form of KS is rare in the United States. Among persons with AIDS or immune deficiency, KS is common.

MOST OFTEN AFFECTED

KS affects individuals between 16 and 75 years of age. It tends to occur more often in males than females.

RISK FACTORS

- Infection with the human immunodeficiency virus (HIV)
- Treatment with immunosuppressant medications
- Transplantation and chemotherapy

 ## Diagnosis

WHAT THE DOCTOR LOOKS FOR

Other possible causes of similar lesions of the skin, such as abnormal blood vessel growth

TESTS

- A computed tomography (CT) scan of the chest and abdomen may be done to assess internal organs.
- A biopsy of a sarcoma or lymph node may be obtained to assist in diagnosis.
- Lesions may be examined by bronchoscopy if the airway is affected.

 ## Treatment

GENERAL MEASURES

- KS is usually managed on an outpatient basis.
- If KS is caused by immunosuppressant medications, dosages may be modified.
- If KS is related to HIV, drug therapy may be initiated.
- Treatment is otherwise determined by the extent of the disease.
- Lesions may be surgically removed, typically as an outpatient.
- Other treatments include radiation therapy, chemotherapy, immunotherapy, and anti-viral therapy.
- The person with KS should be observed for a return of lesions or other change in condition.

ACTIVITY

Remain active as long as possible

DIET

No special diet

Medications

COMMONLY PRESCRIBED DRUGS

- Chemotherapy agents: doxorubicin, bleomycin, vinblastine, vincristine
- Anti-viral: interferon

CONTRAINDICATIONS

Refer to manufacturer's literature.

PRECAUTIONS

Refer to manufacturer's literature. Chemotherapy may suppress the function of bone marrow.

POSSIBLE DRUG INTERACTIONS

Refer to manufacturer's literature.

OTHER DRUGS

Uncontrolled studies indicate that some individuals respond to anti-herpes medications.

 Followup

PATIENT MONITORING

Among those with HIV, other opportunistic infections must be aggressively treated.

PREVENTION

Safe sex practices reduce the risk of HIV transmission.

COMPLICATIONS

An aggressive form of KS affects at least 1/3 of those infected with HIV.

WHAT TO EXPECT

- Better treatments may result in improved HIV-related KS survival.
- Individuals with the indolent form of KS typically survive for 10 years after diagnosis.

 Miscellaneous

OTHER FACTORS

N/A

PEDIATRIC

N/A

GERIATRIC

Indolent form most often occurs among elderly men.

OTHERS

N/A

PREGNANCY

N/A

FURTHER INFORMATION

N/A

Kidney Stones

 Basics

DESCRIPTION

Kidney stones, also called urolithiasis or renal colic, are the formation of hard mineral deposits called calculi within the urinary system.

SIGNS AND SYMPTOMS

- Usually sudden onset
- Severe agonizing pain, which may be felt from the rib cage to the groin, depending on the location of stone
- Patient is unable to obtain relief from discomfort.
- Nausea with or without vomiting
- Sweating
- Rapid heartbeat
- Abdominal distension
- Tenderness to deep abdominal examination
- Frequent, urgent, or difficult urination
- Fever
- Blood or pus in the urine
- May be asymptomatic if stone stays within kidney

CAUSES

Kidney stones may be caused by a wide range of factors related to the body's water and mineral balance.

SCOPE

About 2–5% of the U.S. population can expect to have kidney stones, which affect 70–210 per 100,000 of the population in their lifetime.

MOST OFTEN AFFECTED

Kidney stones affect people ranging from 20–60 years of age. Incidence peaks at 20–30 years of age. Males are affected four times as often as females. The tendency to develop kidney stones tends to run in families.

RISK FACTORS

- Family history
- Hot climate
- Work in hot environment
- Inadequate fluid intake
- Diet high in minerals and vitamins
- Cancer
- Gout
- Use of diuretics (water pills)
- Bowel or kidney disease

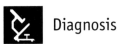 Diagnosis

WHAT THE DOCTOR LOOKS FOR

- Other medical disorders, such as kidney disease, diabetes, infection, intestinal conditions, or gynecological problems

TESTS AND PROCEDURES

- Urinalysis and culture
- Blood tests for electrolytes, chemistry, and hormones
- Stone may be analyzed to determine its chemical composition
- Urinary system may be assessed by x-rays or ultrasound
- A special procedure called intravenous pyelogram (IVP) may be performed to evaluate the urinary system.

 Treatment

GENERAL MEASURES

- Most stones pass within 24 hours.
- About 80% of individuals with kidney stones are managed as outpatients.
- About 20% require hospitalization and treatment by a specialist.
- The doctor should provide reassurance to the patient.
- Patient should be instructed to strain urine to recover stone for analysis.
- It is important to maintain adequate fluid intake.
- Doctor should make sure pain is controlled appropriately.
- The patient may be seen by a specialist for intractable pain, obstruction of the urinary tract, stones of large size, infection, or other complicated conditions.
- Surgical measures include:
  - ▶ Extracorporeal shock wave lithotripsy, which uses sound waves to shatter kidney stones
  - ▶ Urethroscopy, in which a stone is crushed and removed through an instrument inserted into the bladder
  - ▶ Minimally invasive techniques
  - ▶ Open surgery, which is performed on less than 5% of patients

Kidney Stones

ACTIVITY

Bed rest during acute phase if necessary. No restrictions after stone passes.

DIET

- Normal diet
- Drink 8 oz. water every 1 hour while awake, and, if possible, every 2 hours during sleep hours.
- If stones consist of uric acid, eat less protein and take sodium bicarbonate to alkalinize urine.

 Medications

COMMONLY PRESCRIBED DRUGS

- Acute therapy:
  - ▶ Pain control: meperidine (Demerol) or morphine or buprenorphine (Buprenex), etc.
  - ▶ 3-day supply pain control: oxycodone-acetaminophen (Percocet), pentazocine (Talwin), hydrocodone-acetaminophen (Vicodin), etc.
  - ▶ Uric acid stones: potassium citrate (Urocit-K)
  - ▶ Cystine stones: penicillamine (Cuprimine, Depen)
  - ▶ Infected stones: antibiotics
- Maintenance therapy:
  - ▶ Hypercalciuria: sodium cellulose phosphate, hydrochlorothiazide (HCTZ), K-citrate
  - ▶ Uric acid: allopurinol (Zyloprim), K-citrate
  - ▶ Cystine: K-citrate, penicillamine

CONTRAINDICATIONS

Penicillamine should not be given to those who are pregnant or have renal failure, aplastic anemia, or known allergic reactions.

PRECAUTIONS

Penicillamine requires regular blood tests and urinalysis.

DRUG INTERACTIONS

Read drug product information.

OTHER DRUGS

N/A

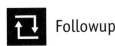 Followup

PATIENT MONITORING

- Strain urine until stone passes or 72 hours after symptoms cease.
- Repeat urinalysis every 2–3 days.
- Urinary system x-ray studies should be repeated if no stone is passed.
- Stone should be analyzed when passed.
- X-rays should be repeated at 3–6 months and at 1 year. If no new stone develops, no further followup is needed.
- Further urinalysis and blood tests may be required for recurring kidney stones.

PREVENTION

Maintain adequate water intake to produce more than 2 liters of urine a day, including one trip to the bathroom at night. Keep dietary calcium below 1 gram per day.

COMPLICATIONS

- Kidney damage
- Infection

WHAT TO EXPECT

- In about 80% of cases, stones pass within 48–72 hours with outpatient therapy.
- About 60% of persons have no recurrence of kidney stones at 10 years.

 Miscellaneous

OTHER FACTORS

N/A

PEDIATRIC

May be caused by inherited disorders

GERIATRIC

N/A

OTHERS

N/A

PREGNANCY

Pregnant women with kidney stones should be seen by a urology specialist.

Section L

Laryngitis

Basics

DESCRIPTION

Laryngitis is an inflammation of the lining of the larynx. It is most common during late fall, winter, and early spring. It can be acute (of short duration) or chronic (long-lasting).

SIGNS AND SYMPTOMS

- Hoarseness
- Abnormal sounding voice
- Inability to speak
- Throat tickling
- Feeling of rawness in throat
- Constant urge to clear the throat
- Fever
- Malaise
- Painful or difficult swallowing
- Throat pain
- Cough
- Enlarged lymph glands in neck

CAUSES

- Infections, viral or bacterial
- Excessive use of voice
- Inhaling irritating substances
- Aspiration of caustic chemical
- Aging
- Damage during surgery
- Esophageal reflux

SCOPE

Laryngitis is common.

PREDOMINANT AGE

Laryngitis affects all ages, males and females in equal numbers.

RISK FACTORS

- Upper respiratory tract infection
- Bronchitis
- Pneumonia
- Influenza (flu)
- Pertussis (whooping cough)
- Measles
- Allergy
- Chronic rhinitis
- Chronic sinusitis
- Voice abuse
- Reflux of gastric contents
- Smoking
- Alcohol abuse
- Constant exposure to dust or other irritants

Diagnosis

WHAT THE DOCTOR LOOKS FOR

- The doctor will evaluate the patient for the presence of laryngitis.
- Other conditions that can cause similar signs and symptoms include croup, measles, diphtheria, vocal cord nodules, and throat cancer.

TESTS AND PROCEDURES

- Blood tests
- A sample of fluid from the throat may be obtained for laboratory analysis.
- The throat may be examined by laryngoscopy.
- A sample of tissue may be obtained by biopsy to assist in diagnosis.

Treatment

GENERAL MEASURES

- Laryngitis is usually managed in the outpatient setting.
- Acute laryngitis
  - ▶ Usually a self-limited illness and not severe
  - ▶ Rest voice
  - ▶ Steam inhalations or cool-mist humidifier
  - ▶ Increase fluid intake
  - ▶ Pain relievers
  - ▶ Avoid smoking (or second-hand smoke) during acute phase
- Chronic
  - ▶ Symptomatic treatment as above
  - ▶ Voice therapy
  - ▶ Stop smoking
  - ▶ Reduce alcohol intake
  - ▶ Occupational change or modification, if needed
  - ▶ For reflux laryngitis: elevate head of bed, other antireflux management
- Surgery may be necessary.

ACTIVITY

Rest until fever subsides, then no restrictions.

DIET

No special diet

 ## Medications

- Usually none are required

COMMONLY PRESCRIBED DRUGS (IF NEEDED)

- Pain relievers
- Antifever drugs
- Cough suppressants
- Penicillin, erythromycin

CONTRAINDICATIONS

Read drug product information.

PRECAUTIONS

Read drug product information.

DRUG INTERACTIONS

Read drug product information.

OTHER DRUGS

N/A

 ## Followup

PATIENT MONITORING

No followup is usually needed.

PREVENTION

- Avoid overuse of voice.
- Prompt treatment of respiratory infections
- Flu vaccine for high-risk individuals

COMPLICATIONS

Chronic hoarseness

WHAT TO EXPECT

Complete clearing of the inflammation without long-term effects

 ## Miscellaneous

OTHER FACTORS

N/A

PEDIATRIC

Laryngitis is common in children.

GERIATRIC

The elderly may have more severe symptoms and may be slower to heal.

OTHERS

N/A

PREGNANCY

Use antibiotics with caution.

FURTHER INFORMATION

N/A

Lazy Eye

 ## Basics

DESCRIPTION

Amblyopia, also called "lazy eye," is a reduction in visual acuity in one eye that cannot be corrected by eyeglasses or contact lenses, in the absence of other disease.

SIGNS AND SYMPTOMS

Decreased visual acuity in one eye

CAUSES

Multiple causes

SCOPE

Amblyopia affects about 2.5% of the U.S. population.

MOST OFTEN AFFECTED

Amblyopia may be present from birth or may be detected at any age. Males and females are affected in equal proportions. There is an increased incidence in children with one parent who has a history of amblyopia.

RISK FACTORS

None known

 ## Diagnosis

WHAT THE DOCTOR LOOKS FOR

- A thorough eye examination should be performed.
- Other causes of visual acuity loss in one eye should be considered.

TESTS AND PROCEDURES

Examination by an ophthalmologist may include slit lamp and fundoscopic examination of eye structures.

 ## Treatment

GENERAL MEASURES

- All children should have complete visual examinations prior to starting school.
- Children from families with a history of amblyopia or strabismus should have special examinations by an ophthalmologist.
- Correction of the underlying disorder should be instituted at the earliest opportunity.
- Glasses and/or patching of the stronger eye to encourage visual development may be helpful.
- Amblyopia never corrects itself spontaneously and always requires treatment.
- Children do not outgrow amblyopia.
- Surgical correction of an abnormal eye position may be required.

ACTIVITY

No restrictions

DIET

No special diet

Medications

COMMONLY PRESCRIBED DRUGS

N/A

CONTRAINDICATIONS

N/A

PRECAUTIONS

N/A

DRUG INTERACTIONS

N/A

OTHER DRUGS

N/A

 Followup

PATIENT MONITORING

The doctor should be seen as often as needed until the problem is resolved.

PREVENTION

None

COMPLICATIONS

Permanent and profound visual loss can develop if proper therapy is not begun early.

WHAT TO EXPECT

- In most cases, amblyopia is a treatable condition if the diagnosis is made early.
- Patching therapy, eyeglasses, and surgical correction of abnormal eye positions can result in nearly normal vision when performed early.
- Visual development occurs during the first several years of life; amblyopia therapy can be effective until approximately age 12.

 Miscellaneous

OTHER FACTORS

N/A

PEDIATRIC

Commonly seen in young children

GERIATRIC

When seen among the elderly population, the diagnosis has usually been made early in childhood.

OTHERS

N/A

PREGNANCY

N/A

FURTHER INFORMATION

N/A

Lead Poisoning

Basics

DESCRIPTION

Lead poisoning is a toxic condition that results from exposure to lead, an element with no known function in the human body.

SIGNS AND SYMPTOMS

- Often no symptoms
- Mild to moderate toxicity:
  - ▶ May cause muscle or joint pain, loss of sensation, fatigue, irritability, lethargy, abdominal discomfort, difficulty concentrating, headache, tremor, vomiting, weight loss
- Severe toxicity:
  - ▶ Causes loss of appetite, metallic taste in mouth, constipation, severe abdominal cramps
  - ▶ Neuromuscular type: peripheral neuritis
  - ▶ Seizures; coma; and long-term effects including brain damage, retarded mental development, hyperactivity
  - ▶ Chronic exposure to lead may cause renal failure.

CAUSES

Inhalation of lead dust or fumes or ingestion of lead

SCOPE

17% of preschoolers in the United States have lead poisoning. Sporadic cases have been reported in adults.

MOST OFTEN AFFECTED

- Children 1–5 years old; adult workers in industries that use lead
- Males and females are affected in equal numbers.

RISK FACTORS

- Children who eat nonfood items (e.g., dirt)
- Children with iron deficiency anemia
- Residence or frequent visitor in deteriorating, pre-1960 housing with lead-paint surfaces
- Children with seizures
- Children with hyperkinetic or autistic behavior
- Sibling or playmate with lead poisoning

- Dust from clothing of lead worker
- Lead dissolved in water from lead or lead-soldered plumbing
- Lead-glazed ceramics, especially with acidic food or drink
- Food stored in inverted plastic bread bags printed with colored ink
- Colored comics
- Soil near lead industries and roads
- Folk remedies
- Hobbies
- Occupational exposure
- Dietary: zinc or calcium deficiency

Diagnosis

WHAT THE DOCTOR LOOKS FOR

The doctor will perform a physical examination to identify the signs and symptoms of lead poisoning.

TESTS AND PROCEDURES

- Blood tests
- X-ray of the abdomen or long bones

Treatment

GENERAL MEASURES

- Lead poisoning is often managed in the outpatient setting.
- Hospitalization may be required for chelation therapy.
- Local health department may be notified.

ACTIVITY

Avoid activity at any site of potential lead contamination.

DIET

- If symptomatic, avoid excessive fluids.
- Consume adequate calcium and iron.
- Eat a low-fat diet to reduce absorption and retention of lead.

Lead Poisoning

 Medications

COMMONLY PRESCRIBED DRUGS

- Oral chelation: succimer (Chemet, dimercapto-succinic acid, DMSA)
- Intravenous (IV) chelation: dimercaprol (British anti-Lewisite, BAL), Ca EDTA (edetate calcium disodium)
- Diazepam (Valium)

CONTRAINDICATIONS

BAL should not be given to persons allergic to peanuts (the drug solution contains peanut oil).

PRECAUTIONS

Chelation drugs have many precautions; read drug product information.

DRUG INTERACTIONS

Vitamins should not be given concurrently with oral chelation.

OTHER DRUGS

- Penicillamine (d-penicillamine, Depen, Cuprimine)

 Followup

PATIENT MONITORING

- The doctor should be seen after 7–10 days and then 1–2 times per month.
- Testing should be periodically repeated; e.g., every 3 months.

PREVENTION

- Identify potential sources of lead and decrease lead exposure. Wet mopping and dusting with a high-phosphate solution (e.g., powdered automatic dishwasher detergent, 1/4 cup per gallon of water) will help control lead-bearing dust.
- If the source is in the home (e.g., lead paint), the patient must reside elsewhere until lead removal is completed.

COMPLICATIONS

- Toxicity may be long-lasting or permanent.
- Long-term lead exposure may cause chronic renal failure and gout.

WHAT TO EXPECT

- Symptomatic lead poisoning without brain damage generally improves with chelation, but subtle effects may be long-lasting or permanent.
- If brain damage occurs, permanent effects (mental retardation, seizure disorder, blindness, paralysis) are seen in 25 to 50% of patients.

 Miscellaneous

OTHER FACTORS

N/A

PEDIATRIC

- Increasing evidence exists that low-lead level exposure may be toxic to children.
- Children are at increased risk because of incomplete development of the brain.
- Common childhood behaviors such as frequent hand-to-mouth activity and pica (ingestion of nonfood products) greatly increase the risk of ingesting lead.

GERIATRIC

N/A

OTHERS

N/A

PREGNANCY

- Lead exposure in pregnancy is associated with reduced birth weight and premature birth.
- Lead causes birth defects in animals.

FURTHER INFORMATION

- The Inside Story: A Guide to Indoor Air Quality, EPA/400/1-88/004. EPA and Consumer Product Safety Commission, 1988. Lead and Your Drinking Water. EPA, 1988, OPA-87-006
- Because there is too much lead in your child's body . . . , Bock Pharmacal Co., (800) 727-2625

Leukemia, Acute Lymphoblastic In Adults (ALL)

 Basics

DESCRIPTION

Acute lymphoblastic leukemia (ALL) is a cancerous proliferation and accumulation of immature white blood cells.

SIGNS AND SYMPTOMS

- Anemia: fatigue, shortness of breath, light-headedness, chest pain, headache
- Insufficient platelets: pinpoint red spots, bruising, nosebleed, retinal bleeding
- Insufficient white blood cells: fever, infection
- Lymphatic disorder: enlarged glands, enlarged spleen and/or liver, bone pain
- Immune system suppression
- Metabolic disturbances: kidney failure
- Central nervous system: confusion, nerve disorder

CAUSES

Unknown. Epstein-Barr virus is suspected.

SCOPE

About 1,000 adult cases of ALL occur annually in the United States.

MOST OFTEN AFFECTED

The average age of patients is 35–40 years, but incidence increases with age. Males are affected slightly more frequently than females.

RISK FACTORS

- Age over 60
- Exposure to agents such as benzene or radiation
- May follow aplastic anemia

 Diagnosis

WHAT THE DOCTOR LOOKS FOR

- The doctor will perform a physical examination to identify the presence of ALL.
- Other diseases may cause similar signs and symptoms, including other forms of leukemia or other cancers, immune system disorders, and noncancerous conditions.

TESTS AND PROCEDURES

- Blood tests
- A sample of bone marrow may be obtained for laboratory analysis.
- Special genetic testing may be done.
- Chest x-ray, ultrasound
- A sample of lymph node tissue may be obtained by biopsy for laboratory analysis.
- A sample of spinal fluid may be obtained by lumbar puncture (spinal tap).

 Treatment

GENERAL MEASURES

- Treatment of ALL requires hospitalization for chemotherapy.
- Management after therapy is given on an out-patient basis.
- Access to the resources and expertise of a major oncology center is important for appropriate support.
- The person with ALL must be isolated from infection.
- Surgery may be required.
- Bone marrow transplantation may be required.

ACTIVITY

Physical activity as tolerated

DIET

- Nutritional support
- Avoid alcohol

Leukemia, Acute Lymphoblastic In Adults (ALL)

 Medications

COMMONLY PRESCRIBED DRUGS

- Optimal therapy is not yet known. Although all treatment regimens are still experimental, they are clearly effective for some patients.
- Drugs include cyclophosphamide, daunorubicin, vincristine, asparaginase (L-asparaginase), prednisone, methotrexate, hydrocortisone, mercaptopurine (6-mercaptopurine), cytarabine, doxorubicin, dexamethasone, thioguanine (6-thioguanine), and cytarabine.

CONTRAINDICATIONS

N/A

PRECAUTIONS

N/A

SIGNIFICANT POSSIBLE INTERACTIONS

N/A

OTHER DRUGS

Other experimental drugs

 Followup

PATIENT MONITORING

The doctor should be seen daily or weekly during chemotherapy, monthly during maintenance therapy, and every 3 months thereafter.

PREVENTION

N/A

COMPLICATIONS

- Infections
- Bleeding
- Need for transfusions
- Sterility from treatment
- Severe drug side effects
- Relapse of leukemia

WHAT TO EXPECT

- 80–90% of patients younger than 60 years old will achieve a complete remission, and 35–60% will remain free of disease at 5 years.
- Some patients may receive bone marrow transplantation.

 Miscellaneous

OTHER FACTORS

N/A

PEDIATRIC

Bone growth and mental development may be affected by treatment.

GERIATRIC

N/A

OTHERS

N/A

PREGNANCY

Many chemotherapy drugs cause birth defects.

FURTHER INFORMATION

N/A

Light Sensitivity

 ## Basics

DESCRIPTION

Light sensitivity, also called sun poisoning, is a skin rash induced by exposure to sunlight. It is often a side effect of medication.

SIGNS AND SYMPTOMS

- Reddening
- Rash
- Blisters
- Usually develops shortly after sun exposure.
- Pain
- Itching

CAUSES

- Sunlight
- Phenothiazines
- Diuretics
- Tetracyclines
- Sulfonamides
- Oral contraceptives
- Topicals: psoralens, coal tars, photoactive dyes (eosin, acridine orange)

SCOPE

Unknown

MOST OFTEN AFFECTED

All ages; males and females affected equally

RISK FACTORS

Propensity to light sensivity may be inherited in some inbred populations (e.g., Pima Indians).

 ## Diagnosis

WHAT THE DOCTOR LOOKS FOR

The doctor will perform a physical examination to identify light sensitivity.

TESTS AND PROCEDURES

- Blood tests
- A sample of skin may be obtained by biopsy for laboratory analysis.
- Allergy testing may be done.

 ## Treatment

GENERAL MEASURES

- Avoid or limit exposure to sunlight.
- Use protective clothing and sunscreens.
- Cold packs/cold water compresses.

ACTIVITY

Avoid sunlight.

DIET

No special diet

Medications

COMMONLY PRESCRIBED DRUGS

- Topical corticosteroids
- Nonsteroidal anti-inflammatory drugs (NSAIDs)
- Prednisone
- Antihistamines
- Sunscreens

CONTRAINDICATIONS

Read drug product information.

PRECAUTIONS

Read drug product information.

DRUG INTERACTIONS

Read drug product information.

OTHER DRUGS

N/A

 Followup

PATIENT MONITORING

The doctor should be seen as often as necessary for persistent light allergy or recurrence of the condition.

PREVENTION

- Sunlight avoidance
- Wear protective clothing.
- Identification and avoidance of drugs that cause light sensitivity
- Sunscreens: apply before exposure to sunlight

COMPLICATIONS

N/A

WHAT TO EXPECT

Good outcome with avoidance and proper protection measures.

 Miscellaneous

OTHER FACTORS

N/A

PEDIATRIC

N/A

GERIATRIC

More likely to experience light sensitivity caused by drugs

OTHERS

N/A

PREGNANCY

N/A

FURTHER INFORMATION

N/A

Low Back Pain

 ## Basics

DESCRIPTION

Low back pain is generally a self-limited condition of the aging spine that responds to conservative measures, including rest and pain management. Pain is typically at the belt line, occasional involving the buttocks and/or posterior thighs. Low back pain is often the result of the stresses and demands placed on the low back area by everyday activities. In the vast majority of cases, the condition is of short duration and recovery is complete.

SIGNS AND SYMPTOMS

- Onset of low back pain begins suddenly after an injury or gradually over the next 24 hours.
- Variable pain at posterior belt-line, typically on both sides
- Pain may radiate to buttocks and/or posterior thighs
- Pain is aggravated by back motion, sitting, standing, lifting, bending, and twisting.
- Pain relieved by rest

CAUSES

- Normal aging process of musculoskeletal system
- Acute event (injury)

SCOPE

80% of Americans experience mechanical low back pain at some point in their life.

MOST OFTEN AFFECTED

Individuals 25–45 years of age, males and females in equal numbers

RISK FACTORS

- Age
- Activity
- Smoking
- Obesity
- Vibration, e.g., driving motor vehicles
- Sedentary lifestyle
- Psychosocial factors

 ## Diagnosis

WHAT THE DOCTOR LOOKS FOR

- The doctor will perform a thorough physical examination, in particular evaluating the function of the back.
- Numerous other medical conditions that may be responsible for the symptoms should be investigated and ruled out.

TESTS AND PROCEDURES

- Blood tests
- X-rays, bone scans may be done to assist in diagnosis.
- Magnetic resonance imaging (MRI) or computed tomography (CT scan) may be done.

 ## Treatment

GENERAL MEASURES

- Low back pain is managed in the outpatient setting.
- Initial short-term bed rest (2–3 days)
- Short-term pain relievers
- Nonsteroidal anti-inflammatory drugs (NSAIDs)
- Muscle relaxants
- Physical therapy
- Manipulation

ACTIVITY

- Restricted activities for 3–6 weeks
- Resume activities of daily living as tolerated.

DIET

Weight reduction, if needed

Medications

COMMONLY PRESCRIBED DRUGS

NSAIDs: ibuprofen, naproxen, salsalate

CONTRAINDICATIONS

Read drug product information.

PRECAUTIONS

- History of ulcer disease
- Elderly patients
- Kidney disease
- Heart disease

DRUG INTERACTIONS

Read drug product information.

OTHER DRUGS

N/A

 Followup

PATIENT MONITORING

- The doctor should be seen as often as necessary.
- Duration of care is 1–6 weeks.

PREVENTION

- Smoking cessation
- Weight reduction
- General physical condition
- Avoid aggravating tasks; e.g., heavy lifting, bending, twisting, sudden unexpected movements

COMPLICATIONS

- Incorrect diagnosis: missed disease
- Chronic low back pain
- Narcotic addiction
- Persistent psychosocial impairment

WHAT TO EXPECT

Normal activity without lasting symptoms in most cases

 Miscellaneous

OTHER FACTORS

N/A

PEDIATRIC

N/A

GERIATRIC

N/A

OTHERS

N/A

PREGNANCY

Pregnancy is commonly associated with low back pain and/or sciatica. Treatment is conservative.

FURTHER INFORMATION

N/A

Lumbar Disk Disorders

 Basics

DESCRIPTION

Many patients with low back pain have lumbar disc disease and involvement of surrounding spinal ligaments, muscles, and bones. Over time, disc degeneration, herniation, and arthritic changes may develop.

SIGNS AND SYMPTOMS

- Variable pain; usually dull, originating in back, extending below knee
- Back pain decreases at night. Bed rest usually improves symptoms at least temporarily.
- Pain increases with walking.
- Sciatica can occur without back pain.
- Tingling, numbness, loss of sensation in legs and feet
- Muscle weakness
- Muscle spasm

CAUSES

- Injury
- Frequent lifting of heavy objects, especially if improper technique is used
- Vibration; e.g., driving motor vehicles

SCOPE

- 60–90% of Americans experience lumbar back disorder in their lifetime. It is one of the most common reasons for seeking medical attention.

MOST OFTEN AFFECTED

Individuals 25–45 years of age, with the first episode in 20s and 30s; infrequent before 20 years of age or after age 65. Males and females are affected with equal frequency.

RISK FACTORS

- Normal aging process after age 20
- Cigarette smoking
- Spine disorders
- Stress, muscle tension
- Obesity
- Osteoporosis

 Diagnosis

WHAT THE DOCTOR LOOKS FOR

- The doctor will perform a complete physical examination to evaluate back function.
- Numerous other disorders can cause similar symptoms, including strains, arthritis, fracture, poor posture, bursitis, cancers, infection, and other conditions.

TESTS AND PROCEDURES

- Blood tests
- X-rays of affected area of back
- A special procedure called electromyography may be done to assess nerve and muscle function.
- Other special radiology procedures that may be done include myelography, computed tomography (CT scan), and magnetic resonance imaging (MRI).

 Treatment

GENERAL MEASURES

- Most cases of lumbar disk disorders are managed in the outpatient setting.
- Severe disability or surgery may require hospitalization.
- Initial: ordinary activities as tolerated, local heat, pelvic traction, sedation, physical therapy
- Following bed rest: activity with support
- For chronic pain: Improve physical fitness with low impact aerobic exercise. Manipulation and physical therapy have shown to be beneficial.
- Transcutaneous electrical nerve stimulation (TENS): very short-term benefit
- Surgery may be required.

Lumbar Disk Disorders

ACTIVITY

- After pain is controlled (7–10 days), begin progressive walking program. Short walks initially 4 times a day and lengthen as tolerated.
- Return to work as soon as possible but avoid high-risk activities, e.g., heavy lifting, vibration, smoking.

DIET

Weight reduction if appropriate

 ## Medications

COMMONLY PRESCRIBED DRUGS

- Pain relievers
- Nonsteroidal anti-inflammatory medication (NSAIDs)
- Muscle relaxants
- Mild sedatives

CONTRAINDICATIONS

Read drug product information.

PRECAUTIONS

Elderly, hypertension, peptic ulcer disease or bleeding, kidney disease, liver disease, cardiac dysfunction

DRUG INTERACTIONS

Read drug product information.

OTHER DRUGS

N/A

 ## Followup

PATIENT MONITORING

- The doctor should be seen about 10 days following initial visit.
- Thereafter, the doctor should be seen every 2 weeks until full function returns.

PREVENTION

- Modification of jobs to reduce exposure to known risk factors.
- Selection of workers by strength testing for certain jobs
- Avoid smoking
- Use proper lifting technique.
- Use good posture.

COMPLICATIONS

- Foot drop, weakness of leg muscles
- Bladder and rectum weakness with retention or incontinence
- Limitation of movement and restricted activity
- Narcotic addiction

WHAT TO EXPECT

- Expect to recover spontaneously with conservative therapy.
- Chronic pain: Most patients respond to conservative management such as manipulation, fitness, weight reduction, and good back care habits. Surgery produces good results in selected cases.

 ## Miscellaneous

OTHER FACTORS

N/A

PEDIATRIC

N/A

GERIATRIC

N/A

OTHERS

N/A

PREGNANCY

Pregnancy is commonly associated with low back pain and/or sciatica. Treatment is conservative.

FURTHER INFORMATION

N/A

Lyme Disease

 ## Basics

DESCRIPTION

Lyme disease is a multisystem infection caused by a microbe transmitted by deer ticks.
- Stage 1 includes a characteristic expanding ringlike skin rash and flulike symptoms.
- Stage 2 may involve one or more organ systems; neurologic and cardiac disease are most common.
- Stage 3, chronic Lyme disease, involves arthritis and chronic neurological symptoms.

SIGNS AND SYMPTOMS

- Stage 1
  - ▶ Expanding bull's-eye rash
  - ▶ Fever
  - ▶ Headache
  - ▶ Muscle and joint pain
  - ▶ May be no symptoms
- Stage 2:
  - ▶ Multiple ringlike rashes
  - ▶ Inflammation of facial nerves
  - ▶ Meningitis
  - ▶ Heart disorders
  - ▶ Inflammation of the testicles or liver
  - ▶ Arthritis
- Stage 3:
  - ▶ Recurring joint and muscle inflammation
  - ▶ Brain disorders (psychosis, dementia, memory loss, depression, stroke-like symptoms)
  - ▶ Nerve disorders
  - ▶ Eye disorders

CAUSES

Infection with *Borrelia burgdorferi,* transmitted by the bite of deer tick

SCOPE

Lyme disease affects 5.2 out of 100,000 persons in the United States. It is most prevalent in Connecticut, Rhode Island, New York, New Jersey, Pennsylvania, Wisconsin, and Maryland.

MOST OFTEN AFFECTED

Lyme disease can occur in all ages, but it is most common in children under age 15 and in 25–44 year olds. Males and females are affected in equal frequency.

RISK FACTORS

Exposure to tick-infested area; most common from May to September

 ## Diagnosis

WHAT THE DOCTOR LOOKS FOR

- The doctor will perform a physical examination to identify the presence of Lyme disease.
- Similar signs and symptoms may be caused by juvenile rheumatoid arthritis, viral infection, or many other diseases.

TESTS AND PROCEDURES

- Blood tests
- A sample of spinal fluids may be obtained by lumbar puncture (spinal tap).

 ## Treatment

GENERAL MEASURES

- Early stages of Lyme disease can be treated in the outpatient setting.
- Management of Stages 2 and 3 may require more intensive treatment, based on symptoms.

ACTIVITY

No restriction

DIET

No special diet

Lyme Disease

 ## Medications

COMMONLY PRESCRIBED DRUGS

- Doxycycline (Vibramycin)
- Amoxicillin
- Ceftriaxone (Rocephin), cefotaxime (Claforan), penicillin G
- Steroids

CONTRAINDICATIONS

- Allergy to drug
- Doxycycline is contraindicated in children and in women who are pregnant or breast feeding.

PRECAUTIONS

Read drug product information.

DRUG INTERACTIONS

- May cause sensitivity to sunlight; use sunscreen
- The dosage of oral blood thinners (anticoagulants) may need to be reduced.
- Oral contraceptives may be less effective.

OTHER DRUGS

Cefuroxime (Ceftin)

 ## Followup

PATIENT MONITORING

Individuals with Stages 2 and 3 disease should see the doctor often over a period of months to years, based on the severity of symptoms.

PREVENTION

- Prevention of infection is possible by careful examination of skin for ticks after outdoor activities. Deer ticks are extremely small.
- Remove ticks promptly.
- Wear clothing that covers the ankles in endemic areas.
- Use insect repellant.

COMPLICATIONS

- Recurrent inflammation
- Chronic neurological symptoms
- See signs and symptoms of Stage 3 disease

WHAT TO EXPECT

- Early treatment with antibiotics can shorten the duration of symptoms and prevent later disease.
- Response of late-stage disease is variable.

 ## Miscellaneous

OTHER FACTORS

N/A

PEDIATRIC

N/A

GERIATRIC

N/A

OTHERS

Ticks are commonly found on deer. Hunters may be at increased risk.

PREGNANCY

Pregnant patients with active disease should receive intravenous (IV) antibiotics. Doxycycline should not be used in pregnancy.

FURTHER INFORMATION

Lyme Borreliosis Foundation, P.O. Box 462, Tolland, CT, 06084, (203) 871-2900

Lymphoma, Burkitt's

 Basics

DESCRIPTION

Burkitt's lymphoma is a cancer of the lymphatic system that may involve sites other than lymph nodes, particularly bone marrow and the central nervous system.

SIGNS AND SYMPTOMS

- Mouth pain
- Loose teeth
- Jaw mass
- Anemia
- Abdominal mass
- Abdominal pain

CAUSES

Unknown; association with Epstein-Barr virus

SCOPE

Burkitt's lymphoma is rare in the United States.

MOST OFTEN AFFECTED

Individuals 3 months to 16 years of age, more often in males than females

RISK FACTORS

Living in area where Burkitt's lymphoma occurs

 Diagnosis

WHAT THE DOCTOR LOOKS FOR

N/A

TESTS AND PROCEDURES

- Blood tests
- Specialized laboratory testing may be done.
- Tissue from a lymph node may be obtained by biopsy for laboratory analysis.
- Spinal fluids may be obtained by lumbar puncture (spinal tap).
- A sample of bone marrow may be obtained to assist in diagnosis.
- Computed tomography (CT scan) may be done to assess internal structures.

 Treatment

GENERAL MEASURES

- Staging surgery and chemotherapy requires hospitalization.
- After treatment, Burkitt's lymphoma is managed in the outpatient setting.
- Surgery is usually necessary.

ACTIVITY

As tolerated

DIET

- Patients may have difficulty swallowing or chewing; small meals of soft foods (protein milk shakes) help prevent malnutrition.
- Adequate fluid intake

Medications

COMMONLY PRESCRIBED DRUGS

Combination chemotherapy according to most recent protocols

CONTRAINDICATIONS

Read drug product information.

PRECAUTIONS

Read drug product information.

DRUG INTERACTIONS

Read drug product information.

OTHER DRUGS

Intensive chemotherapy with or without bone marrow transplantation

 Followup

PATIENT MONITORING

The doctor should be seen as often as needed to monitor chemotherapy and detect recurrence of disease.

PREVENTION

Avoid areas where Burkitt's lymphoma is endemic.

COMPLICATIONS

Kidney failure

WHAT TO EXPECT

- 70–90% of patients experience long-term remission and possible cure.
- With newer treatments, some patients with more advanced disease have also been cured.
- Without treatment, prognosis is grave.

 Miscellaneous

OTHER FACTORS

N/A

PEDIATRIC

Common age group for Burkitt's lymphoma

GERIATRIC

Burkitt's lymphoma is unusual in the elderly.

OTHERS

N/A

PREGNANCY

N/A

FURTHER INFORMATION

Leukemia Society of America, 733 3rd Avenue, New York, NY 10017, (212) 573-8424

Lymphoma, Non-Hodgkin's

 Basics

DESCRIPTION

Non-Hodgkin's lymphoma is a varied group of lymphatic cancers, distinct from Hodgkin's disease. Characteristics include widespread disease, painless enlargement of one or more lymph nodes. Usual course is progressive.

SIGNS AND SYMPTOMS

N/A

CAUSES

Malignant tumors of lymph tissues

SCOPE

N/A

MOST OFTEN AFFECTED

N/A

RISK FACTORS

N/A

 Treatment

GENERAL MEASURES

- Radiotherapy
- Chemotherapy

ACTIVITY

N/A

DIET

N/A

Medications

N/A

COMMONLY PRESCRIBED DRUGS

N/A

CONTRAINDICATIONS

N/A

PRECAUTIONS

N/A

DRUG INTERACTIONS

N/A

OTHER DRUGS

N/A

 Followup

PATIENT MONITORING

N/A

PREVENTION

N/A

COMPLICATIONS

N/A

WHAT TO EXPECT

N/A

 Miscellaneous

OTHER FACTORS

N/A

PEDIATRIC

N/A

GERIATRIC

N/A

OTHERS

N/A

PREGNANCY

N/A

FURTHER INFORMATION

N/A

Section M

Macular Degeneration, Age-Related (ARMD)

 Basics

DESCRIPTION

Age-related macular degeneration (ARMD) is a deterioration of a portion of the retina (the "screen" at the back of the eye that is responsible for vision), leading to progressive vision loss. ARMD is the leading cause of irreversible severe visual loss in persons over 65 years of age. Stages include dry (nonexudative) and wet (exudative).

SIGNS AND SYMPTOMS

- Formation of small yellowish-white spots on the retina (drusen)
- Atrophy of retinal pigment
- Distortion of central vision; straight lines (e.g., telephone poles) appear crooked

SCOPE

- About 25% of individuals 52 years or older have signs of ARMD.
- About 2.2% of patients over 65 years of age are blind in one or both eyes from ARMD.

MOST OFTEN AFFECTED

- The prevalence of severe visual loss from ARMD increases with age.
- Primarily affects those 50 or more years of age
- Females affected more frequently than males

CAUSES

Exposure to light

RISK FACTORS

- Excess sunlight exposure
- Blue or light eye color
- Far-sightedness
- History of cardiovascular disease
- Short height
- History of lung infection
- Cigarette smoking

 Diagnosis

WHAT THE DOCTOR LOOKS FOR

The doctor will perform a physical examination to identify the presence of macular degeneration.

TESTS AND PROCEDURES

Blood vessels of the eye may be assessed with a special radiology procedure called angiography.

 Treatment

GENERAL MEASURES

- Macular degeneration is managed in the out-patient setting, including laser surgery.
- Hospitalization may be required for some surgical procedures.
- No specific treatment alters the course of de-terioration.
- Vitamins A, E, C and beta-carotene may be useful in preventing cellular damage.
- Oral zinc may retard visual loss.
- Laser treatment or other surgery may be an option.
- Low-vision aids may be helpful.

ACTIVITY

N/A

DIET

- A diet high in vitamins A, E, C and beta-carotene along with zinc may be helpful.
- Eating dark green, leafy vegetables (spinach or collard greens), which are rich in caroti-noids, may decrease the risk of developing the wet stage.

Macular Degeneration, Age-Related (ARMD)

 Medications

COMMONLY PRESCRIBED DRUGS

- Zinc and anti-oxidants may be beneficial.
- Interferon (experimental)

CONTRAINDICATIONS

N/A

PRECAUTIONS

Excess zinc ingestion can be associated with anemia and worsening of cardiovascular disease.

SIGNIFICANT POSSIBLE INTERACTIONS

N/A

OTHER DRUGS

N/A

 Followup

PATIENT MONITORING

- After laser treatment, contact doctor promptly if there are any new visual symptoms.
- The Amsler grid can aid in discovering visual disturbances.
- Is important to monitor vision, such as by Amsler grid.
- If there are no new symptoms, see the doctor every 6–12 months.

PREVENTION

- Protect eyes from ultraviolet (UV) light.
- Eat a well-balanced diet which includes zinc and vitamins A, E, C, and beta-carotene.
- Routine visits to an ophthalmologist
- Use an Amsler grid daily.
- Have eye examination every 2–4 years for individuals between 40 and 64 years of age and every 1–2 years for individuals 65 years or older.

COMPLICATIONS

Blindness

WHAT TO EXPECT

Increased risk of visual loss; individual outcomes vary

 Miscellaneous

OTHER FACTORS

N/A

PEDIATRIC

N/A

GERIATRIC

Prevalence increases with age.

OTHERS

N/A

PREGNANCY

N/A

FURTHER INFORMATION

American Academy of Ophthalmology, 655 Beach Street, San Francisco, CA 94109-1336

Meniere's Disease

 ## Basics

DESCRIPTION

Meniere's disease is an inner ear disorder resulting in recurrent attacks of hearing loss, tinnitus (ringing in the ears) and vertigo.
- Usually occurs in one ear, but 10–50% of cases may later involve the second ear
- Severity and frequency of symptoms may diminish over the years but with increasing loss of hearing.

SIGNS AND SYMPTOMS

- Ringing in the ears (tinnitus)
- Hearing loss
- Vertigo: spontaneous attacks, lasting 20 minutes to several hours
- Sensation of fullness in the ear
- Occurs as attacks, with intervening remission
- During severe attacks:
  - ▶ Pallor
  - ▶ Sweating
  - ▶ Nausea and vomiting
  - ▶ Falling
  - ▶ Prostration
  - ▶ All symptoms aggravated by motion.

CAUSES

Unknown

SCOPE

There are about 1,150 cases of Meniere's disease per 100,000 persons in the United States.

MOST OFTEN AFFECTED

Usual age of onset 20–60; males and females affected in equal proportion

RISK FACTORS

- Caucasian race
- Stress
- Allergy
- Increased salt intake
- Noise

 ## Diagnosis

WHAT THE DOCTOR LOOKS FOR

- The doctor will perform a physical examination to assess the presence of Meniere's disease.
- Conditions that can cause similar signs and symptoms should be investigated, such as acoustic tumor, multiple sclerosis, and other ear disorders.

TESTS AND PROCEDURES

- The ear may be examined by otoscopy.
- Hearing testing may be done.
- Magnetic resonance imagine (MRI) may be done to assist with diagnosis.

 ## Treatment

GENERAL MEASURES

- Meniere's disease is usually managed in the outpatient setting
- Surgery may involve hospitalization
- Medications are given primarily for symptomatic relief of vertigo and nausea. There is no medication available that influences the disease process.
- For attacks, bed rest with eyes closed and protection from falling. Attacks rarely last longer than 4 hours.
- Surgery may be required.

ACTIVITY

- Limit activity during attacks
- Between attacks, patient may be fully active.

DIET

Limit total intake during attacks because of nausea. Otherwise, diet is usually not a factor, unless attacks are brought on by certain foods. A restricted salt diet may be useful in some cases.

Medications

COMMONLY PRESCRIBED DRUGS

- Atropine
- Diazepam (Valium)
- Transdermal (skin patch) scopolamine
- Meclizine (Antivert, Bonine)
- Ergotamine-belladonna-phenobarbital (Bellergal Spacetabs)

CONTRAINDICATIONS

- Atropine: cardiac disease, especially supraventricular tachycardia and other arrhythmias
- Scopolamine: use with caution in children and elderly

PRECAUTIONS

- Sedating drugs should be used with caution, particularly in the elderly.
- Don't operate motor vehicles while taking sedating drugs.
- Read drug product information.

DRUG INTERACTIONS

- Bellergal: oral anticoagulants, tricyclic antidepressants, phenothiazines, narcotics, beta blockers, estrogens, and others
- Transdermal scopolamine: anticholinergics, belladonna products, antihistamines, tricyclic antidepressants, and others

OTHER DRUGS

- Droperidol
- Promethazine (Phenergan)
- Diphenhydramine (Benadryl)
- Carbogen
- Diphenidol (Vontrol)
- Chlorothiazide (Diuril)

 ## Followup

PATIENT MONITORING

- The doctor should be seen as often as necessary.
- Hearing status should be monitored frequently.

PREVENTION

- Reduce stress.
- Reduce salt intake.
- Don't smoke.
- Avoid significant noise exposure, or use ear protectors.

COMPLICATIONS

- Failure to diagnose acoustic tumor
- Loss of hearing
- Injury during attack
- Inability to work

WHAT TO EXPECT

- Alternating attacks and remission
- Over time, balance improves but hearing worsens.
- The majority of cases can be managed successfully with medication.
- About 5–10% of patients require surgery for incapacitating vertigo.

 ## Miscellaneous

OTHER FACTORS

N/A

PEDIATRIC

Unusual, but occasionally occurs among children

GERIATRIC

Meniere's disease is less likely to occur in the elderly. Patients exposed to loud noise levels over many years are more susceptible.

OTHERS

Usual onset age 20–60

PREGNANCY

Not a common problem, but medications pose risk of birth defects

FURTHER INFORMATION

N/A

Meningitis, Bacterial

 Basics

DESCRIPTION

Bacterial meningitis is an inflammation of the lining of the brain and spinal cord caused by a bacterial infection. This condition must be identified and treated promptly. It constitutes a medical emergency.

SIGNS AND SYMPTOMS

- Upper respiratory tract infection
- Fever
- Headache
- Vomiting
- Sensitivity to light
  - ▶ Seizures
- Nausea
- Profuse sweating
- Weakness
- Altered mental function
  - ▶ Excess Lethargy
  - ▶ Confusion
- Rash

CAUSES

Bacterial infection

SCOPE

There are 3–10 cases of bacterial meningitis per 100,000 persons in the United States.

MOST OFTEN AFFECTED

Newborns, infants and the elderly; males and females affected in equal proportion

RISK FACTORS

- Immune system disorder
- Alcoholism
- Neurosurgery procedure or head injury
- Abdominal surgery

 Diagnosis

WHAT THE DOCTOR LOOKS FOR

The doctor will perform a physical examination to identify the signs and symptoms of bacterial meningitis.

TESTS AND PROCEDURES

- A sample of spinal fluids may be obtained by lumbar puncture (spinal tap).
- Blood may be cultured for microbiological analysis.
- X-ray of head, computed tomography (CT scan) may be done to assist with diagnosis.

 Treatment

GENERAL MEASURES

- Management of bacterial meningitis usually requires hospitalization, often in intensive care unit.
- Antibiotic therapy

ACTIVITY

As tolerated in hospital and on discharge

DIET

Regular as tolerated

Medications

COMMONLY PRESCRIBED DRUGS

- Ampicillin
- Cefotaxime, ceftriaxone
- Aminoglycoside (Tobramycin)
- Chloramphenicol
- Steroids: dexamethasone

CONTRAINDICATIONS

Allergies to antibiotics

PRECAUTIONS

- Ear damage
- Hearing loss
- Developmental abnormalities related to meningitis

DRUG INTERACTIONS

Read drug product information.

OTHER DRUGS

- Vancomycin
- Penicillin
- Aztreonam
- Quinolones (e.g., ciprofloxacin)

 ## Followup

PATIENT MONITORING

The doctor should be seen as often as necessary.

PREVENTION

Prompt medical treatment for infections

COMPLICATIONS

- Seizures
- Brain damage
- Nerve disorders

WHAT TO EXPECT

- Overall death rate is 14%.
- Patients often make a complete recovery with prompt diagnosis and treatment.

 ## Miscellaneous

OTHER FACTORS

N/A

PEDIATRIC

N/A

GERIATRIC

May be less evident in elderly patients

OTHERS

N/A

PREGNANCY

N/A

FURTHER INFORMATION

American Academy of Pediatrics, 141 Northwest Point Blvd., P.O. Box 927, Elk Grove Village, IL 60009-0927, (800) 433-9016

Meningitis, Viral

 ## Basics

DESCRIPTION

Viral meningitis is a viral infection of the layer covering the brain and spinal cord. It is usually acute (of short duration) but may be relapsing. Incidence peaks in the summer.

SIGNS AND SYMPTOMS

- Fever
- Headache, often severe
- Stiff neck
- Nausea and vomiting
- Sensitivity to light
- Generalized aches and pains
- Rash

CAUSES

Viral infection

SCOPE

An average of 10,000 cases of viral meningitis are reported annually in the United States.

MOST OFTEN AFFECTED

May affect all ages, but most common in young adults; males and females affected in equal numbers

RISK FACTORS

- No specific risk factors are known.
- Immune system disorders

 ## Diagnosis

WHAT THE DOCTOR LOOKS FOR

- The doctor will perform a physical examination to identify the presence of viral meningitis.
- Other conditions that cause similar signs and symptoms will be investigated, such as bacterial meningitis and other central nervous system disorders.

TESTS AND PROCEDURES

- A sample of spinal fluid may be obtained by lumbar puncture (spinal tap).
- An electroencephalograph (EEG) may be done to evaluate brain function.
- Computed tomography (CT scan) or magnetic resonance imaging (MRI) may be done to assist in diagnosis.

 ## Treatment

GENERAL MEASURES

- Viral meningitis is usually managed with hospitalization.
- Fever control
- Intravenous (IV) fluids if oral intake is poor or vomiting is present.

ACTIVITY

Bed rest initially, then activity as tolerated

DIET

Determined by symptoms; may be nothing by mouth due to nausea or vomiting, advancing to clear fluids and regular diet as tolerated

Medications

COMMONLY PRESCRIBED DRUGS

- Meperidine (Demerol), nalbuphine (Nubain), morphine
- Promethazine (Phenergan), prochlorperazine (Compazine)
- Acetaminophen-codeine, oxycodone-acetaminophen (Percocet)
- Antifever drugs: acetaminophen (Tylenol)
- Antibiotics

CONTRAINDICATIONS

Read drug product information.

PRECAUTIONS

- Aspirin should be avoided in children and adolescents due to a possible association with Reye's syndrome.
- Phenothiazines may produce a reaction, especially in adolescents.

DRUG INTERACTIONS

Read drug product information.

OTHER DRUGS

Symptomatic relief may be provided by a variety of anti-emetics and analgesics (e.g., nonsteroidal anti-inflammatory drugs).

 Followup

PATIENT MONITORING

The doctor should be seen as often as necessary once the acute illness begins to resolve.

PREVENTION

N/A

COMPLICATIONS

- Deafness
- Fatigue
- Irritability
- Muscle weakness
- Seizures (rare)

WHAT TO EXPECT

Complete recovery in 2–7 days; headaches and other uncomfortable symptoms may persist for 1–2 weeks.

 Miscellaneous

OTHER FACTORS

N/A

PEDIATRIC

N/A

GERIATRIC

Viral meningitis is rarely seen in the elderly.

OTHERS

N/A

PREGNANCY

N/A

FURTHER INFORMATION

American Academy of Pediatrics, 141 Northwest Point Blvd., P.O. Box 927, Elk Grove Village, IL 60009-0927, (800) 433-9016

Menopause

 Basics

DESCRIPTION

Menopause is the cessation of spontaneous menstrual cycles.

- Climacteric or perimenopausal period is the period of time during which ovarian function declines. Although a woman may continue to have periodic uterine bleeding, such cycles may be without ovulation. During this time, hormone production diminishes and a woman may experience early signs of estrogen deficiency, such as "hot flashes."
- Postmenopause is the period after menopause usually accounting for more than a third of a women's total life.

SIGNS AND SYMPTOMS

- Cessation of menstruation: either abruptly or preceded by a period of irregular cycles and/or diminished bleeding
- Vasomotor symptoms: hot flashes, sweating
- Psychological symptoms: depression, nervousness, insomnia
- Painful intercourse
- Urinary incontinence
- Skin atrophy: wrinkles
- Osteoporosis: fractures
- Arteriosclerosis: coronary artery disease

CAUSES

- Physiologic: normal depletion of ovary
- Surgical: removal of ovaries, hysterectomy
- Medical: may result from treatment of endometriosis or breast cancer. May occur after chemotherapy and be permanent or reversible.

SCOPE

Menopause is becoming more common as life span increases; currently affects more than 30 million American women.

MOST OFTEN AFFECTED

- Average age is 51; virtually all women will be postmenopausal by age 58.
- Premature menopause occurs before age 30 and may be associated with abnormalities of the sex chromosomes.

RISK FACTORS

- Increasing age
- Pelvic surgery
- Sex chromosome abnormalities

Diagnosis

WHAT THE DOCTOR LOOKS FOR

- The doctor will take a history and perform a physical examination to identify the presence of menopause.
- Other conditions that may appear similar include pregnancy, ovarian disease, hormone disorders, and urinary tract disorders.
- The doctor should check for conditions known to be associated with menopause, such as osteoporosis and atherosclerosis.

TESTS AND PROCEDURES

- Blood tests
- A sample of tissue from the uterus may be obtained by biopsy for laboratory analysis.
- The reproductive tract may be examined by endoscopy.
- Computed tomography (CT scan) may be done to assist in diagnosis.
- Special test may be done to measure bone density.
- Pap smear

Treatment

GENERAL MEASURES

- Menopause is managed by periodic office visits with primary care provider.
- To retard development of osteoporosis: adequate calcium intake; exercise; avoid smoking, excessive alcohol or caffeine intake
- Estrogen replacement therapy

ACTIVITY

Active exercise to the extent possible. Some type of weight-bearing exercise is recommended.

DIET

Increased calcium intake

Menopause

 Medications

COMMONLY PRESCRIBED DRUGS

- Estrogens: conjugated estrogen (Premarin)
- Progestogen: medroxyprogesterone acetate (Provera)
- Combinations: Prempro, Premphase

CONTRAINDICATIONS

- Estrogen-sensitive cancer
- Unexplained uterine bleeding
- History of clotting disorders
- Active liver disease

PRECAUTIONS

Read drug product information.

DRUG INTERACTIONS

Read drug product information.

OTHER DRUGS

- Oral: estropipate (Ogen), estradiol (Estrace)
- Transdermal (patch): estradiol (Estraderm, Vivelle, Climara)
- Vaginal: conjugated estrogens (Premarin cream)
- Progestogens (Depo-Provera)
- Clonidine (Catapres)
- Osteoporosis: alendronate (Fosamax)

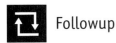 Followup

PATIENT MONITORING

- The doctor should be seen as often as necessary.
- Annual Pap smear and pelvic and breast examinations
- Annual mammography

PREVENTION

Menopause is a physiological process that cannot be avoided, but the negative effects can be moderated or eliminated by estrogen replacement therapy.

COMPLICATIONS

- Vasomotor symptoms (flushing, sweating)
- Psychological symptoms
- Vaginal atrophy
- Skin wrinkles
- Osteoporosis
- Arteriosclerosis

WHAT TO EXPECT

- If untreated:
  - ▶ Flushing and sweating resolve over several years
  - ▶ Atrophy of reproductive and urinary systems
  - ▶ Osteoporosis: possible fractures especially of the hip, vertebrae, and wrists
  - ▶ Mortality associated with hip fractures is 15%.
  - ▶ Coronary artery disease
- If treated:
  - ▶ Minimal effects of menopause
  - ▶ Slower development of bone loss, reduced risk of coronary artery disease
  - ▶ Therapy may be continued indefinitely.

 Miscellaneous

OTHER FACTORS

N/A

PEDIATRIC

N/A

GERIATRIC

N/A

OTHERS

N/A

PREGNANCY

N/A

FURTHER INFORMATION

- American College of Obstetricians and Gynecologists (ACOG), 409 12th St. S.W., Washington, D.C. 20024, (800) 673-8444
- American Academy of Family Physicians Foundation, P.O. Box 8418, Kansas City, MO 64114, (800) 274-2237, ext. 4400

Menorrhagia

 Basics

DESCRIPTION

Menorrhagia is an excessive amount or duration of menstrual flow, at more or less regular intervals.

SIGNS AND SYMPTOMS

- "Excessive" menstrual flow varies greatly from woman to woman.
- Bleeding substantially heavier than the patient's usual flow
- Bleeding lasting more than 7 days
- Passage of significant clots
- Anemia

CAUSES

- Hypothyroidism
- Uterine disorders
- Blood-clotting disorders

SCOPE

Abnormal bleeding is common in the United States.

MOST OFTEN AFFECTED

- Women between menarche and menopause; about 50% of cases occur after 40 years of age.
- Abnormal bleeding is common in adolescence and near menopause.

RISK FACTORS

- Obesity
- Lack of ovulation
- Estrogen therapy

 Diagnosis

WHAT THE DOCTOR LOOKS FOR

- The doctor will perform a complete physical examination to identify the cause of heavy menstrual flow.
- Other conditions, such as pregnancy and bleeding disorders, should be investigated and ruled out.

TESTS AND PROCEDURES

- Pregnancy test
- Blood tests
- A sample of uterine tissue may be obtained by biopsy for laboratory analysis.
- Ultrasound and computed tomography (CT scan) may be used to assist with diagnosis.
- Pap smear
- The uterus may be examined by hysteroscopy.

 Treatment

GENERAL MEASURES

- Most women with menorrhagia can be managed as outpatients in the doctor's office or emergency department.
- Severe bleeding may require hospitalization.
- Pregnancy complications and nonuterine bleeding must be ruled out.

ACTIVITY

As tolerated. Resting with feet elevated may be helpful.

DIET

Iron supplementation may be needed to offset increased blood loss.

Medications

COMMONLY PRESCRIBED DRUGS

- Estrogen, conjugated (Premarin)
- Medroxyprogesterone acetate (Provera)

CONTRAINDICATIONS

Pregnancy, breast or endometrial cancer, clotting disorder, liver failure

PRECAUTIONS

Nausea and vomiting are common.

DRUG INTERACTIONS

Read drug product information.

OTHER DRUGS

- Norethindrone acetate (Norlutin, Norlutate)
- Megestrol acetate (Megace)
- Naproxen sodium, mefenamic acid, ibuprofen

 ## Followup

PATIENT MONITORING

The doctor should be seen as often as necessary.

PREVENTION

Annual Pap smear and pelvic examination

COMPLICATIONS

Anemia

WHAT TO EXPECT

- The outcome varies with the cause of bleeding.
- Most patients with hormonal causes will respond to hormone therapy.

 ## Miscellaneous

OTHER FACTORS

N/A

PEDIATRIC

Genital bleeding before puberty can result from trauma, foreign bodies, vaginal infection, or hormonal disorders.

GERIATRIC

Genital atrophy may predispose to bleeding with minimal trauma.

OTHERS

- In adolescence, irregular bleeding is common.
- After age 35–40, endometrial dysplasia and cancer are significant causes of bleeding.

PREGNANCY

N/A

FURTHER INFORMATION

N/A

Middle Ear Infection

 Basics

DESCRIPTION

Otitis media is an inflammation of the middle ear. Acute otitis media (AOM) is usually a bacterial infection that is accompanied by an viral upper respiratory infection.

SIGNS AND SYMPTOMS

- Earache
- Fever
- Nasal discharge
- Cough common
- Decreased hearing
- Bleeding or discharge from ear
- Irritability

SCOPE

By 7 years of age, 93% of American children have had 1 or more episodes of AOM; 39% have 6 or more episodes of AOM.

MOST OFTEN AFFECTED

Peak incidence is 6–12 months. Incidence declines after 7 years of age. AOM is rare in adults; males and females are affected in equal numbers.

CAUSES

- Bacterial, viral infection
- Allergy

RISK FACTORS

- Day care
- Formula feeding
- Smoking in household
- Male gender
- Family history of middle ear disease

 Diagnosis

WHAT THE DOCTOR LOOKS FOR

The doctor will perform a physical examination to identify the presence of otitis media.

TESTS AND PROCEDURES

Hearing tests may be performed.

 Treatment

GENERAL MEASURES

- Acute otitis media is managed in the outpatient setting except for infants with fever and those who require surgery.
- Antibiotics
- Surgery (tubes in eardrum, removal of adenoids) may be recommended.

ACTIVITY

No restrictions

DIET

No special diet

 Medications

COMMONLY PRESCRIBED DRUGS

Amoxicillin

CONTRAINDICATIONS

Allergy to penicillins

PRECAUTIONS

Read drug product information.

DRUG INTERACTIONS

Read drug product information.

OTHER DRUGS

- Amoxicillin-clavulanate (Augmentin)
- Cefaclor (Ceclor)
- Cefixime (Suprax)
- Cefpodoxime (Vantin)
- Ceftriaxone (Rocephin)
- Clarithromycin (Biaxin)
- Trimethoprim-sulfamethoxazole (Septra, Bactrim)
- Erythromycin-sulfisoxazole (Pediazole)
- Sulfisoxazole

 Followup

PATIENT MONITORING

The doctor should be seen 2–4 weeks after diagnosis; for persistent otitis media, the doctor should be seen monthly.

PREVENTION

- Breast-feeding decreases incidence of AOM.
- Eliminate cigarette smoking in the household.

COMPLICATIONS

- Perforation of eardrum
- Bleeding from ear
- Nerve, bone, brain involvement
- Hearing loss

WHAT TO EXPECT

- The symptoms of acute otitis media usually improve in 48 to 72 hours; residual symptoms resolve within 3 months in 90% of cases.
- Recurring infections usually resolve by school age; only a small number of children have complications.

 Miscellaneous

OTHER FACTORS

N/A

PEDIATRIC

Otitis media is primarily a disease of childhood.

GERIATRIC

Otitis media in adults is rare: consider full evaluation to exclude tumors impinging on the eustachian tube.

OTHERS

N/A

PREGNANCY

N/A

FURTHER INFORMATION

N/A

Migraine

 Basics

DESCRIPTION

Migraine is an attack of headache lasting 4–72 hours. Frequency of episodes vary from more than once a week to less than 1 per year, with symptoms abating completely between attacks. Nonspecific symptoms, called prodromal symptoms, may be felt hours to days before headache.

SIGNS AND SYMPTOMS

- Symptoms of migraine vary from person to person or from attack to attack within the same individual.
- Five phases of a migraine:
  - ▶ Prodrome: warning signs preceding migraine, such as mood disruptions (e.g., euphoria, irritability, depression), fatigue, muscle tension, food craving, bloating, yawning
  - ▶ Aura: visual disruptions, such as spots, geometric patterns, and occasionally hal-lucinations. Headache typically begins within 1 hour after aura.
  - ▶ Headache: one-sided, throbbing pain lasting 4–72 hours, intensified by movement; accompanied by nausea, vomiting, diarrhea, light sensitivity, sound sensitivity, muscle tenderness, lighthead-edness, dizziness
  - ▶ Headache termination: untreated, usually occurs with sleep
  - ▶ Postdrome: Headache pain resolved but other symptoms linger, such as food intol-erance, impaired concentration, fatigue, muscle soreness.

CAUSES

Exact cause is unknown.

SCOPE

In the United States, 17.6% of female adults and 5.6% of male adults suffer from migraine. Childhood prevalence is unknown but may be significant.

MOST OFTEN AFFECTED

- Often begins in childhood and increases in early adolescence, through 30s and 40s; decreases with age but attacks may persist into mature adulthood.
- May be more common among males in childhood, more common among females adolescents and adults.
- May be inherited; more than 80% of patients have a family history of migraines.

RISK FACTORS

- Specific foods, alcohol, missing meals, menstrual cycle, excessive sleep, fatigue, emotional stress
- Medications (estrogen replacement, vasodila-tors)
- Family history of migraine
- Female gender
- Young age
- History of childhood vomiting, abdominal pain, motion sickness

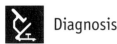 Diagnosis

WHAT THE DOCTOR LOOKS FOR

- The doctor will take a history and do a physical examination to identify the presence of migraine.
- Other causes of similar symptoms include other types of headache, tumor, infection, epilepsy and other conditions.

TESTS AND PROCEDURES

Blood tests

 Treatment

GENERAL MEASURES

- Migraine is usually managed in the outpatient setting.
- Severe cases and individuals with complications may require hospitalization
- Compression to temple artery or tender areas of scalp or neck on affected side
- Cold compresses to area of pain
- Rest with pillows comfortably supporting head or neck in quiet, darkened area.
- Withdrawal from stressful surroundings
- Sleep
- Biofeedback and early psychologic intervention in appropriate cases or when pain behaviors are first identified
- Most attacks of migraine are managed with self-care.

ACTIVITY

Rest in bed in a dark, quiet environment

DIET

Maintain fluid intake. Avoid dietary triggers of migraine.

Migraine

 ## Medications

COMMONLY PRESCRIBED DRUGS

- Sumatriptan (Imitrex)
- Dihydroergotamine (DHE), metoclopramide, prochlorperazine
- Ergotamine-caffeine (Cafergot)
- Aspirin
- Acetaminophen
- Ibuprofen (Nuprin, Motrin)
- Naproxen (Naprosyn)
- Ketoprofen (Orudis)
- Ketorolac (Toradol)
- Isometheptene—dichloralphenazone—aceta-minophen (Midrin)
- Acetaminophen-butalbital (Phrenilin)
- Acetaminophen-butalbital (Fioricet), aceta-minophen-butalbital-codeine (Fiorinal)

CONTRAINDICATIONS

Drugs have many contraindications; read drug product information.

PRECAUTIONS

Read drug product information.

SIGNIFICANT POSSIBLE INTERACTIONS

Other sedatives, analgesics, alcohol, decongestants

OTHER DRUGS

- Butorphanol (Stadol)
- Zolmitriptan, naratriptan, eletriptan, rizatrip-tan

Followup

PATIENT MONITORING

The doctor should be seen as often as necessary to monitor symptoms and drug therapy.

PREVENTION

- Avoid triggers of attacks.
- Biofeedback and psychologic intervention may be helpful.
- Preventive therapy: If attacks significantly interfere with lifestyle or are not adequately controlled, daily preventive therapy with one of the following may be appropriate:
  - ▶ Propranolol (Inderal)
  - ▶ Atenolol (Tenormin)
  - ▶ Nadolol (Corgard)
  - ▶ Timolol (Blocadren)
  - ▶ Metoprolol (Lopressor)
  - ▶ Amitriptyline (Elavil)
  - ▶ Nortriptyline (Pamelor)
  - ▶ Verapamil (Calan, Isoptin)
  - ▶ Isradipine (DynaCirc)
  - ▶ Methysergide (Sansert)
  - ▶ Cyproheptadine (Periactin)
  - ▶ Valproic acid (Depakene) or divalproex (Depakote)
- A referral to a specialist may be of benefit for patients who do not respond to standard treatment.

COMPLICATIONS

- Severe, persistent migraine (rare)
- Mini-strokes (rare)
- Side effects of treatment

WHAT TO EXPECT

- With age: reduction in severity, frequency, and disability of attacks
- Most attacks subside within 72 hours.

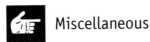 Miscellaneous

OTHER FACTORS

N/A

PEDIATRIC

Recurring abdominal pain and vomiting may be main symptoms; attacks may be of shorter duration. Headache not typical.

GERIATRIC

N/A

OTHERS

Migraine affects all races, social classes, and intelligence levels.

PREGNANCY

Attacks often diminish during pregnancy. No treatment drug has FDA approval in pregnancy; ergotamines are contraindicated.

FURTHER INFORMATION

N/A

Miscarriage

 ## Basics

DESCRIPTION

Miscarriage, or spontaneous abortion, is the loss of a fetus prior to survival outside the womb. Miscarriage is "threatened" when vaginal bleeding occurs early in pregnancy, with or without uterine contractions

SIGNS AND SYMPTOMS

- In a previously diagnosed pregnancy:
  - ▶ Vaginal bleeding (pink or brownish discharge)
  - ▶ Cramping
  - ▶ Cervical dilation
  - ▶ Ruptured membranes
  - ▶ Passage of nonviable products of conception
  - ▶ Fever
  - ▶ Shock

CAUSES

The cause of most spontaneous abortions is unknown.

SCOPE

- 30–50% of all fertilized ova spontaneously miscarry. Most are not recognized.
- 10–15% of all recognized pregnancies end in clinically apparent miscarriage.

MOST OFTEN AFFECTED

- Young women, less than 15 years of age
- Advancing age: Women over 35 years of age have 3 times the risk of miscarriage compared with women less than 30 years of age.

RISK FACTORS

- Fetal chromosomal abnormalities
- Uterine abnormalities
- Maternal alcohol/drug ingestion
- Increasing maternal age
- Deteriorating health status (i.e., diabetes/thyroid disease)
- Infections
- Previous abortions

 ## Diagnosis

WHAT THE DOCTOR LOOKS FOR

- The doctor will perform a thorough physical examination to assess reproductive status, including a pelvic examination.
- Cervical polyps, cancer, and/or inflammatory conditions can cause vaginal bleeding.

TESTS AND PROCEDURES

- Cultures: for group B Streptococcus, gonorrhea and chlamydia
- Blood tests
- The products of conception may be retained for analysis.
- Ultrasound may be used to assist in diagnosis.
- Fluid or tissue from the reproductive tract may be sampled for laboratory analysis.

 ## Treatment

GENERAL MEASURES

- Miscarriage may be managed in the outpatient setting or require hospitalization, depending on the nature of the condition.
- Threatened miscarriage: bed rest (usually at home) and insert nothing in the vagina. If bleeding is severe (i.e., more than a heavy period), hospitalization and close observation may be required.
- Surgical procedures (dilatation and curettage [D&C]) may be required.

ACTIVITY

If appropriate, bed rest until resolution

DIET

No special diet

Medications

COMMONLY PRESCRIBED DRUGS

- Oxytocin (Pitocin)
- Methylergonovine (Methergine)
- Analgesics if needed
- Rho(D) immune globulin if mother is Rh negative
- Beta-agonists (e.g. isoxsuprine)
- Progesterone

CONTRAINDICATIONS

None

PRECAUTIONS

Read drug product information.

SIGNIFICANT POSSIBLE INTERACTIONS

Read drug product information.

OTHER DRUGS

N/A

Followup

PATIENT MONITORING

- The doctor should be seen as often as necessary.
- Subsequent pregnancy will require special care and attention.
- Counseling may be helpful for coping with emotional issues.

PREVENTION

- Any vaginal bleeding during pregnancy is abnormal and should be considered a "threatened" miscarriage until proven otherwise. In reality, vaginal bleeding in early pregnancy is common and often the bleeding source eludes diagnosis.
- Surgery for habitual miscarriage

COMPLICATIONS

- Complications of surgery include uterine perforation, infection, and bleeding.
- Recurrent miscarriage
- Depression and feelings of guilt

WHAT TO EXPECT

- In cases of threatened miscarriage where bleeding stops and pregnancy continues to progress normally, maternal prognosis is excellent.
- First-trimester bleeding is associated with preterm delivery, delivery of low-birth-weight infants, and neonatal death.
- After surgery for incomplete or inevitable miscarriage and after complete miscarriage, the outcome is excellent.

Miscellaneous

OTHER FACTORS

N/A

PEDIATRIC

N/A

GERIATRIC

N/A

OTHERS

N/A

PREGNANCY

A complication of pregnancy

FURTHER INFORMATION

American College of Obstetricians & Gynecologists, 409 12th St., SW, Washington, DC 20024-2188, (800) 762-ACOG

Mitral Valve Prolapse

 Basics

DESCRIPTION

Mitral valve prolapse is a bulging that occurs to the mitral valve as the heart pumps, producing a distinctive sound that can be heard with a stethoscope. Mitral valve prolapse is usually harmless, causes no symptoms, and is not progressive. A small group of people with mitral valve develop related conditions, such as irregular heart rhythms, other cardiac disorders, or sudden death. Some have chest pain, palpitations, fatigue, shortness of breath, dizziness, anxiety, and panic attacks.

SIGNS AND SYMPTOMS

- May have no symptoms
- Chest pain: recurring, located on left or beneath breastbone, varies from moments to hours in duration
- Fatigue
- Fainting
- Shortness of breath
- Psychiatric symptoms including anxiety and panic attacks

CAUSES

- Inherited
- Caused by any number of medical conditions

SCOPE

Mitral valve prolapse affects about 5% of the U.S. population.

MOST OFTEN AFFECTED

Mitral valve prolapse is uncommon before adolescence and is usually detected in young adulthood. It is more common in females under age 20 and more common in males after age 50.

RISK FACTORS

- Family history
- Connective tissue disorder

 Diagnosis

WHAT THE DOCTOR LOOKS FOR

The doctor will perform a physical examination, in particular assessing heart sounds with a stethoscope.

TESTS AND PROCEDURES

- Chest x-ray
- An electrocardiogram (EKG) and echocardiogram may be done to assist in diagnosis.
- Other specialized tests may be done, such as the tilt-table studies, EKG stress test, and 24-hour Holter monitoring of cardiac activity.

 Treatment

GENERAL MEASURES

- Mitral valve prolapse is usually managed in the outpatient setting.
- 75% of cases are not associated with any increase in illness or death, and no treatment is required.
- Complications tend to occur after age 50 (in men more than women) and include irregular heart rhythms and other conditions requiring surgery.
- People with mitral valve prolapse have an increased risk of developing infection of the mitral valve. Because dental procedures can release bacteria from dental plaque into the bloodstream, preventive antibiotics should be taken before and after dental procedures.
- Surgical repair or replacement of the valve may be necessary.

ACTIVITY

- Generally unrestricted
- Vigorous sports and dehydration may cause fainting.
- Competitive sports should be avoided in patients with severe symptoms.

DIET

- Adequate salt intake
- Caffeine, alcohol, and cigarettes should be avoided by individuals with palpitations.

Medications

COMMONLY PRESCRIBED DRUGS (IF NEEDED)

- Beta-blockers
- Aspirin
- Antibiotics

CONTRAINDICATIONS

Read drug product information.

PRECAUTIONS

Beta-blockers will increase fatigue and dizziness.

DRUG INTERACTIONS

Read drug product information.

OTHER DRUGS

None

Followup

PATIENT MONITORING

- The doctor should be seen as often as necessary.

PREVENTION

- Preventive antibiotics before dental procedures

POSSIBLE COMPLICATIONS

- Complications are uncommon.
- Heart inflammation
- Stroke, mini-stroke
- Heart failure
- Irregular heart rhythms
- Sudden death
- Fainting

WHAT TO EXPECT

- 75% of people with mitral valve prolapse have an excellent outcome.
- 25% of cases become progressively worse, with a long (25-year) period without symptoms followed by rapid deterioration requiring surgery.

Miscellaneous

OTHER FACTORS

N/A

PEDIATRIC

Mitral valve is rarely seen in young children.

GERIATRIC

Complications occur mostly in men over 50.

OTHERS

N/A

PREGNANCY

- Mitral valve prolapse itself is not a contraindication to pregnancy.
- Connective tissue diseases may be a contraindication to pregnancy.
- Symptoms of mitral valve prolapse may improve during pregnancy.

FURTHER INFORMATION

American Heart Association, 7320 Greenville Avenue, Dallas, TX 75231, (214) 373-6300

Molluscum Contagiosum

 ## Basics

DESCRIPTION

Molluscum contagiosum is a common, harmless viral skin disorder consisting of small elevations of skin that tend to occur on the face, trunk and extremities in children, and on the groin and genitalia in adults. The lesions can be extensive in a person with immune system disorder.

SCOPE

Molluscum contagiosum is common in the United States.

MOST OFTEN AFFECTED

Children and young adults, males and females in equal proportions

SIGNS AND SYMPTOMS

- Pearly to flesh-colored, firm elevations of skin
- Diameter 2 to 6 millimeters
- Usually grouped in 1 or 2 areas
- Lesions may be itchy or tender.
- Distribution: anywhere on the body; predilection for face, trunk, and extremities in children, and groin and genitalia in adults.

CAUSES

Viral infection

RISK FACTORS

- Close contact with infected persons
- In children, transmission can occur in swimming pools.
- In adults, sexual transmission is common.
- Immune system disorders

 ## Diagnosis

WHAT THE DOCTOR LOOKS FOR

- The doctor will perform a physical examination to identify the presence of molluscum contagiosum.
- Similar signs may be caused by skin cancer, warts, and numerous other skin conditions.

TESTS AND PROCEDURES

- A lesion may be sampled by biopsy for laboratory analysis.

 ## Treatment

GENERAL MEASURES

- Molluscum contagiosum is managed in the outpatient setting.
- Spontaneous resolution is common in 6–12 months. Individual lesions resolve in 2 months.
- Lesions may be surgically removed.
- Cryotherapy is also effective.

ACTIVITY

No restrictions

DIET

No special diet

Medications

COMMONLY PRESCRIBED DRUGS

N/A

CONTRAINDICATIONS

N/A

PRECAUTIONS

N/A

DRUG INTERACTIONS

N/A

OTHER DRUGS

N/A

 Followup

PATIENT MONITORING

- The doctor should be seen 2–4 weeks after treatment.
- 2–4 visits are often required for complete course of treatment.

PREVENTION

In adults, avoid sexual contact with infected individuals.

COMPLICATIONS

- Disease may persist or spread.
- May be transmitted to others
- People with immune system disorders may have extensive infections.

WHAT TO EXPECT

- Untreated, the condition is usually self-limited. Individual lesions spontaneously heal in 2 months. Total resolution usually takes 6–12 months.
- Recurrences are uncommon.

 Miscellaneous

OTHER FACTORS

N/A

PEDIATRIC

Commonly seen on face, trunk and extremities; may be spread in swimming pools

GERIATRIC

N/A

OTHERS

Often a sexually transmitted disease in adults

PREGNANCY

N/A

FURTHER INFORMATION

N/A

Mononucleosis

 ## Basics

DESCRIPTION

Mononucleosis, or "mono," is a viral illness caused by the Epstein-Barr virus (EBV). The illness is characterized by fatigue, fever, enlarged spleen, enlarged lymph nodes, and sore throat.

SIGNS AND SYMPTOMS

- Malaise
- Fatigue
- Headache
- Fever
- Enlarged lymph nodes
- Tonsillitis
- Swelling around eyes
- Rash

CAUSES

EBV

SCOPE

14–90% of the population has been exposed to EBV.

MOST OFTEN AFFECTED

High school and college students, males and females in equal proportions

RISK FACTORS

- College and high school students
- Kissing
- 70–90% of people with mononucleosis continue to shed virus 2–6 months after initial infection.

 ## Diagnosis

WHAT THE DOCTOR LOOKS FOR

- The doctor will perform a physical examination to identify the presence of mononucleosis.

TESTS AND PROCEDURES

Blood tests

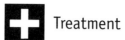 ## Treatment

GENERAL MEASURES

- Mononucleosis is managed in the outpatient setting.
- No specific treatment
- Quarantine not indicated
- General supportive measures
- Gargling
- Surgery may be required.

ACTIVITY

- Rest
- Avoid contact sports, heavy lifting, strenuous athletics.

DIET

- Healthy diet is important.
- Drink milk shakes, fruit juices, and consume soft foods to ease sore throat.

 ## Medications

COMMONLY PRESCRIBED DRUGS

- Antibiotics
- Pain relievers: acetaminophen (Tylenol), codeine
- Prednisone

CONTRAINDICATIONS

Aspirin should not be taken because of the risk of Reye's syndrome.

PRECAUTIONS

Read drug product information.

DRUG INTERACTIONS

Read drug product information.

OTHER DRUGS

N/A

Followup

PATIENT MONITORING

- The doctor should be seen as often as necessary.
- See the doctor before resuming contact sports.

PREVENTION

Most likely spread by saliva

COMPLICATIONS

- Chronic infections (chronic fatigue syndrome; very controversial)
- Rupture of the spleen (rare)
- Anemia
- Blood-clotting disorders
- Seizures
- Brain damage
- Nerve disorders
- Coma
- Psychosis
- Heart disorders
- Airway obstruction
- Lung disorders
- Liver failure
- Digestive disorders
- Dermatitis
- Rash
- Kidney disorders
- Infection

WHAT TO EXPECT

- Fever subsides in about 10 days.
- Enlarged lymph nodes and enlarged spleen subside in about 4 weeks.
- Children should be able to return to school when signs of infection have decreased; appetite returns; and alertness, strength, and sense of well-being allow.

 Miscellaneous

OTHER FACTORS

N/A

PEDIATRIC

Children have mild infections.

GERIATRIC

N/A

OTHERS

N/A

PREGNANCY

N/A

FURTHER INFORMATION

N/A

Motion Sickness

 Basics

DESCRIPTION

Motion sickness is not a true illness, but a normal response to an abnormal situation in which there is a sensory conflict about body motion and position. A mismatch between the visual, balance, and body-position senses results in motion sickness.

SIGNS AND SYMPTOMS

- Nausea
- Vomiting
- Profuse sweating
- Pallor
- Excessive production of saliva
- Yawning
- Rapid breathing
- Anxiety, panic
- Malaise
- Fatigue
- Weakness
- Confusion

CAUSES

Motion (auto, plane, boat, amusement rides)

SCOPE

N/A

MOST OFTEN AFFECTED

N/A

RISK FACTORS

- Travel
- Visual stimuli (e.g., moving horizon)
- Poor ventilation (fumes, smoke, carbon monoxide)
- Emotions (fear, anxiety)
- Low or zero gravity (amusement park ride)
- Other illness or poor health

 Diagnosis

WHAT THE DOCTOR LOOKS FOR

Conditions with similar signs and symptoms of motion sickness include mountain sickness, vestibular disease, gastroenteritis, metabolic disorders, and toxic exposure.

TESTS AND PROCEDURES

N/A

 Treatment

GENERAL MEASURES

- Remove triggers or stimuli of motion sickness.
- Minimize exposure (sit in middle of plane or boat)
- Improve ventilation

ACTIVITY

- Semi-reclined position
- Fix vision at 45 angle above horizon.
- Avoid fixation of vision on moving objects (e.g., waves).
- Avoid reading.

DIET

- Decrease oral intake or take frequent small feedings.
- Avoid alcohol.

Medications

COMMONLY PRESCRIBED DRUGS

Scopolamine

CONTRAINDICATIONS

Glaucoma

PRECAUTIONS

- Use Scopolamine cautiously in:
  - ▶ Young children
  - ▶ Elderly
  - ▶ Pregnancy
  - ▶ Urinary obstruction
  - ▶ Pyloric obstruction

DRUG INTERACTIONS

- Sedatives (antihistamines, alcohol, antide-pressants)
- Belladonna alkaloids

OTHER DRUGS

- Dimenhydrinate (Dramamine)
- Meclizine (Antivert)

Followup

PATIENT MONITORING

N/A

PREVENTION

- Minimize exposure (sit in middle of plane or boat).
- Improve ventilation.
- Semi-reclined position
- Fix vision at 45 angle above horizon.
- Avoid fixation of vision on moving objects (e.g., waves).
- Avoid reading.
- Minimize food intake prior to travel.

COMPLICATIONS

- Low blood pressure
- Dehydration
- Depression
- Panic

WHAT TO EXPECT

- Symptoms should resolve when motion exposure ends.
- Resistance to motion sickness seems to increase with age.

Miscellaneous

OTHER FACTORS

N/A

PEDIATRIC

Children are more susceptible to motion sickness.

GERIATRIC

Age confers some resistance to motion sickness.

OTHERS

N/A

PREGNANCY

N/A

FURTHER INFORMATION

N/A

Multiple Sclerosis

 Basics

DESCRIPTION

Multiple sclerosis (MS) is an inflammatory progressive disease of the brain and spinal cord resulting in multiple and varied neurologic symptoms and signs. It is usually intermittent, progressive, and relapsing. It may be acute (of short duration) or slowly progressive. MS is a major cause of disability in young adults.

SIGNS AND SYMPTOMS

- Incoordination
- Neurological disturbances
- Blurred, double or loss of vision in a single eye
- Muscle spasm
- Clumsiness
- Difficulty moving
- Mood swings
- Fatigue
- In women, loss of sensation in genital area
- Paralysis of the hands
- Paralysis of the right or left half of the body
- Loss of position sense
- Monoparesis
- Eye paralysis
- Loss of sensation, tingling
- Erectile dysfunction in men
- Urinary frequency, hesitancy, incontinence

CAUSES

Unknown; may be result of autoimmune disorder or viral infection

SCOPE

There are 25,000 new cases of multiple sclerosis annually in the United States.

MOST OFTEN AFFECTED

Young adult (16–40 years of age); more frequent in females than males; may be genetic component

RISK FACTORS

- Living in temperate climate
- Northern European descent
- Family history of multiple sclerosis

 Diagnosis

WHAT THE DOCTOR LOOKS FOR

- The doctor will perform a physical examination to identify the signs and symptoms of MS.
- Conditions that may appear similar to MS include tumors, infections, and other nervous system disorders.

TESTS AND PROCEDURES

- A sample of spinal fluids may be obtained by lumbar puncture (spinal tap).
- Blood tests
- Special diagnostic procedures may be done to assess the nervous system, including visual evoked response (VER), somatosensory evoked potentials, and brain stem auditory evoked responses.
- Magnetic resonance imaging (MRI) and computed tomography (CT scan) may be done to assist in diagnosis.

 Treatment

GENERAL MEASURES

- MS should be managed in the outpatient setting for as long as possible.
- A long-term care facility may be required for physical therapy or complications.
- There is no specific treatment for multiple sclerosis. Remissions occur spontaneously.
- Emotional support, encouragement, and reas-surances are necessary to help avoid a hopeless outlook.
- Occupational therapy
- Urologic evaluation including any sexual dys-function problems (erectile dysfunction common in male patients)
- Self-catheterizations for inadequate bladder emptying
- Custodial care, if there is cognitive impairment
- Physical therapy to maintain range of movement and strength and to avoid compli-cations

ACTIVITY

- Maintain activity, avoid overwork and fatigue.
- Rest during periods of acute relapse.

DIET

If constipation a problem, high-fluid intake plus a high-fiber diet

Medications

COMMONLY PRESCRIBED DRUGS

Drug therapy is used to relieve symptoms:
- Methylprednisolone
- Baclofen, diazepam
- Stool softeners, bulk producing agents, laxative suppositories
- Propantheline, oxybutynin chloride
- Antibiotics
- Primidone, clonazepam
- Haloperidol, lithium, amitriptyline
- Nonsteroidal anti-inflammatory drugs (NSAIDs)
- Carbamazepine
- Azathioprine, ACTH (adrenocorticotropic hormone), methylprednisolone, cyclophosphamide, interferons, cyclosporine still experimental

CONTRAINDICATIONS

Read drug product information.

PRECAUTIONS

Read drug product information.

SIGNIFICANT POSSIBLE INTERACTIONS

Read drug product information.

OTHER DRUGS
- Amantadine (no specific evidence that this works)
- Interferon (approved for limited cases)
- Copolymer-1, cladribine (experimental)

Followup

PATIENT MONITORING

Physicians and other health care providers should be seen as often as necessary to maintain optimal health status.

PREVENTION

No known preventive measures. Avoid factors that may precipitate an attack, particularly stress from hot weather.

COMPLICATIONS
- Coma
- Delirium
- Mood swings
- Vision disturbances
- Paraplegia
- Sexual impotence (men)
- Urinary tract infections

WHAT TO EXPECT
- The outcome of MS is highly variable and unpredictable.
- About 70% of people with MS lead active, productive lives with prolonged period of good health.
- MS may be disabling by early adulthood or cause death within months of onset.
- Average duration of the illness exceeds 25 years.
- 30% of individuals with MS relapse in one year, 20% in 5 to 9 years, 10% in 10 to 30 years.

Miscellaneous

OTHER FACTORS

N/A

PEDIATRIC

Multiple sclerosis is unlikely before puberty.

GERIATRIC

Remissions less frequent among the elderly

OTHERS

N/A

PREGNANCY

A triggering factor for multiple sclerosis in some cases

FURTHER INFORMATION

National Multiple Sclerosis Society, 205E 42nd Street, New York, NY 10017, (800) 624-8236

Mumps

 Basics

DESCRIPTION

Mumps is an acute infection usually presenting with inflammation of one or both parotid glands, which are located just behind the corner of the jaw. The swollen parotid glands can get quite large, obscuring the normal contour of the cheek. Epidemics of mumps occur in late winter and spring. The virus that causes mumps is transmitted in the air. The incubation period is approximately 14–24 days.

SIGNS AND SYMPTOMS

- Pain and swelling in one or both parotid glands at the corner of the jaw
- Pre-illness syndrome of fever, neck muscle ache, malaise
- Swelling peaks in 1–3 days, lasts 3–7 days.
- Sour foods cause pain.
- Moderate fever, usually not above 104° F (40.0° C)
- May affect joints, testicles (orchitis), thyroid, breasts, pancreas
- Rash
- Up to 50% of cases have no symptoms.

CAUSES

Viral infection

SCOPE

Mumps is common in the United States.

MOST OFTEN AFFECTED

80% of mumps cases occur in people younger than 15 years of age. The illness is more severe in adults. Males and females are affected with equal frequency

RISK FACTORS

- Urban epidemics, nonvaccinated population
- Usual contagious period is 2 days before to 6–10 days after onset.

 Diagnosis

WHAT THE DOCTOR LOOKS FOR

- The doctor will perform a physical examination to determine the presence of mumps.
- Numerous other medical conditions can cause signs and symptoms similar to mumps.

TESTS AND PROCEDURES

- Blood tests
- Body fluids may be cultured for laboratory analysis.
- A sample of spinal fluids may be obtained by lumbar puncture (spinal tap).

 Treatment

GENERAL MEASURES

- Mumps is managed in the outpatient setting if there are no complications.
- General care is supportive and symptomatic.
- For orchitis, cold packs to scrotum can help relieve pain.
- Scrotal support with adhesive bridge while lying down and/or athletic supporter while walking

ACTIVITY

Mumps orchitis: bed rest and local supportive clothing, such as wearing 2 pairs of briefs or adhesive-tape bridge

DIET

Liquids if the patient cannot chew

Medications

COMMONLY PRESCRIBED DRUGS

- Corticosteroids
- Nonsteroidal anti-inflammatory drugs (NSAIDs)
- Acetaminophen

CONTRAINDICATIONS

Read drug product information.

PRECAUTIONS

Avoid aspirin for pain in children because of the risk of Reye's syndrome.

DRUG INTERACTIONS

Read drug product information.

OTHER DRUGS

N/A

 ## Followup

PATIENT MONITORING

Most cases of mumps are mild. Monitor fluid intake to prevent dehydration.

PREVENTION

- Mumps vaccine is recommended for active immunization at 15 months of age and at entry to middle school.

COMPLICATIONS

May affect the brain, heart, pancreas, kidneys, ears, eyes, testicles, ovaries, and other body systems.

WHAT TO EXPECT

- Complete recovery is usual, immunity is permanent.
- Temporary hearing loss occurs in 4% of adults.
- Rarely recurs

 ## Miscellaneous

OTHER FACTORS

N/A

PEDIATRIC

- In adolescents, orchitis is more common.
- Most cases of acute epidemic mumps occur in children 5–15 years of age. It is unusual in children less than 2 years of age. Most infants less than 1 year are immune.
- Less likely to develop complications

GERIATRIC

Most elderly persons are immune to mumps.

OTHERS

Most complications occur in postpubertal group.

PREGNANCY

- Although no complications of vaccine administration to pregnant women have been noted, theoretically it should not be given in pregnancy as it is a "live" vaccine.
- Disease may increase rate of miscarriage in first trimester.

FURTHER INFORMATION

N/A

Section N

Nail Fungus

 ## Basics

DESCRIPTION

Infectious inflammation of the folds of skin surrounding the fingernail or toenail can be caused by a fungus. This condition is also called paronychia. It may be acute (of short duration) or chronic (long-lasting).

SIGNS AND SYMPTOMS

- Separation of nail fold from nail plate
- Red, painful swelling of skin around nail plate
- Pus, drainage
- Changes of nail plate
- Greenish tint to nail

CAUSES

Infection by bacteria, *Candida albicans,* other fungi, or molds

SCOPE

Common

MOST OFTEN AFFECTED

All ages; three times more frequent in females than males

RISK FACTORS

- Trauma to skin surrounding nail
- Ingrown nails
- Frequent immersion of hands in water
- Diabetes mellitus

 ## Diagnosis

WHAT THE DOCTOR LOOKS FOR

The doctor will identify the presence of nail fungus.

TESTS AND PROCEDURES

Nail tissue may be sampled for laboratory analysis.

 ## Treatment

GENERAL MEASURES

- Acute: warm compresses or soaks, elevation
- Chronic: keep fingers dry
- Surgical incision and drainage of abscess, if present.
- Partial or complete removal of nail may be necessary.

ACTIVITY

Full activity

DIET

No special diet

Medications

COMMONLY PRESCRIBED DRUGS

- Dicloxacillin
- Cloxacillin
- Erythromycin
- Cephalexin (Keflex)
- Mupirocin
- Limidazoles (econazole, ketoconazole)
- Itraconazole
- Fluconazole

CONTRAINDICATIONS

Allergy to antibiotic

PRECAUTIONS

Erythromycin may cause significant gastrointestinal upset.

DRUG INTERACTIONS

Numerous interactions; read drug product information.

OTHER DRUGS

N/A

 ## Followup

PATIENT MONITORING

The doctor should be seen routinely until the condition has healed.

PREVENTION

- Avoid frequent wetting of hands, wear rubber gloves with cloth liner.
- Good diabetic control

COMPLICATIONS

- Acute: abscess under nail
- Chronic: ridging, thickening and discoloration of nail; nail loss

WHAT TO EXPECT

With adequate treatment and prevention, healing can be expected.

 ## Miscellaneous

OTHER FACTORS

N/A

PEDIATRIC

May be related to thumb/finger sucking

GERIATRIC

N/A

OTHERS

N/A

PREGNANCY

N/A

FURTHER INFORMATION

N/A

Nosebleed

 Basics

DESCRIPTION

Nosebleed, or epistaxis, is a hemorrhage from the nostril, nasal cavity, or nasal portion of the throat.

SIGNS AND SYMPTOMS

Usually bleeding from the nostril. However, nose can bleed to the back of the throat and not be apparent, resulting in nausea, the spitting or vomiting of blood, or the appearance of dark, tarry stool.

CAUSES

- Unknown (most common)
- Injury: nose picking, low humidity, foreign body
- Infection
- Vascular abnormalities
- Cancer
- High blood pressure
- Blood clotting disorders
- Deviation or perforation of the nasal septum

SCOPE

Unknown

MOST OFTEN AFFECTED

Children younger than 10 years or adults older than 50 years of age. Males and females are affected with equal frequency.

RISK FACTORS

- Hay Fever

 Diagnosis

WHAT THE DOCTOR LOOKS FOR

Epistaxis is a symptom or a sign, not a disease; the underlying cause of nosebleed should be identified and treated.

TESTS AND PROCEDURES

- Blood tests
- X-rays of the sinuses
- Special imaging of blood vessels may be done, called angiography (rare).

 Treatment

GENERAL MEASURES

- Nosebleed is usually managed in the outpatient setting.
- Nasal packing may be required.
- Management of severe bleeding may require hospitalization.
- Elderly patient may require hospitalization.
- Provide first aid as needed
- Pinch nostrils together to help reduce bleeding.
- If nosebleeds persist, the doctor may stop prescribing sedation, pain relievers, or high blood pressure medication.

ACTIVITY

Bed rest with head at 45° to 90° angle

DIET

No alcohol or hot liquids

Medications

COMMONLY PRESCRIBED DRUGS

Antibiotics, decongestants, iron supplements

CONTRAINDICATIONS

Drug allergies

PRECAUTIONS

Read drug product information.

DRUG INTERACTIONS

Read drug product information.

OTHER DRUGS

N/A

 Followup

PATIENT MONITORING

The doctor should be seen as often as needed.

PREVENTION

- Application of petroleum jelly (Vaseline) to nostril to prevent drying and picking
- Humidification at night
- Cut fingernails.

COMPLICATIONS

- Sinusitis
- Airway obstruction
- Injury to nasal structures by treatment
- Drug side effects

WHAT TO EXPECT

The outcome is good with proper treatment.

 Miscellaneous

OTHER FACTORS

N/A

PEDIATRIC

N/A

GERIATRIC

N/A

OTHERS

N/A

PREGNANCY

N/A

FURTHER INFORMATION

N/A

Section 0

Obesity

 ## Basics

DESCRIPTION

Obesity is a condition of increased body weight (consisting of both lean and fat tissue) that leads to increased illness and death. Obesity is also defined as weight 20% greater than an individual's desirable weight.

SIGNS AND SYMPTOMS

Increased body weight and adipose tissue

CAUSES

- Multiple factors
- May have genetic cause
- Imbalance between food intake and energy expenditure
- Medical conditions (pancreatic disease, thalamus disorder, Cushing's syndrome)
- Drug side effect

SCOPE

20–30% of adult men and 30–40% of adult women in the United States are overweight.

MOST OFTEN AFFECTED

Obesity affects all ages; females affected more frequently than males; 20–25% of weight tendency is inherited.

RISK FACTORS

- Parental obesity
- Pregnancy
- Sedentary lifestyle
- High-fat diet
- Low socioeconomic status

 ## Diagnosis

DIFFERENTIAL DIAGNOSIS

N/A

TESTS AND PROCEDURES

- Blood tests
- Body mass index (BMI) may be calculated.

 ## Treatment

GENERAL MEASURES:

- Health care providers should assess the degree of health risk from obesity; help set goals for therapy; counsel or refer to a registered dietician or weight loss program for in-depth work on diet, exercise, and behavior modification.
- Behavior modification can improve dietary adherence and longterm results of weight loss and should be included in any weight-loss program.
- Many reputable commercial and community programs offer weight reduction treatment. Look for programs with diets that meet the Recommended Daily Allowance (RDA) for nutrients, include exercise counseling, behavior modification, and provisions for longterm maintenance.
- Occasionally, patients with severe obesity are treated with a gastric bypass or stapling procedure. This complex procedure should only be done in a center skilled in this treatment. Surgical treatment is the most effective longterm weight loss treatment available for morbid obesity.

ACTIVITY

Exercise alone rarely causes significant weight loss. It may improve longterm results of weight loss treatment and should be an integral part of any weight loss program.

DIET

- Diet restriction is the cornerstone of obesity management (low-fat, high-complex carbohydrate and high-fiber).
- A 500 kilocalorie (kcal) reduction in calorie intake per day will result in approximately 1 pound of weight loss per week.
- Very low-calorie diets (400–800 kcal per day) are usually based on liquid formulas and cause more rapid weight loss. However, they can cause serious medical complications, and medical supervision is important.
- Avoid fad diets and miracle cures.

Medications

COMMONLY PRESCRIBED DRUGS

- Drug treatment is not usually recommended.
- Appetite suppressants may be indicated for short-term use (few weeks) along with a weight-loss regimen:
  ▶ Diethylpropion
  ▶ Phentermine
  ▶ Fenfluramine
  ▶ Mazindol
  ▶ Dexfenfluramine (Redux)
  ▶ Phendimetrazine
  ▶ Benzphetamine

CONTRAINDICATIONS

Advanced atherosclerosis, cardiovascular disease, hypertension, hyperthyroidism, glaucoma, history of drug abuse, agitated states, use of monoamine oxidase (MAO) inhibitors

PRECAUTIONS

- Abuse potential
- Weight gain after discontinuation of drug

DRUG INTERACTIONS

N/A

OTHER DRUGS

Phenylpropanolamine (PPA) is used in over-the-counter weight-loss preparations.

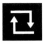
Followup

PATIENT MONITORING

Longterm followup and management is crucial to prevent further weight gain or regain after weight loss.

PREVENTION

Regular exercise and prudent diet with regular followup, especially in children and young adults and individuals with a family history of obesity or diabetes mellitus

COMPLICATIONS

- Increased risk of death due largely to cardiovascular disease
- Diabetes mellitus
- High blood pressure
- High levels of lipids in the bloodstream
- Gallbladder disease with stone formation
- Osteoarthritis
- Gout
- Blood clot formation
- Breathing problems and sleep apnea
- Poor self-esteem
- Discrimination

WHAT TO EXPECT

- Longterm maintenance of weight loss is extremely difficult.
- If person is not motivated, successful weight loss is unlikely.

Miscellaneous

PEDIATRIC

Prevalence of obesity is increasing in children, due, in part, to decreased physical activity and increased television viewing.

GERIATRIC

Acceptable weight ranges increase with age.

OTHERS

Prepuberty and young adulthood appear to be sensitive periods for development of obesity.

PREGNANCY

Pregnancy is a common time for onset of or increase in obesity.

FURTHER INFORMATION

N/A

Obsessive-Compulsive Disorder

 Basics

DESCRIPTION

Obsessive-compulsive disorder (OCD) is a psychiatric condition characterized by intrusive thoughts (obsessions) and compulsions. Compulsions are ritualistic behaviors that relieve the anxiety of obsessions.
- Common obsessive themes:
  ▶ Violence, such as harming a child
  ▶ Doubt, such as whether doors or windows are locked or iron turned off
  ▶ Blasphemous thoughts, such as in a devoutly religious person
  ▶ Contamination, dirt, or disease
  ▶ Symmetry or orderliness
- Common rituals or compulsions:
  ▶ Hand washing
  ▶ Checking
  ▶ Counting
  ▶ Hoarding
  ▶ Repeating, such as dressing rituals

SIGNS AND SYMPTOMS

- Obsessions and/or compulsions that consume more than 1 hour a day and cause significant distress or impairment
- Neither obsessions nor compulsions are related to another mental disorder.
- Compulsions (actions) are repetitive, purposeful behaviors that are performed in an attempt to neutralize intrusive thoughts, e.g., checking in response to doubt (locks, doors, windows, or driving back over route to check for any possible damage inadvertently done while driving one's car)
- Repeated hand washing or ritualistic hand washing in response to fear of contamination
- 80–90% of patients have obsessions and compulsions.
- 10–19% of patients are purely obsessional.
- 5% perform rituals until they "feel right" and may not have an identifiable obsession.

CAUSES

Disorder of neurotransmitter serotonin

SCOPE

About 2.5% of Americans will experience obsessive-compulsive behavior in their lifetime.

MOST OFTEN AFFECTED

- Average age of 20 years
- One-third of cases present by age 15.
- New cases after age 50 rare
- 20% of cases have family history.
- Males and females affected in equal proportions

RISK FACTORS

Family history of OCD

 Diagnosis

WHAT THE DOCTOR LOOKS FOR

The doctor will evaluate for the presence of obsessive-compulsive behavior or other mental health disorders.

TESTS AND PROCEDURES

- Psychological testing may be done.
- Positron emission tomography (PET) may be done to assist in diagnosis.

 Treatment

GENERAL MEASURES

- Counseling by psychiatrist or other mental health professional
- Drug therapy
- Psychosurgery (last resort)

ACTIVITY

No restriction

DIET

N/A

Medications

COMMONLY PRESCRIBED DRUGS

Fluoxetine (Prozac)

CONTRAINDICATIONS

Read drug product information.

PRECAUTIONS

Many precautions; read drug product information.

DRUG INTERACTIONS

Drugs have many possible interactions; read drug product information.

OTHER DRUGS

Clomipramine

Followup

PATIENT MONITORING

The doctor should be seen as often as necessary to monitor disorder and drug therapy.

PREVENTION

N/A

COMPLICATIONS

- Depression
- Phobias
- Anxiety and paniclike episodes

WHAT TO EXPECT

Chronic waxing and waning course for most people

Miscellaneous

OTHER FACTORS

N/A

PEDIATRIC

Adolescent onset in 15%; at this age, males outnumber females 3:1.

GERIATRIC

OCD is not usually diagnosed after age 50.

OTHERS

N/A

PREGNANCY

- Onset of obsessive compulsive disorder has been noted after delivery.
- Safety of fluoxetine and clomipramine has not been established in pregnancy or lactation.

FURTHER INFORMATION

- OCD Foundation, P.O. Box 9573, New Haven, CT 06535, (203) 772-0565
- Obsessive-Compulsive Anonymous, P.O. Box 215, New Hyde Park, NY 11040, (516) 741-4901

Osteoporosis

 Basics

DESCRIPTION

Osteoporosis is a skeletal disease characterized by severe bone loss sufficient to predispose to fractures of the vertebral column, leg, arm, pelvis, or ribs.

SIGNS AND SYMPTOMS

- Back ache, pain
- Curvature of the spine
- Fractures in the absence of trauma
- Loss of height

CAUSES

Multiple factors; in many cases, the exact cause is unknown

SCOPE

30–40% of women and 5–15% of men will develop osteoporosis.

MOST OFTEN AFFECTED

Osteoporosis can be diagnosed in individuals from 8 years of age to the elderly. It is more common in females than males and in Caucasians and Asians than in African-Americans or Latinos.

RISK FACTORS

- Dietary: inadequate calcium, excessive phosphate/protein; inadequate vitamin D
- Physical: immobilization, sedentary lifestyle
- Alcohol, smoking, caffeine
- Medical: chronic diseases, malabsorption, hormone disorders
- Drug therapy: corticosteroids, thyroid hormone replacement, heparin, chemotherapy, diuretics, anticonvulsants, radiation therapy
- Heredity

 Diagnosis

WHAT THE DOCTOR LOOKS FOR

- The doctor will assess the presence and degree of osteoporosis.
- Numerous diseases can cause similar signs and symptoms, including cancers and other bone disorders.

TESTS AND PROCEDURES

- Blood tests
- Urinalysis
- X-rays
- Specialized radiology procedures may be done, including bone mineral density (BMD) measurement.
- A sample of bone tissue may be obtained for laboratory analysis (rare).

 Treatment

GENERAL MEASURES

- Osteoporosis is usually managed in the outpatient setting.
- Acute back pain may require hospitalization, especially for vertebral fractures and upper leg and pelvic fractures.
- Nursing home or home care may be needed following fractures.
- Treatment is directed at relief of pain and disability, e.g., heat, pain relievers, physical therapy.

ACTIVITY

- Walk 1 mile twice a day. If possible, try swimming and bicycling.
- Avoid exercises and maneuvers that increase compressive forces and mechanical stress on bone.
- Rehabilitation may be prescribed for back-muscle spasm and walking.

Osteoporosis

DIET

- Reducing diet if overweight.
- Calcium intake 1500 milligrams per day (mg/day) from all sources, if not contraindicated.
- Avoid excess phosphate or protein intake, i.e., avoid phosphoric-acid-containing beverages and excess meat intake.
- 600–800 international units (IU) of vitamin D daily from all sources

 ## Medications

COMMONLY PRESCRIBED DRUGS

- Hormone replacement therapy (HRT) [estrogen/progesterone]
- Synthetic salmon calcitonin nasal spray (Miacalcin)
- Oral synthetic salmon calcitonin (Osteocalcin, Calcimar, Miacalcin)
- Alendronate (Fosamax)

CONTRAINDICATIONS

Numerous contraindications; read product information.

PRECAUTIONS

Numerous precautions; read drug product information.

DRUG INTERACTIONS

None

OTHER DRUGS

- Etidronate disodium
- Sodium fluoride (experimental)
- Tamoxifen (experimental)
- Raloxifene (experimental)
- Hormones (experimental)

 ## Followup

PATIENT MONITORING

- The doctor should be seen monthly during start of therapy, every 2–4 months thereafter.

- Annual gynecological examination, breast examination, and mammography
- Repeat x-rays every 3 years, more often when indicated

PREVENTION

- Diet, exercise, and hormone replacement at menopause
- Increased calcium intake and adequate vitamin D intake
- Correction of treatable medical conditions and other risk factors

COMPLICATIONS

- Severe disabling pain
- Nerve disorder caused by vertebral fracture (rare)
- Disability or death due to complications of upper leg fractures

WHAT TO EXPECT

- In 70% patients, treatment will lead to stabilization.
- Small increases in bone mass occur in many cases.
- Reduced pain, increased mobility

 ## Miscellaneous

OTHER FACTORS

N/A

PEDIATRIC

A juvenile form of osteoporosis exists.

GERIATRIC

N/A

OTHERS

N/A

PREGNANCY

Osteoporosis of pregnancy exists but is rare.

FURTHER INFORMATION

National Osteoporosis Foundation, 2100 M St., Suite 602, Washington, DC 20037

Ovarian Cancer

 Basics

DESCRIPTION

Ovarian cancer comprises a variety of malignancies that arise from the ovary.

SIGNS AND SYMPTOMS

- Vague gastrointestinal symptoms
- Bloating, heartburn
- Abdominal swelling, pain, and distention
- Occasional vaginal discharge
- Irregular vaginal bleeding
- Pelvic mass
- Painful intercourse
- Weight loss

CAUSES

Unknown

SCOPE

Ovarian cancer is responsible for 12,000 deaths each year in the United States. It is the 5th leading cause of cancer death in women.

MOST OFTEN AFFECTED

- The most common form of ovarian cancer affects women 40–75 years of age.
- Other types of ovarian cancer affect women 12–40 years of age.
- May have a genetic component

RISK FACTORS

- Risk decreases as the number of childbirths increases.
- Late pregnancies (over 30 years of age)
- Family history

 Diagnosis

WHAT THE DOCTOR LOOKS FOR

The doctor will perform a physical examination to identify the presence of ovarian cancer and associated conditions.

TESTS AND PROCEDURES

- Blood tests
- Other radiological procedures may be used, including mammogram, barium enema, computed tomography (CT scan) and upper gastrointestinal (GI) series.
- Pelvic ultrasound may be used to assist in diagnosis.
- A sample of ovarian tissue may be obtained for laboratory analysis.
- Surgery may be necessary for diagnosis and staging.

 Treatment

GENERAL MEASURES

- Ovarian cancer is usually managed by hospitalization.
- Surgical staging and debulking are critical.
- Chemotherapy and/or radiotherapy may be recommended by oncologist.
- Other surgical procedures (e.g. hysterectomy) may be necessary.

ACTIVITY

As tolerated

DIET

High-protein diet

Medications

COMMONLY PRESCRIBED DRUGS

- Platinum-based regimen (cisplatin or carboplatin)
- Cyclophosphamide (Cytoxan)
- Paclitaxel (Taxol)
- Other drugs based on current protocol

CONTRAINDICATIONS

Cisplatin: impaired kidney function, hearing loss, nerve disease

PRECAUTIONS

All drugs cause bone marrow suppression. Cisplatin is toxic to the eyes, kidney, and peripheral nerves.

DRUG INTERACTIONS

Read drug product information.

OTHER DRUGS

- Etoposide
- 5-Fluorouracil
- Doxorubicin (Adriamycin)
- Melphalan, hexamethylmelamine, ifosfamide, thiotepa
- Ondansetron (Zofran), dronabinol (Marinol), metoclopramide (Reglan), and others for nausea

 ## Followup

PATIENT MONITORING

The doctor should be seen as often as needed to assess health and monitor drug therapy.

PREVENTION

Oral contraceptive agents may provide some protection.

COMPLICATIONS

- Lung disorders
- Thyroid disorder
- Accumulation of fluid in the abdomen
- Radiotherapy and chemotherapy adverse reactions
- Bowel obstruction

WHAT TO EXPECT

- Five-year survival rate depends on cancer cell type, stage, and residual disease:
  - ▶ Stage I, 80%
  - ▶ Stage II, 60%
  - ▶ Stage III, 15–30%
  - ▶ Stage IV, 10%

 ## Miscellaneous

OTHER FACTORS

N/A

PEDIATRIC

N/A

GERIATRIC

N/A

OTHERS

N/A

PREGNANCY

N/A

FURTHER INFORMATION

N/A

Section P

Painful Intercourse

 Basics

DESCRIPTION

Painful intercourse (dyspareunia) is recurring and persistent genital pain associated with intercourse, in either the male or female.

SIGNS AND SYMPTOMS

Pelvic/genital pressure, aching, tearing, and/or burning

CAUSES

- Vaginal or pelvic disorders (e.g., decreased lubrication, infection)
- Gastrointestinal disorders (e.g., inflammatory bowel disease, constipation)
- Urinary tract disorders (e.g., cystitis)
- Male reproductive disorder (e.g., muscle spasm, infection, prostate condition)
- Psychologic disorders (e.g., fear, anxiety, phobias)

SCOPE

- Most women who are sexually active will experience dyspareunia at some time in their lives. Approximately 15% of adult women will have dyspareunia on a few occasions during a year. About 1–2% of women will have painful intercourse on a more-than-occasional basis.
- Prevalence among males is unknown.

MOST OFTEN AFFECTED

All ages, females more frequently than males

RISK FACTORS

- Diabetes
- Estrogen deficiency
- Alcohol/marijuana use
- Menopause
- Medroxyprogesterone use

 Diagnosis

WHAT THE DOCTOR LOOKS FOR

- The doctor will take a history and perform a physical examination.
- Causes of dysfunction should be identified and treated, such as vaginismus (spasm of muscles of the vaginal opening).

TESTS AND PROCEDURES

- Urinalysis
- Fluid from the urinary or reproductive tract may be sampled for laboratory analysis.
- For female patient, Pap smear may be done.
- The urinary system may be assessed with a test called voiding cystourethrogram.
- X-rays of the digestive system may be done to assist in diagnosis.
- The reproductive, urinary, or intestinal systems may be visually examined by endoscopy.

 Treatment

GENERAL MEASURES

- Dyspareunia is managed in the outpatient setting.
- The first step in treatment is to educate the patient and partner about the nature of the problem and reassure them the problem can be solved.
- Referral for long-term therapy may be necessary, e.g., behavioral therapy, individual therapy, couple therapy.

ACTIVITY

Routine

DIET

Regular

Medications

COMMONLY PRESCRIBED DRUGS

Depends on the cause. May include antibiotics, estrogen, pain relievers, and lubricants.

CONTRAINDICATIONS

Read drug product information.

PRECAUTIONS

Read drug product information.

DRUG INTERACTIONS

Read drug product information.

OTHER DRUGS

N/A

 ## Followup

PATIENT MONITORING

The doctor should be seen as frequently as needed for therapy, every 6–12 months once resolved.

PREVENTION

Avoid alcohol and tobacco products.

COMPLICATIONS

N/A

WHAT TO EXPECT

The majority of cases respond to treatment.

 ## Miscellaneous

OTHER FACTORS

N/A

PEDIATRIC

N/A

GERIATRIC

The incidence of dyspareunia increases dramatically in the postmenopausal woman who is not receiving hormone replacement therapy (HRT). Over half of all sexually active women report dyspareunia.

OTHERS

N/A

PREGNANCY

Episiotomy may result in dyspareunia.

FURTHER INFORMATION

N/A

Pancreatitis

 Basics

DESCRIPTION

Pancreatitis is an inflammation of the pancreas, which may be acute or chronic.

SIGNS AND SYMPTOMS

- Abdominal pain: upper abdomen, may radiate to back
- Nausea and/or vomiting
- Mild abdominal distention
- Fever (100–101°F [37.7–38.3°C])
- Shock
- Jaundice
- Discoloration of the flank or navel
- Discoloration around the navel

CAUSES

- Gallstones
- Alcoholism and acute intoxication
- Medications
- Metabolic disorders
- Peptic ulcer (rare)
- Trauma/surgery
- Infection
- Tumor
- Systemic lupus erythematosus
- Mumps
- Cystic fibrosis
- AIDS
- Insect/animal sting

SCOPE

There are 10–22 cases of pancreatitis per 100,000 persons in the United States.

MOST OFTEN AFFECTED

Acute pancreatitis can affect all ages; chronic pancreatitis primarily affects individuals 35–45 years of age (usually related to alcohol). Males and females are affected in equal numbers.

RISK FACTORS

Listed with Causes

 Diagnosis

WHAT THE DOCTOR LOOKS FOR

The doctor will assess for the presence of pancreatitis and other conditions that can cause similar signs and symptoms.

TESTS AND PROCEDURES

- Blood tests
- X-rays of abdomen
- Ultrasound
- Computed tomography (CT scan)
- The pancreas may be examined by endoscopy.

 Treatment

- Acute pancreatitis: hospitalization, unless very mild and the patient is able to maintain oral intake
- Chronic pancreatitis: outpatient treatment except for complications

GENERAL MEASURES

- Acute pancreatitis usually requires hospitalization but may be managed on an outpatient basis if mild.
- Chronic pancreatitis is managed on an outpatient basis except for complications.
- Surgery may be required.

ACTIVITY

- Acute pancreatitis: usually bed rest, although sitting in a chair may be more comfortable.
- Chronic pancreatitis: not restricted

DIET

- Acute pancreatitis: small amounts of high-carbohydrate, low-fat, and low-protein foods
- Chronic pancreatitis: small meals high in protein

Medications

COMMONLY PRESCRIBED DRUGS

- Meperidine (Demerol)
- Analgesics: acetaminophen (Tylenol), oxycodone-acetaminophen (Tylox), hydrocodone-acetaminophen (Vicodin), propoxyphene napsylate
- Pancreatic enzyme (Pancrease MT, Creon)
- H_2-blockers

CONTRAINDICATIONS

Read drug product information.

PRECAUTIONS

Narcotic addiction

DRUG INTERACTIONS

Read drug product information.

OTHER DRUGS

N/A

 ## Followup

PATIENT MONITORING

- The doctor should be seen as often as needed.
- The cause of pancreatitis should be identified and treated.

PREVENTION

Avoid alcohol.

COMPLICATIONS

Pancreas damage with subsequent diabetes mellitus

WHAT TO EXPECT

- Acute pancreatitis: In 85–90% of patients, the condition resolves spontaneously; 3–5% mortality rate.
- Chronic pancreatitis: Patients may have recurrent acute episodes.

 ## Miscellaneous

OTHER FACTORS

N/A

PEDIATRIC

Pancreatitis can sometimes accompany mumps.

GERIATRIC

N/A

OTHERS

N/A

PREGNANCY

N/A

FURTHER INFORMATION

National Digestive Diseases Information Clearinghouse, Box NDDIC, Bethesda, MD 20892, (301) 468-6344

Parkinson's Disease

 ## Basics

DESCRIPTION

Parkinson's disease is a degenerative disorder of the central nervous system that affects adults. The condition is marked by tremors at rest, rigidity, and slow movement.

SIGNS AND SYMPTOMS

- Tremor
- Slow movement
- Rigidity
- Speech is poorly enunciated, low volume, clipped
- Eye abnormalities: decreased blinking, spasm of eye lid
- Seborrhea
- Constipation, incontinence, sexual dysfunction
- Depression
- Dementia
- Walking disturbances: no arm swing, problems standing up from chair
- Neglect of swallowing with drooling

CAUSES

Unknown

SCOPE

Parkinson's disease affects 50,000 persons annually in the United States.

MOST OFTEN AFFECTED

Individuals 60 years of age and older; slightly more common in males; may be inherited

RISK FACTORS

Unknown

 ## Diagnosis

WHAT THE DOCTOR LOOKS FOR

- The doctor will perform a physical examination to identify the signs and symptoms of Parkinson's disease.
- Numerous other conditions that can appear similar to Parkinson's disease should be ruled out.

TESTS AND PROCEDURES

Computed tomography (CT scan), magnetic resonance imaging (MRI) or positron emission tomography (PET) may be done to assist in diagnosis.

 ## Treatment

GENERAL MEASURES

- Parkinson's disease is managed in the outpatient setting except for complications or elective surgery.
- Drugs have therapeutic and toxic effects.
- Worsening symptoms may indicate noncompliance with drug therapy, depression, or another illness.
- Course is progressive with or without drugs. Life-long therapy is directed toward control of symptoms and treatment of disability.
- Physical, occupational, and speech therapy may be useful.
- Patient's physical limitations may require many adjustments in the home; e.g., special chairs, elevated toilet seat, eating utensils, assistance with dressing.
- Surgery may be recommended.

ACTIVITY

Maintain activity to whatever degree possible; use cane for walking.

DIET

- Small frequent meals if eating is difficult
- High liquid intake important; high bulk foods
- Reduced protein diet is unnecessary.

Parkinson's Disease

 Medications

COMMONLY PRESCRIBED DRUGS

- Selegiline, 5 milligrams in the morning and at noon
- Levodopa-carbidopa (Sinemet, Sinemet SR)
- Bromocriptine
- Pergolide
- Trihexyphenidyl (Artane)
- Benztropine (Cogentin)
- Amantadine

CONTRAINDICATIONS

Read drug product information.

PRECAUTIONS

Numerous precautions; read drug product information.

DRUG INTERACTIONS

Most of the drugs have additive therapeutic and side effects.

OTHER DRUGS

- Tricyclic antidepressants
- Apomorphine
- Clozapine

 Followup

PATIENT MONITORING

The doctor should be seen frequently to monitor health status, drug therapy, and physical therapy.

PREVENTION

Avoid drugs known to cause tardive dyskinesia, such as fluphenazine, perphenazine, prochlorperazine, thiopropazate, trifluoperazine, promazine, thioridazine, haloperidol, droperidol, benperidol, fluspirilene, pimozide, trifluperidol, chlorprothixene, clopenthixol, and thiothixene.

WHAT TO EXPECT

Parkinson's disease is slowly progressive.

COMPLICATIONS

Dementia, depression, pneumonia, falls, freezing, movement difficulty; also associated with a 2-fold increase in risk of death

 Miscellaneous

OTHER FACTORS

N/A

PEDIATRIC

N/A

GERIATRIC

Common among elderly

OTHERS

N/A

PREGNANCY

N/A

FURTHER INFORMATION

- United Parkinson Foundation, 360 W. Superior St., Chicago, IL 60610, (312) 664-2344
- Parkinson's Education Program—USA, 3900 Birch Street, 105, Newport Beach, CA 92660, (800) 344-7872

Parvovirus B19 Infection

 Basics

DESCRIPTION

Human parvovirus B19 is the primary cause of erythema infectiosum (EI, or fifth disease). It can cause arthritis and joint pain, and in some persons can cause aplastic anemia. In a pregnant woman, the virus can cross the placenta and infect the fetus.

SIGNS AND SYMPTOMS

- Rash on the face ("slapped cheek appearance") followed 1–4 days later by a second-stage rash on the trunk and limbs
- Itching and mild joint pain
- Headache, sore throat, runny nose, joint and muscle aches, and gastrointestinal disturbances are more frequent and severe in adults.
- 80% of adults may experience arthritis or joint pain.
- In children, joint symptoms are less common.

CAUSES

Viral infection; virus can be transmitted to fetus during pregnancy

SCOPE

Parvovirus is extremely common. 50% of adults have evidence of prior infection. Parvovirus infection is most common as community epidemics in winter and spring in nontropical regions.

MOST OFTEN AFFECTED

- Infection is common in childhood.
- Peak age for illness is 4–12 years of age.
- Males and females are affected in equal numbers.

RISK FACTORS

- Anemia
- Immune system disorders
- Intrauterine infection

 Diagnosis

WHAT THE DOCTOR LOOKS FOR

- The doctor will perform a physical examination to identify the presence of parvovirus infection.
- Numerous other conditions that can cause similar signs and symptoms should be ruled out, including rubella (german measles), other viral infections, systemic lupus erythematosus, drug reaction, Lyme disease, and rheumatoid arthritis.

TESTS AND PROCEDURES

- Blood tests
- If patient is pregnant, fetal ultrasound, amniocentesis, or chorionic villus sampling (CVS) may be done.

 Treatment

GENERAL MEASURES

- Parvovirus infection is usually managed in the outpatient setting.
- Individuals with severe symptoms may require hospitalization

ACTIVITY

- Unrestricted
- Individuals with arthritis may require physical therapy or an exercise program.

DIET

No special diet

Medications

- Usually, no treatment is needed.

COMMONLY PRESCRIBED DRUGS (IF NEEDED)

- Intravenous immune globulin (IVIG)
- Blood transfusions
- Anti-inflammatory agents may alleviate arthritic symptoms.

CONTRAINDICATIONS

Read drug product information.

PRECAUTIONS

Read drug product information.

DRUG INTERACTIONS

Read drug product information.

OTHER DRUGS

None

 ## Followup

PATIENT MONITORING

The doctor should be seen often for repeat blood tests.

PREVENTION

- Standard hygienic practices can minimize spread.
- Because the illness is so common, it is not possible to avoid exposure completely.
- Pregnant health care workers should avoid caring for patients with bone marrow disorders.
- Pregnant child care workers are at some increased risk; however, exclusion from the work place will not eliminate this risk, and exclusion is not recommended.

COMPLICATIONS

- Complications are rare, but they are more commonly seen in adults than children.
- Arthritis
- Persistent anemia
- Blood disorders
- Lung inflammation
- Brain disease
- Reports of birth defects, but no clear-cut association

WHAT TO EXPECT

- Usually self-limited
- Joint symptoms subside in weeks
- Full recovery in 2 to 3 weeks

 ## Miscellaneous

OTHER FACTORS

N/A

PEDIATRIC

N/A

GERIATRIC

None known

OTHERS

N/A

PREGNANCY

See above

FURTHER INFORMATION

N/A

Pelvic Inflammatory Disease (PID)

 Basics

DESCRIPTION

Pelvic inflammatory disease (PID) is caused by bacterial infection of the female reproductive tract. PID is a broad term that includes a variety of upper genital tract infections unrelated to pregnancy or surgical procedures.

SIGNS AND SYMPTOMS

- May cause no symptoms
- Lower abdominal pain
- Fever and malaise
- Vaginal discharge
- Irregular bleeding
- Urinary discomfort
- Bowel inflammation
- Nausea and vomiting
- Abdominal tenderness
- Tender cervix

CAUSES

Bacterial infection

SCOPE

An estimated 1 million women are treated for PID annually in the United States.

MOST OFTEN AFFECTED

Females 16–40 years of age

RISK FACTORS

- Sexually active, reproductive age
- Most common in adolescents
- Multiple sexual partners
- Use of an intrauterine device (IUD)
- Previous history of PID
- Cervicitis
- Gonorrhea
- Condoms and vaginal spermicides lessen the risks of PID.
- Oral contraceptives may reduce the risk of PID.

 Diagnosis

WHAT THE DOCTOR LOOKS FOR

- The doctor will perform a physical examination to identify PID.
- Other possible causes of similar signs and symptoms should be ruled out, such as ectopic pregnancy, appendicitis, or other medical disorders.

TESTS AND PROCEDURES

- Pregnancy test
- Blood tests
- Urinalysis
- The uterus may be sampled for culture.
- Pelvic ultrasound may be done.
- The reproductive tract may be examined by laparoscopy.

 Treatment

GENERAL MEASURES

- PID is usually managed in the outpatient setting.
- Hospitalization may be required for severe cases or other special factors.
- Avoid sex until treatment is completed.
- Sex partners should be evaluated and treated.
- Surgery may be required.

ACTIVITY

According to severity of illness

DIET

According to severity of illness

Pelvic Inflammatory Disease (PID)

Medications

COMMONLY PRESCRIBED DRUGS

Antibiotics

CONTRAINDICATIONS

Read drug product information.

PRECAUTIONS

Read drug product information.

DRUG INTERACTIONS

Read drug product information.

OTHER DRUGS

N/A

Followup

PATIENT MONITORING

- Individuals with fever or other severe symptoms should be followed closely.
- The doctor should be seen as often as necessary.
- Ultrasonography should be repeated.

PREVENTION

- Use safe sex practices.
- Use barrier contraceptives, especially condoms, and spermicidal creams or sponges.
- Evaluation and treatment of sex partners
- Comply with management instructions.
- Seek medical care early when genital lesions or discharge appear.
- Seek routine check-ups for sexually transmitted diseases (STDs) if in nonmutually monogamous relationship

COMPLICATIONS

- Abscess
- Recurrent infection
- Increased risk of ectopic pregnancy
- Tubal infertility
- Chronic pelvic pain

WHAT TO EXPECT

- PID has a wide variation in outcome with good prognosis if early, effective therapy is instituted and further infection is avoided.
- Poor prognosis is related to late therapy and continued unsafe lifestyle.

Miscellaneous

OTHER FACTORS

N/A

PEDIATRIC

- PID is rare before puberty.
- Adolescents are highly vulnerable to STDs including PID.

GERIATRIC

PID is rare after menopause.

OTHERS

N/A

PREGNANCY

PID is rare during pregnancy but occurs occasionally.

FURTHER INFORMATION

Information Services, Centers for Disease Control, E06, Atlanta, GA 30333, (404) 639-1819

Peptic Ulcer Disease

 ## Basics

DESCRIPTION

A peptic ulcer is an ulcer in the lining of the gastrointestinal tract.

SIGNS AND SYMPTOMS

- Gnawing or burning upper abdominal pain 1–3 hours after meals, relieved by food or antacids
- Nocturnal pain causing early morning awakening
- Dyspepsia: belching, bloating, abdominal distention, food intolerance
- Heartburn
- Dizziness, fainting, blood in vomit, tarry stool
- Feeling full early in meal
- Weight loss

CAUSES

The cause of ulcers involves multiple factors. The bacteria *Heliobacter pylori* is found in 75–90% or more of ulcer patients. Other physiological factors are involved.

SCOPE

There are 200,000–500,000 new cases of peptic ulcer disease annually in the United States.

MOST OFTEN AFFECTED

Individuals 25–75 years of age; slightly more common in males than females

RISK FACTORS

- Cigarette smoking
- Drugs (e.g., nonsteroidal anti-inflammatory drugs [NSAIDs])
- Family history of ulcer
- Stress
- Lower socioeconomic status
- Manual labor
- Poorly or not associated: dietary spices, alcohol, caffeine, acetaminophen

 ## Diagnosis

WHAT THE DOCTOR LOOKS FOR

- The doctor will perform a history and physical examination to identify the presence of peptic ulcer.
- Numerous other conditions that can cause similar signs and symptoms should be investigated.

TESTS AND PROCEDURES

- Blood tests
- Special tests may be done to assess gastric function.
- The stomach may be examined by endoscopy.
- A sample of the digestive tract lining may be obtained by biopsy for laboratory analysis.
- Exploratory surgery may be recommended.

 ## Treatment

GENERAL MEASURES

- Hospitalization and surgery may be required for perforation or bleeding.
- Avoid cigarette smoking.
- Reduce use of NSAIDs.
- Reduce stress.

ACTIVITY

Fully active for uncomplicated disease, exercise to tolerance after hemorrhage

DIET

Three regular meals daily with avoidance of dietary irritants

Medications

COMMONLY PRESCRIBED DRUGS

- H_2-blockers: ranitidine, nizatidine, cimetidine, famotidine
- Omeprazole, lansoprazole
- Antibiotics to treat *H. pylori*

CONTRAINDICATIONS

Allergies to antibiotics

PRECAUTIONS

Antibiotic-related side effects include diarrhea, nausea/vomiting, unpleasant taste in mouth, rash, colitis, and severe allergic reaction.

DRUG INTERACTIONS

Many drug interactions; read drug product information.

OTHER DRUGS

- Sucralfate
- Antacids: magnesium hydroxide, aluminum hydroxide

 ## Followup

PATIENT MONITORING

The doctor should be seen as often as needed to asses health status and monitor treatment.

PREVENTION

- Eradication of *H. pylori*
- Maintenance therapy
- Bleeding ulcers may require continued maintenance therapy even if *H. pylori* is eradicated.

COMPLICATIONS

- Hemorrhage
- Perforation
- Intestinal obstruction

WHAT TO EXPECT

- Relapse rates after antibiotic treatment is low.
- Re-infection rate is less than 1% per year.

 ## Miscellaneous

OTHER FACTORS

N/A

PEDIATRIC

Peptic ulcers are uncommon before puberty.

GERIATRIC

N/A

OTHERS

N/A

PREGNANCY

Use medications with caution in pregnancy.

FURTHER INFORMATION

National Digestive Diseases Information Clearinghouse, Box NDDIC, Bethesda, MD 20892, (301) 468-6344

Pink Eye

 ## Basics

DESCRIPTION

Conjunctivitis, also called "pink eye," is the inflammation of the inner surface of the eye lid or the "white" of the eye.

SIGNS AND SYMPTOMS

- Red eyes
- Burning sensation
- Foreign body sensation
- Itching
- Excessive tearing
- Matting of eye lashes
- Swelling
- Drooping of the eye lid
- Sensitivity to light
- Visual impairment does not occur

CAUSES

- Bacteria, including Chlamydia
- Viral
- Allergic reaction
- Irritation (home/industrial chemicals, wind, smoke, ultraviolet light)
- Other infections

SCOPE

Conjunctivitis is common in the United States.

MOST OFTEN AFFECTED

Affects all ages, males and females in equal proportion

RISK FACTORS

Numerous, including trauma from wind, cold and heat; chemicals; and foreign body

 ## Diagnosis

WHAT THE DOCTOR LOOKS FOR

The doctor will examine the eye for signs of conjunctivitis, as well as for a foreign body or other conditions.

TESTS AND PROCEDURES

Fluid from eye may be obtained for laboratory analysis.

 ## Treatment

GENERAL MEASURES

- Conjunctivitis is managed in the outpatient setting.
- See Medications
- Ophthalmologic referral may be needed for the presence of an ulcer or herpes or if the condition worsens after 24 hours of treatment.
- Compresses: warm if infective, cold if allergic or irritative
- Remove material and debris (may require frequent irrigation).
- Discontinue use of contact lenses.

ACTIVITY

No restrictions

DIET

No restrictions

Medications

COMMONLY PRESCRIBED DRUGS

- Antibiotics: tobramycin, gentamicin, sodium sulfacetamide, erythromycin ophthalmic ointment
- Antivirals: trifluridine, acyclovir
- Chlamydial: doxycycline
- Allergic: naphazoline, antazoline (Albalon-A, Vasocon-A), oral antihistamines

CONTRAINDICATIONS

Read drug product information.

PRECAUTIONS

- Read drug product information.
- It is important to avoid contamination of medication eye droppers. Do not touch the eye with the eye dropper.

DRUG INTERACTIONS

Read drug product information.

OTHER DRUGS

Other antibiotics

 Followup

PATIENT MONITORING

The doctor should be seen if eye is worse after 24 hours of treatment.

PREVENTION

- Avoid listed causes when possible.
- Wash hands often.

COMPLICATIONS

- Scarring and other eye conditions
- Bacterial superinfection

WHAT TO EXPECT

- Bacterial: resolves within 10–14 days without treatment, 2–4 days with treatment
- Some forms of conjunctivitis may take 3–9 months to resolve without treatment, 3–5 weeks with treatment.

 Miscellaneous

OTHER FACTORS

N/A

PEDIATRIC

N/A

GERIATRIC

The elderly are more likely to have the diseases or problems listed in Causes.

OTHERS

N/A

PREGNANCY

N/A

FURTHER INFORMATION

N/A

Pinworms

 Basics

DESCRIPTION

Pinworms are parasites that infect the gastrointestinal tract and cause anal itching. Itching is usually worse at night.

SIGNS AND SYMPTOMS

- Perianal itching
- Perineal itching
- Vulvovaginitis
- Bed-wetting
- Abdominal pain
- Insomnia

CAUSES

The intestinal parasite *Enterobius* (Oxyuris) *vermicularis*

SCOPE

Pinworms affect about 20% of children 5–10 years of age.

MOST OFTEN AFFECTED

Children 5–14 years of age; females affected more often than males

RISK FACTORS

- Institutionalization (50–90% of institutionalized children have pinworms.)
- Crowded living conditions
- Poor hygiene
- Warm climate

 Diagnosis

WHAT THE DOCTOR LOOKS FOR

- The doctor will perform a physical examination to identify pinworms.
- Numerous skin conditions can appear similar to pinworms.

TESTS AND PROCEDURES

Pinworms may be directly observed; tape test may be done to identify parasite.

 Treatment

GENERAL MEASURES

- All symptomatic family members should be treated simultaneously.
- Bedclothes and underwear of infected individuals should be washed in hot water at the time of treatment (eggs can remain viable for 2 to 3 weeks in a moist environment).
- Strict hand washing can help prevent transmission.
- Practice good hygiene (showers, nail cleaning)
- Topical use of anti-itch creams or ointments may help relieve itch.

ACTIVITY

No restrictions

DIET

No restrictions

Medications

COMMONLY PRESCRIBED DRUGS

- Mebendazole (Vermox)
- Pyrantel pamoate (Antiminth)
- Thiabendazole (Mintezol)

CONTRAINDICATIONS

Read drug product information.

PRECAUTIONS

- All family members should be treated.
- Take medicine on empty stomach.
- Medication may cause diarrhea and/or nausea.

DRUG INTERACTIONS

Read drug product information.

OTHER DRUGS

N/A

 ## Followup

PATIENT MONITORING

Unnecessary unless symptoms persist after drug therapy

PREVENTION

- Careful hand washing, keep nails short and clean.
- Wash anus and genitals at least once a day, preferably in a shower.
- Don't scratch anus or put fingers near nose or mouth.

COMPLICATIONS

- Perianal scratching may cause infection.
- Young girls: infection of reproductive tract
- Urinary tract infections

WHAT TO EXPECT

- Carriers of pinworms often have no symptoms.
- Infections are cured more than 90% of the time with drug therapy.
- Re-infection is common.

 ## Miscellaneous

OTHER FACTORS

N/A

PEDIATRIC

Pinworms are more common in children.

GERIATRIC

N/A

OTHERS

N/A

PREGNANCY

Drug therapy is contraindicated in pregnancy.

FURTHER INFORMATION

Centers for Disease Control, Dept. of Health and Human Services, Office of Public Affairs, Atlanta, GA 30333, (404) 329-3534

Pneumonia, Bacterial

 Basics

DESCRIPTION

Bacterial pneumonia is an acute (of short duration) bacterial infection of the lung.

SCOPE

- There are about 1,200 cases of bacterial pneumonia per 100,000 persons annually in the United States. Among hospitalized individuals, there are 800 cases of hospital-acquired bacterial pneumonia per 100,000 patients annually.

MOST OFTEN AFFECTED

Extremes of age: the very young and the very old; more frequent in males

SIGNS AND SYMPTOMS

- Cough and fever
- Chest pain (pleuritic)
- Chill, with sudden onset
- Dark, thick or rusty (bloody) sputum
- Rapid (or slow) heart rate
- Rapid breathing rate
- Bluish discoloration around eyes, lips and nail beds
- Changes in the level of consciousness
- Anxiety, confusion, restlessness, and meningeal signs
- Abdominal pain
- Loss of appetite
- Profuse sweating
- Muscle aches
- Pinpoint bruises

CAUSES

Bacterial infection, spread by air or blood

RISK FACTORS

- Recent viral infections
- Extremes of age
- Alcoholism
- Acquired Immune Deficiency Syndrome (AIDS) or other immune system disorders
- Smoking
- Kidney failure
- Cardiovascular disease
- Lung disease
- Diabetes mellitus
- Malnutrition
- Cancer
- Occupational exposure

 Diagnosis

WHAT THE DOCTOR LOOKS FOR

- The doctor will perform a physical examination to identify pneumonia.
- Bacterial pneumonia may be caused by a number of different organisms; many other respiratory diseases may appear similar to pneumonia.

TESTS AND PROCEDURES

- Blood tests
- Blood culture
- Chest x-ray
- Fluid from the airway may be sampled for culture.
- The lower airway may be examined by bronchoscopy.
- The fluids from the chest cavity may be obtained by thoracentesis for laboratory analysis.

Pneumonia, Bacterial

 Treatment

GENERAL MEASURES

- Mild cases of bacterial pneumonia are managed in the outpatient setting.
- Severe cases require hospitalization.
- Antibiotic therapy
- Respiratory support as needed
- Maintain fluid and salt balance.
- Pain relievers
- Respiratory isolation if tuberculosis suspected

ACTIVITY

Bed rest and/or reduced activity during acute phase

DIET

- Nothing by mouth if there is risk of respiratory failure.
- Consider soft, easy-to-eat foods

 Medications

COMMONLY PRESCRIBED DRUGS

Antibiotics

CONTRAINDICATIONS

Allergy to prescribed drugs

PRECAUTIONS

Read drug product information.

DRUG INTERACTIONS

Read drug product information.

OTHER DRUGS

Other antibiotics

 Followup

PATIENT MONITORING

- The doctor should be seen every day during the acute phase. Contact primary care provider if no improvement or getting worse in 48 to 72 hours.
- Repeat chest x-rays

PREVENTION

- Reduce risk factors where possible.
- Avoid use of antibiotics during minor viral infections.
- Annual flu vaccine for high-risk individuals
- Pneumococcal vaccine

COMPLICATIONS

- Severe infection
- Multiple organ failure
- Adult respiratory distress syndrome (ARDS)

WHAT TO EXPECT

- Usual course in otherwise healthy individual is improvement and fever resolution in 1–3 days.
- Overall death rate is about 5%.
- Poorest prognosis: extremes of age, spread of infection to blood, presence of other medical disease, immune system disorders

 Miscellaneous

OTHER FACTORS

N/A

PEDIATRIC

The risk of illness and death is high in children under 1 year of age.

GERIATRIC

The risk of illness and death is high among those over 70 years of age, especially if there are other disease or risk factors.

OTHERS

N/A

PREGNANCY

N/A

FURTHER INFORMATION

American Lung Association, 1740 Broadway, New York, NY 100019 (212) 315-8700

Peumonia, Viral

 Basics

DESCRIPTION

Viral pneumonia is an inflammatory disease of the lungs caused by viral infection.

SIGNS AND SYMPTOMS

- Fever
- Chills
- Cough (with or without sputum production)
- Difficulty breathing
- Noisy breathing
- Altered breath sounds
- Chest pain
- Headache
- Muscle ache
- Malaise
- Gastrointestinal symptoms

CAUSES

Viral infection

SCOPE

- About 90% of childhood pneumonia is viral.
- 4–39% of pneumonia in adults is caused by a virus.
- Prevalence is unknown and variable due to seasonal variation, although it is more common in winter months.
- Mixed infections with bacteria is common.

MOST OFTEN AFFECTED

More common in children than in adults; males and females affected in equal frequency

RISK FACTORS

- Immune system disorders
- Living in close quarters
- Seasonal: epidemic upper respiratory illness
- Elderly
- Heart disease
- Chronic lung disease
- Recent upper respiratory infection

 Diagnosis

WHAT THE DOCTOR LOOKS FOR

- The doctor will perform a physical examination to assess the presence of viral pneumonia.
- Similar signs and symptoms can be caused by other forms of pneumonia, cancer, and other lung diseases.

TESTS AND PROCEDURES

- Blood tests
- Sputum culture
- Chest x-ray
- The throat may be swabbed for laboratory analysis.
- The lower airway may be examined by bronchoscopy.

 Treatment

GENERAL MEASURES

- Most cases of viral pneumonia are managed in the outpatient setting.
- Infants under 4 months of age, the elderly, and individuals with severe infection are managed by hospitalization.
- Encourage coughing and deep breathing exercises to clear secretions.
- Careful disposal of secretions/body fluids
- Maintain adequate fluid intake.
- Respiratory isolation for highly contagious viruses

ACTIVITY

Rest

DIET

Increase fluids; eat a high-calorie, high-protein, soft diet

Medications

COMMONLY PRESCRIBED DRUGS

- Amantadine (Symmetrel)
- Acyclovir (Zovirax)
- Ganciclovir (Cytovene)
- Ribavirin (Virazole)

CONTRAINDICATIONS

Read drug product information.

PRECAUTIONS

- Amantadine should be used cautiously in patients with liver disease, epilepsy, kidney disease, or eczema and individuals with a history of psychotic illness.
- Ribavirin causes birth defects and should not be taken by pregnant women.

DRUG INTERACTIONS

Read drug product information.

OTHER DRUGS

- Rimantadine (Flumadine)
- Antibiotics
- Foscarnet (Foscavir)
- Immune globulin, intravenous (IVIG)

Followup

PATIENT MONITORING

The doctor should be seen as often as necessary.

PREVENTION

- Influenza A and B vaccine
- For those patients unable to receive influenza vaccine (egg allergy or other) and are at high risk, amantadine or rimantadine can be given.
- Health care workers who are pregnant need to take proper precautions to avoid infectious patients.
- Measles vaccine
- Varicella zoster vaccine

COMPLICATIONS

- Bacterial infections
- Respiratory failure
- Adult respiratory distress syndrome (ARDS)

WHAT TO EXPECT

Usually favorable prognosis with illness lasting several days to a week. Post-viral fatigue is common. However, death can occur, especially in pediatric or bone-marrow transplant infections or among the elderly stricken with influenza.

Miscellaneous

OTHER FACTORS

N/A

PEDIATRIC

Some viral infections in children are serious.

GERIATRIC

The elderly have the greatest risk of illness and death.

OTHERS

N/A

PREGNANCY

Pregnant women should avoid contact with persons who may have viral infections.

FURTHER INFORMATION

American Lung Association, 1740 Broadway, New York, NY 100919, (212) 315-8700

Post-Traumatic Stress Disorder (PTSD)

 Basics

DESCRIPTION

Post-traumatic stress disorder (PTSD) is a condition seen in people who have experienced an event that would be extremely distressing to most human beings; e.g., serious threat to one's life, physical, or psychological integrity; serious threat or harm to one's children, spouse, siblings, parents, or other close relatives or friends; sudden destruction of one's home or community; seeing another person who has recently been (or is being) injured or killed as a result of a man-made violent act or natural disaster.

SIGNS AND SYMPTOMS

- Recurrent and intrusive distressing recollections of the event
- Recurrent distressing dreams of the event
- Acting or feeling as if the traumatic event were recurring
- Reactions such as increased heart rate, changes in blood pressure, discoloration of the skin, blurred vision, nausea, vomiting, diarrhea, urinary urgency, etc.
- Efforts to avoid thoughts, feelings, or conversations associated with the trauma
- Efforts to avoid activities, places, or people that arouse recollections of the trauma
- Inability to recall an important aspect of the trauma (psychogenic amnesia)
- Diminished interest in significant activities
- Feelings of detachment or estrangement from others
- Sense of a foreshortened future (e.g., does not expect to have a career, marriage, or a normal life span)
- Difficulty falling or staying asleep (insomnia)
- Irritability or outbursts of anger
- Difficulty in concentrating
- Hypervigilance
- Exaggerated startle response
- Lasts longer than 1 month
- Causes significant impairment in social, occupational, or other areas of functioning

CAUSES

Events that threaten one's personal integrity, self-esteem, and security are psychologically traumatic and may lead to PTSD.

SCOPE

Up to 30% of victims of disasters develop PTSD. Up to 14% of the U.S. population experience PTSD at some point.

MOST OFTEN AFFECTED

The elderly and the very young are more vulnerable to PTSD.

RISK FACTORS

Individuals with a history of childhood neglect, abuse, or dysfunctional families and children of alcoholic parents are predisposed and more susceptible to developing PTSD in response to trauma.

Post-Traumatic Stress Disorder (PTSD)

 Diagnosis

WHAT THE DOCTOR LOOKS FOR

The doctor will assess the person to determine whether PTSD exists, or whether symptoms are due to some other emotional, mental, or behavioral disorder.

TESTS AND PROCEDURES

- Neuropsychological testing
- Electroencephalograph (EEG) to rule out brain damage
- Sleep studies
- Computed tomography (CT scan) and magnetic resonance imaging (MRI) may be done.

 Treatment

GENERAL MEASURES

- As indicated by the individual's general condition, treatment includes individual psychotherapy, group therapy, hypnotherapy, narcoanalysis and narcosynthesis, and behavior therapy.
- Crisis intervention shortly after the traumatic event is valuable for the immediate distress and may prevent the development of a chronic or delayed form of PTSD.
- Relaxation exercises to help reduce anxiety and improve sleep have been found to be helpful.

ACTIVITY

- As indicated by patient's physical condition
- Restoration of regular sleep at night is essential in cases of insomnia.

DIET

A healthy diet of complex carbohydrates, proteins, and multi-vitamins and minerals. Avoid fatty foods.

Post-Traumatic Stress Disorder (PTSD)

 Medications

COMMONLY PRESCRIBED DRUGS

- Fluoxetine
- Sertraline
- Paroxetine
- Venlafaxine
- Doxepin
- Nortriptyline
- Imipramine
- Desipramine
- Amitriptyline
- Trimipramine
- Protriptyline
- Amoxapine
- Maprotiline
- Phenelzine
- Trazodone
- Nefazodone
- Bupropion
- Neuroleptics
- Benzodiazepines

CONTRAINDICATIONS

- Allergic reactions to specific drugs
- Use with caution in alcoholic patients with poor liver function.

PRECAUTIONS

- Do not mix tricyclic antidepressants with monoamine oxidase (MAO) inhibitors.
- Long-term use of benzodiazepines may lead to increased tolerance and drug dependency.

DRUG INTERACTIONS

MAO inhibitors may interact with other antidepressants. Stimulants, such as pseudoephedrine, and many foods interact with tyramine.

OTHER DRUGS

- Clomipramine, fluvoxamine, fluoxetine
- Buspirone
- Propranolol, clonidine

Post-Traumatic Stress Disorder (PTSD)

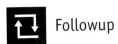 Followup

PATIENT MONITORING

Psychotherapy for at least 1 hour per week is necessary in the first phase of treatment.

PREVENTION

Crisis intervention immediately after the traumatic event involving intensive support and treatment may prevent the development of chronic PTSD later.

COMPLICATIONS

Suicide, self-inflicted violence

WHAT TO EXPECT

- The lack of crisis intervention immediately following the trauma may lead to the persistence of symptoms.
- If symptoms persist over 3 months, patients may develop chronic PTSD which may lead to loss of job, marital conflicts, total disability, and repeated and/or lengthy hospitalizations.
- The onset of symptoms may be 6 months or more after the traumatic event.

 Miscellaneous

OTHER FACTORS

N/A

PEDIATRIC

Young children are susceptible to abuse and neglect and can develop chronic PTSD with failure to progress and grow in a healthy way.

GERIATRIC

The elderly have fewer social support resources and their adjustment to trauma is less flexible. Also, they are more sensitive to medication.

OTHERS

N/A

PREGNANCY

Avoid drugs in the first trimester. Try nondrug treatment techniques such as psychotherapy, hypnotherapy, relaxation therapy, etc.

FURTHER INFORMATION

N/A

Pre-eclampsia

 Basics

DESCRIPTION

Pre-eclampsia is hypertension associated with edema and acute excessive weight gain developing during pregnancy after 20 weeks gestation.

SIGNS AND SYMPTOMS

- Elevated blood pressure
- Swelling
- Rapid excessive weight gain (more than 5 pounds per week)
- Epigastric pain
- Headache
- Visual disturbances
- Apprehension
- Amnesia
- Scant or absent urine

CAUSES

- Altered cardiovascular reaction
- Disorders of blood or blood vessels
- Hypertension

SCOPE

Preeclampsia affects 5–10% of all pregnancies.

MOST OFTEN AFFECTED

- Young women pregnant for the first time
- Women over 35 years of age

RISK FACTORS

- Family history of preeclampsia
- Lower socio-economic status
- Multiple fetuses
- Teenage mother
- Connective tissue disorders
- Age over 35
- First pregnancy
- Diabetes mellitus of pregnancy
- Chronic hypertension
- History of kidney disease

 Diagnosis

WHAT THE DOCTOR LOOKS FOR

- The doctor will assess for the presence of pre-eclampsia.
- Other factors should be considered, such as pre-existing hypertension that may be induced or worsened by pregnancy.

TESTS AND PROCEDURES

- Blood tests
- Urinalysis

 Treatment

GENERAL MEASURES

- A mild case of preeclampsia may be managed in the outpatient setting.
- Moderate or changing case of preeclampsia requires hospitalization.
- If preeclampsia is severe, delivery of fetus as soon as possible

ACTIVITY

- Bed rest on left side
- Walk only to bathroom

DIET

No salt restriction

Medications

COMMONLY PRESCRIBED DRUGS

Magnesium sulfate

CONTRAINDICATIONS

Read drug product information.

PRECAUTIONS

Read drug product information.

DRUG INTERACTIONS

Read drug product information.

OTHER DRUGS

- Hydralazine (Apresoline)
- Diazoxide
- Diazepam (Valium)

 ## Followup

PATIENT MONITORING

The doctor should be seen often to monitor health status.

PREVENTION

- Weight control
- Recent data indicates that low-dose aspirin may sometimes prevent preeclampsia.

COMPLICATIONS

- Eclampsia (seizures)
- Hypertensive crisis
- Acute kidney disease
- Acute liver disease
- Acute lung disease

WHAT TO EXPECT

Prevention of seizures and delivery of viable baby with prompt and appropriate treatment

 ## Miscellaneous

OTHER FACTORS

N/A

PEDIATRIC

There is an increased risk of pre-eclampsia among teenagers.

GERIATRIC

N/A

OTHERS

Older pregnant females (older than 35 years of age) have an increased risk of pre-eclampsia.

PREGNANCY

N/A

FURTHER INFORMATION

N/A

Premature Labor

 Basics

DESCRIPTION

Premature labor is labor occurring prior to the completion of 36 weeks' gestation.

SIGNS AND SYMPTOMS

- Regular uterine contractions, with or without pain, continuing for 1 hour
- Dull, low backache; pressure; or pain
- Intermittent lower abdominal or thigh pain
- Intestinal cramping, with or without diarrhea or indigestion
- Change in vaginal discharge
- Palpable contractions on examination
- Dilatation of the cervix
- Effacement of the cervix
- Signs of ruptured membranes

CAUSES

- Infections
- Uterine abnormalities
- Over-distention of uterus
- Premature rupture of membranes
- Unknown

SCOPE

Premature labor affects 8–12% of all births in the United States.

MOST OFTEN AFFECTED

Women of childbearing age

RISK FACTORS

- Prior preterm delivery
- Multiple gestation
- Three or more first-trimester abortions
- Previous second-trimester abortion
- Abdominal surgery during pregnancy
- Uterine or cervical disorders
- Complications of pregnancy
- Fetal abnormalities
- Serious maternal infection
- Second-trimester bleeding
- Low prepregnancy weight: less than 45 kilograms (100 pounds)
- Single parent
- No prenatal care

 Diagnosis

WHAT THE DOCTOR LOOKS FOR

- The doctor will assess the degree of premature labor.
- The doctor will look for signs and symptoms of associated conditions, such as dehydration, infection, and muscular back pain.

TESTS AND PROCEDURES

- Urinalysis and urine culture
- Testing for infection
- Amniocentesis may be done.
- Ultrasound

 Treatment

GENERAL MEASURES

- Premature labor may be managed in the out-patient setting or by hospitalization, depending on circumstances.
- Underlying risk factors should be treated with appropriate measures (antibiotics, hydration).
- If delivery is inevitable, but not immediate, mother may be transported to a tertiary care center or hospital equipped with a neonatal intensive care unit.
- No sexual intercourse

ACTIVITY

- Bed rest. Discontinue work or other physical activities.
- Hospitalization may be necessary.

DIET

Liquids only, if delivery becomes imminent

Medications

COMMONLY PRESCRIBED DRUGS

- Terbutaline
- Ritodrine
- Magnesium sulfate
- Glucocorticoids: betamethasone, dexamethasone, hydrocortisone

CONTRAINDICATIONS

Read drug product information.

PRECAUTIONS

Read drug product information.

DRUG INTERACTIONS

Read drug product information.

OTHER DRUGS

N/A

Followup

PATIENT MONITORING

Weekly office visits for women at high risk for preterm labor.

PREVENTION

Close observation; call physician or go to the hospital if contractions last for more than an hour or if low back pain, change in vaginal discharge, "menstrual cramping" or intestinal cramping occur.

COMPLICATIONS

Premature birth

WHAT TO EXPECT

- If membranes are ruptured, delivery generally occurs within 3 to 7 days.
- If membranes are intact, the woman is treated until 37 weeks of gestation.

Miscellaneous

OTHER FACTORS

N/A

PEDIATRIC

N/A

GERIATRIC

N/A

OTHERS

N/A

PREGNANCY

Premature labor is a problem of pregnancy.

FURTHER INFORMATION

N/A

Premenstrual Syndrome (PMS)

 Basics

DESCRIPTION

Premenstrual syndrome (PMS) is a constellation of symptoms that occurs prior to menstruation and is severe enough to interfere significantly with the patient's life.

SIGNS AND SYMPTOMS

- Depressed mood
- Mood swings
- Irritability
- Difficulty concentrating
- Fatigue
- Swelling
- Breast tenderness
- Headaches
- Sleep disturbances

CAUSES

Unknown, presumed hormonal

SCOPE

Almost all women have some symptoms prior to menses. A low percentage have actual PMS.

MOST OFTEN AFFECTED

Women in the childbearing years, worse during late 20s and 30s

RISK FACTORS

- Other diseases (i.e., depression)
- Caffeine and high-fluid intake
- Stress
- Increasing age

 Diagnosis

WHAT THE DOCTOR LOOKS FOR

The doctor will take a thorough history and perform an examination to identify the presence of PMS.

TESTS AND PROCEDURES

The individual may be asked to track symptoms for several months.

 Treatment

GENERAL MEASURES

- Increase daily exercise.
- Eat regular, balanced meals.
- Stop smoking.
- Get regular sleep.
- Stress reduction
- Individual or couples counseling
- Support groups

ACTIVITY

- No restrictions
- Exercise is recommended.

DIET

- Frequent, small meals
- Low-salt, high-carbohydrate diet
- Reduce caffeine intake.

Medications

- No single drug works for all women.

COMMONLY PRESCRIBED DRUGS

- Diuretics
- Pain relievers
- Anti-depressants: fluoxetine, sertraline, clomipramine, or nortriptyline
- Alprazolam
- Buspirone
- Magnesium
- Calcium
- Vitamin B6
- Vitamin E
- Evening primrose oil
- Bromocriptine
- Danazol

CONTRAINDICATIONS

Read drug product information.

PRECAUTIONS

Read drug product information.

DRUG INTERACTIONS

Read drug product information.

OTHER DRUGS

- Oral contraceptives may help.
- Progesterone

 ## Followup

PATIENT MONITORING

The doctor should be seen as often as necessary for general support and further patient education.

PREVENTION

N/A

COMPLICATIONS

N/A

WHAT TO EXPECT

Many patients adequately control their symptoms.

 ## Miscellaneous

OTHER FACTORS

N/A

PEDIATRIC

N/A

GERIATRIC

N/A

OTHERS

N/A

PREGNANCY

N/A

FURTHER INFORMATION

N/A

Prostate Cancer

 Basics

DESCRIPTION

Cancer of the prostate, a walnut-sized gland located at the base of the urinary bladder of men

SIGNS AND SYMPTOMS

- May have no symptoms
- Difficulty urination
- Blood in urine (rare)
- Urinary tract infection
- Bone pain
- Weight loss
- Anemia
- Shortness of breath
- Enlarged lymph nodes

CAUSES

Unknown

SCOPE

Prostate cancer affects 69 out of 100,000 persons in the United States.

PREDOMINANT AGE

Primarily affects men 50–60 years of age

RISK FACTORS

- Genetic predisposition
- Hormonal influences
- Exposure to chemical carcinogens
- Sexually transmitted diseases
- Male over 60 years of age
- Increased risk with vasectomy has been newly proposed but is unsupported.

 Diagnosis

WHAT THE DOCTOR LOOKS FOR

The doctor will perform a physical examination, including a rectal exam, to identify the presence of prostate cancer.

TESTS AND PROCEDURES

- Blood tests: prostate specific antigen (PSA)
- Urinalysis
- Computerized tomography (CT scan) and magnetic resonance imaging (MRI) may be done.
- Ultrasound
- A sample of prostate, lymph node, or bone may be obtained for laboratory analysis.

 Treatment

GENERAL MEASURES

- Prostate cancer is managed in the outpatient setting except for surgery requiring hospitalization.
- Conservative or palliative treatment for men over age 70
- Radiation therapy
- Hormone therapy
- Surgery may be required.

ACTIVITY

Full activity

DIET

No special diet

Medications

COMMONLY PRESCRIBED DRUGS

- Flutamide (Eulexin)
- Leuprolide (Lupron)

CONTRAINDICATIONS

None

PRECAUTIONS

- Flare of disease
- Fluid retention
- Nausea
- Vomiting
- Hot flashes
- Liver changes

DRUG INTERACTIONS

Read drug product information.

OTHER DRUGS

None

 ## Followup

PATIENT MONITORING

The doctor should be seen (including blood tests) every 3 months for 1 year, then every 6 months for a year, then annual exams thereafter.

PREVENTION

None

COMPLICATIONS

- Cardiac failure
- Phlebitis
- Fractures

WHAT TO EXPECT

- With early diagnosis and treatment, prostate cancer should be curable.
- Advanced unresponsive disease progresses in an average of 18 months.

 ## Miscellaneous

OTHER FACTORS

N/A

PEDIATRIC

Does not occur in children

GERIATRIC

N/A

OTHERS

N/A

PREGNANCY

N/A

FURTHER INFORMATION

National Kidney & Urologic Diseases Information Clearinghouse, Box NKUDIC, Bethesda, MD 20893, (301) 468-6345

Prostatic Hyperplasia, Benign (BPH)

 Basics

DESCRIPTION

Benign prostatic hypertrophy (BPH) is the over-growth of the prostate gland, which can obstruct the flow of urine from the bladder.

SIGNS AND SYMPTOMS

- Decrease force or caliber of urine stream
- Hesitancy
- Dribbling
- Sensation of incomplete bladder emptying
- Incontinence
- Inability to voluntarily stop stream
- Urinary retention
- Frequent urination
- Urination during sleep hours
- Urgency

CAUSES

Exact cause is unknown, but evidence suggests BPH arises from a hormonal imbalance.

SCOPE

BPH is a universal phenomenon seen in older men.

MOST OFTEN AFFECTED

BPH is rarely seen in men less than 40 years of age; affects 50% of men over age 50 and 80% of men over age 70.

RISK FACTORS

- Aging (rare in men younger than 40 years old)
- No dietary, environmental, or sexual practices implicated yet

 Diagnosis

WHAT THE DOCTOR LOOKS FOR

The doctor will perform a physical examination to identify the presence of BPH.

TESTS AND PROCEDURES

- Blood tests
- Urinalysis, culture
- Tissue from the prostate may be obtained by biopsy for laboratory analysis.
- The urinary system may be evaluated with a special diagnostic procedure, intravenous pyelogram.
- Computed tomography (CT scan) or magnetic resonance imaging (MRI) may be done.
- Ultrasound
- Special tests to measure the flow and pressure of urine may be performed to assist in diagnosis.
- The urinary tract may be examined by cys-toscopy.

 Treatment

GENERAL MEASURES

- BPH is managed in the outpatient setting.
- Surgery may be required.

ACTIVITY

No restriction

DIET

Avoid caffeinated or alcoholic beverages, excessively spiced foods.

Prostatic Hyperplasia, Benign (BPH)

 Medications

COMMONLY PRESCRIBED DRUGS

- Prazosin (Minipress), terazosin, doxazosin
- Flutamide, leuprolide, finasteride (Proscar)

CONTRAINDICATIONS

Read drug product information.

PRECAUTIONS

Read drug product information.

DRUG INTERACTIONS

Read drug product information.

OTHER DRUGS

N/A

 Followup

PATIENT MONITORING

- Symptoms should be monitored every 1–6 months.
- Urine testing every 3–12 months.
- Digital rectal exam yearly
- PSA test yearly

PREVENTION

Prostatic hypertrophy appears to be part of the aging process.

COMPLICATIONS

- Bladder stones
- Prostatitis
- Kidney failure

WHAT TO EXPECT

- Symptoms improve or stabilize in 70–80% of patients; 20–30% require treatment because of worsening symptoms.
- 11–33% of men with BPH have prostate cancer.

 Miscellaneous

OTHER FACTORS

N/A

PEDIATRIC

N/A

GERIATRIC

BPH is much more common in elderly men.

OTHERS

N/A

PREGNANCY

N/A

FURTHER INFORMATION

National Kidney & Urologic Diseases Information Clearinghouse, Box NKUDIC, Bethesda, MD 20893, (301) 468-6345

Psoriasis

 Basics

DESCRIPTION

Psoriasis is a common chronic disease characterized by reddened, dry, scaling patches of skin. The condition tends to recur and improve unpredictably over time, with flares possibly related to systemic or environmental factors.

SCOPE

There are 1,000–2,000 cases of psoriasis per 100,000 people in the United States.

MOST OFTEN AFFECTED

Individuals 16–22 and 57–60 years old; can develop in infants; males and females affected in equal numbers; may be inherited

SIGNS AND SYMPTOMS

- Arthritis
- Itching
- Silvery scales on red plaques
- Affects the knees, elbows, and scalp
- Finger and toe nails may appear stippled and pitted.

CAUSES

Possible genetic defect

RISK FACTORS

- Trauma or irritation of skin
- Infection
- Hormone changes
- Stress (physical and emotional)
- Sudden withdrawal of psoriasis drugs
- Alcohol use
- Obesity

 Diagnosis

WHAT THE DOCTOR LOOKS FOR

- The doctor will perform a physical examination to identify the signs and symptoms of psoriasis.
- Numerous other conditions may appear similar to psoriasis.

TESTS AND PROCEDURES

Blood tests

 Treatment

GENERAL MEASURES

- Psoriasis is usually managed in the outpatient setting.
- Hospitalization may be required for severe or resistant cases.
- Medication to soften scales, followed by soft brush while bathing.
- Oatmeal baths for itching
- Tar shampoos
- Avoid excessive sun exposure.
- Desert climates provide a favorable effect for some patients.
- Wet dressings may help relieve itching.
- Ultraviolet light including sunlight is effective and may be best treatment option during pregnancy or in young children. Lamps are available for home use.
- For severe psoriasis that resists treatment, a referral to a specialist in psoriatic therapy is suggested.

ACTIVITY

No restrictions

DIET

No special diet

Psoriasis

 Medications

COMMONLY PRESCRIBED DRUGS

- Emollients: soft yellow paraffin or aqueous cream; petrolatum or aquaphor cream
- Corticosteroids
- Coal tar (Estar, PsoriGel)
- Salicylic acid
- Anthralin ointment
- Methotrexate
- PUVA (psoralen plus ultraviolet light)
- Etretinate
- Isotretinoin
- Triamcinolone
- Vitamin D analogs
- Cyclosporine, tacrolimus

CONTRAINDICATIONS

Read drug product information.

PRECAUTIONS

Read drug product information.

DRUG INTERACTIONS

Read drug product information.

OTHER DRUGS

N/A

 Followup

PATIENT MONITORING

- The doctor should be seen as often as necessary.
- Medications used in treatment require close followup.
- Blood tests may be repeated on a monthly basis.

PREVENTION

- Avoid alcoholic beverages.
- Avoid irritating drugs.
- Avoid stimulating drugs or antimalarial medications.

COMPLICATIONS

- Severe psoriasis or other skin disorders
- Topical corticosteroids may cause skin side effects.

WHAT TO EXPECT

- Psoriasis is usually benign.
- Life-threatening forms do occur.
- May be resistant to to treatment

 Miscellaneous

OTHER FACTORS

N/A

PEDIATRIC

The onset of psoriasis is common before age 10, rare before age 3.

GERIATRIC

- About 3% of psoriasis patients acquire the disease after age 65.
- Elderly patients may have difficulty with application of topicals over all affected body parts.

OTHERS

N/A

PREGNANCY

Pregnancy has an unpredictable effect on psoriasis. Avoid tars, topical corticosteroids, calcipotriene, and systemic therapies. Etretinate is toxic to fetus.

FURTHER INFORMATION

- American Academy of Family Physicians Foundation, P.O. Box 8418, Kansas City, MO 64114, (800) 274-2237, ext. 4400
- National Psoriasis Foundation, Suite 300, 6600 S.W. 92nd Avenue, Portland, OR 97223, (503) 244-7404; toll free (800) 723-9166; fax (503) 245-0626; E-mail 76135.2746@comserve.com

Section R

Rabies

 ## Basics

DESCRIPTION

Rabies is a rapidly progressive infection of the central nervous system caused by a virus. The disease is essentially 100% fatal once symptoms develop. Infection can be prevented by prompt treatment.

SIGNS AND SYMPTOMS

Usually proceed through four stages, although they may overlap:
- Incubation period: often lasts 1–3 months
- Prodrome (2–10 days)
  - ▶ Pain or tingling at bite site
  - ▶ Fever, headache
- Acute neurologic period (2–10 days)
  - ▶ Episodes of hyperactivity
  - ▶ Paralysis
- Coma
- Death

CAUSES

Rabies virus present in saliva of infected animals

SCOPE

There are about 5 cases of rabies per year in humans; about 30,000 people receive treatments after exposure.

MOST OFTEN AFFECTED

Rabies can affect all ages; males and females are affected in equal numbers.

RISK FACTORS

- Professions or activities that may expose a person to wild or domestic animals, e.g., animal handlers, some lab workers, veterinarians, spelunkers (cave explorers)
- International travel to countries where canine rabies is endemic (most common risk factor)
- In the United States, most cases appear due to exposure to bats.

 ## Diagnosis

WHAT THE DOCTOR LOOKS FOR

- The diagnosis of rabies should be considered if an individual has been bitten by an animal capable of transmitting the disease; however, most patients in the United States do not recall exposure.
- Other conditions that can cause similar signs and symptoms should be identified and treated.

TESTS AND PROCEDURES

- Blood tests
- Spinal fluid may be obtained by lumbar puncture (spinal tap).
- The rabies virus may be isolated from saliva or spinal fluid.
- A sample of skin from the bite area may be obtained for laboratory analysis.
- X-rays

 ## Treatment

GENERAL MEASURES

- The management of rabies requires hospitalization.
- Immediate and thorough washing of all bite wounds and scratches with soap and water
- Because there is no treatment for rabies, care is directed at prevention of disease following exposure to potentially rabid animals.

ACTIVITY

As tolerated

DIET

No restrictions

Medications

COMMONLY PRESCRIBED DRUGS

- Rabies immune globulin, human (HRIG)
- Rabies vaccine, human diploid cell (HDCV)
- Rabies vaccine adsorbed (RVA)

CONTRAINDICATIONS

None

PRECAUTIONS

N/A

DRUG INTERACTIONS

N/A

OTHER DRUGS

None

 Followup

PATIENT MONITORING

No followup is required in most cases; see the doctor as often as necessary for wound care.

PREVENTION

- Avoid travel to areas where rabies is endemic.
- Avoid wild or unfamiliar animals that act strange or unusual.
- Seek prompt medical attention after contact with a suspected animal, if bitten or scratched.

COMPLICATIONS

None

WHAT TO EXPECT

There have been no failures of after-exposure treatment in the United States since the 1970's.

 Miscellaneous

OTHER

N/A

PEDIATRIC

N/A

GERIATRIC

N/A

OTHERS

N/A

PREGNANCY

N/A

FURTHER INFORMATION

N/A

Rape (Sexual Assault)

 Basics

DESCRIPTION

- Sexual contact: touching of a person's intimate parts (including thighs) or the clothing covering such areas for the purpose of sexual gratification
- Sexual conduct: vaginal intercourse between a male and female, or anal intercourse, fellatio, or cunnilingus between persons regardless of sex
- Rape: any sexual penetration, however slight, using force or coercion against the person's will
- Corruption of a minor: sexual conduct by an individual 18 years old or greater with an individual less than 15 years of age
- Definitions may vary by state.

SIGNS AND SYMPTOMS

- In adults
  - ▶ History of sexual penetration
  - ▶ Sexual contact or sexual conduct without consent and/or with the use of force
- In children
  - ▶ Actual observation of, or suspicion of, sexual penetration, sexual contact, or sexual conduct
  - ▶ Signs include evidence of the use of force and/or evidence of sexual contact (e.g., presence of semen and/or sperm).

CAUSES

N/A

SCOPE

- Over 100,000 cases of alleged rape are reported in the United States every year.
- It is estimated that only 10–20% adult cases are reported.
- It is estimated that only 5–7% of pediatric cases are reported.

MOST OFTEN AFFECTED

- Majority of adult victims are females in their teens and 20s.
- Child victims may be either gender, with a predominance of females.

- Increasing numbers of adult male victims are presenting for treatment.
- Overall, females are victims more often than males.

RISK FACTORS

- Numerous risk factors
- About 50% of rapes occur in the home, with one-third of these involving a male intruder.

 Diagnosis

WHAT THE DOCTOR LOOKS FOR

The doctor will perform a physical examination to assess the nature of sexual contact and look for signs of penetration, force, and other evidence of sexual assault.

TESTS AND PROCEDURES

- The vagina may be swabbed to test for the presence of semen.
- Pregnancy test

 Treatment

GENERAL MEASURES

- Contact appropriate social services agency or rape crisis center.
- Most adult victims can be treated as outpatients unless associated trauma (physical or mental) requires admission.
- Most pediatric sexual assault/abuse victims will require admission or outside placement until appropriate social agency can evaluate home environment.
- All sexual assault cases must be reported immediately to the appropriate law enforcement agency.
- Sedation and tetanus prevention may be given.
- Sexually transmitted disease prevention for gonorrhea and Chlamydia should be administered.
- Consider possible pregnancy; "morning-after" pills should be offered.

- Testing for exposure to the human immunodeficiency virus (HIV); testing for hepatitis B may be peformed.

ACTIVITY

No restrictions

DIET

No restrictions

 ## Medications

COMMONLY PRESCRIBED DRUGS

- Ceftriaxone, cefixime, spectinomycin, ciprofloxacin, norfloxacin, ampicillin/probenecid, amoxicillin/probenecid
- Zithromycin (Zithromax), doxycycline, tetracycline, erythromycin

CONTRAINDICATIONS

Read drug product information.

PRECAUTIONS

Read drug product information.

DRUG INTERACTIONS

Read drug product information.

OTHER DRUGS

N/A

 ## Followup

PATIENT MONITORING

- The doctor should be seen in 7 to 10 days for followup care, including pregnancy testing and counseling by a gynecologist or appropriate gynecologic clinic.
- Followup tests for pregnancy and sexually transmitted diseases in 5 to 6 weeks and at 6 months after initial treatment
- Referral to agencies that can provide counseling and legal services should be provided.

PREVENTION

Assertiveness training and self-defense training

COMPLICATIONS

- Sexually transmitted disease
- Pregnancy (with the possibility of abortion)
- Trauma (physical and mental)

WHAT TO EXPECT

- Acute phase (usually 1–3 weeks following rape): shaking, pain, wound healing, mood swings, appetite loss, crying. Also feelings of grief, shame, anger, fear, revenge, or guilt.
- Late or chronic phase: Female victim may develop fear of intercourse, fear of men, nightmares, sleep disorders, day-time flashbacks, fear of being alone, loss of self-esteem, anxiety, depression, post-traumatic stress syndrome
- Recovery may be prolonged. Individuals who are able to talk about their feelings seem to have a faster recovery.

 ## Medications

OTHER FACTORS

N/A

PEDIATRIC

Assure the child that he or she is a good person and was not the cause of the incident.

GERIATRIC

N/A

OTHERS

N/A

PREGNANCY

N/A

FURTHER INFORMATION

National Institute of Mental Health, Public Inquiries Branch, Office of Scientific Information, Dept. of Health and Human Services, Parklawn Bldg., Room 15C-05, 5600 Fishers Lane, Rockville, MD 20857, (301) 443-4513

Rash

Basics

DESCRIPTION

A rash consisting of a single or multiple itchy raised bumps on the skin, typically pale with a red halo. The rash may subside rapidly, resulting in no scars or change in pigmentation. Rashes may recur.

- Acute rash:
  - ▶ Reaction to many stimuli
  - ▶ May be unusual response to drug exposure
  - ▶ Subsides over several hours
- Chronic urticaria:
  - ▶ Persists more than 6 weeks in 30% of cases
  - ▶ Cold urticaria: results from cooling and rewarming; can be fatal. Another form may affect several members of a family with fever, chills, joint and muscle pain, and headache.
  - ▶ Heat urticaria: small (5–10 millimeter) spots on upper trunk from overheating, hot shower
  - ▶ Exercise-induced urticaria: from extreme exercise; marked by swelling, wheezing, low blood pressure. Often associated with eating food to which person is allergic
  - ▶ Linear urticaria: results from scratching the skin
  - ▶ Solar urticaria: results from exposure to sunlight. Onset in minutes; subsides in 1 to 2 hours.
  - ▶ Delayed pressure urticaria: occurs 4–6 hours after pressure to skin (elastic, shoes, etc.)
  - ▶ Water urticaria: occurs after contact with water at any temperature; rare

SIGNS AND SYMPTOMS

- Urticaria may appear alone or with swelling.
- May occur with generalized allergic reaction, potentially fatal
- Single or multiple raised, pale spots surrounded by a red halo
- Intense itching
- May occur anywhere on body
- Spots are variably sized.
- Acute urticaria develops rapidly, resolves spontaneously in less than 48 hours

CAUSES

- May be allergic or nonallergic
- Allergy-triggering substance may be inhaled, eaten, or contacted on the skin.
- Drug reaction
- Food or food additive allergy
- Insect bite, sting
- Infection
- Vascular disease
- Physical trauma (heat, cold, sunlight, etc.)
- Emotional stress (reported; little supporting evidence)

SCOPE

Rash affects about 1 in 1000 persons, or 15–20% of the U.S. population at some time during life.

MOST OFTEN AFFECTED

Urticaria can affect all ages. Acute urticaria is mainly seen in children and young adults. Males and females are affected with equal frequency, although chronic rash is more common in older women.

RISK FACTORS

See Causes

Diagnosis

WHAT THE DOCTOR LOOKS FOR

- Conditions known to be associated with rash, such as angioedema and allergic reaction
- Possible causes of urticaria, such as insect bites or skin diseases
- A cause is identified in 10 to 25% of chronic cases.

TESTS AND PROCEDURES

- Urinalysis
- Blood tests may be done to identify signs of infection of inflammation.
- A sample of skin tissue obtained by biopsy may be examined microscopically.
- Tests may be done to evaluate allergies to foods or other substances.
- Special tests include:
  - ▶ Cold urticaria: ice cube test (ice cube placed on skin 5 minutes, observed 10–15 minutes)
  - ▶ Exercise-induced urticaria: exercise challenge; methacholine skin test
  - ▶ Solar urticaria: exposure to defined wavelengths of light.
  - ▶ Delayed pressure urticaria: apply 5–10 pound sandbag for 3 hours, observe
  - ▶ Water urticaria: apply tap water at different temperatures
  - ▶ Vibratory urticaria: apply vibration 4–5 minutes with a lab mixing device, observe

Rash

 Treatment

GENERAL MEASURES

- Acute cases usually do not require a full workup.
- Cool moist compresses help control itching.
- Avoid substances that provoke allergies if they are known. Use antihistamines if accidentally re-exposed.

ACTIVITY

As desired. Avoid overheating.

DIET

As desired. Avoid foods suspected as possible allergy triggers.

 Medications

COMMONLY PRESCRIBED DRUGS

- First-generation antihistamines
  - ▶ Older children and adults: hydroxyzine or diphenhydramine
  - ▶ Children under 6: diphenhydramine
- Second-generation drugs are equally effective as antihistamines and are less sedating but more expensive.
  - ▶ Fexofenadine (Allegra)
  - ▶ Astemizole (Hismanal)
  - ▶ Loratadine (Claritin)
  - ▶ Acrivastine (Semprex)
  - ▶ Cetirizine (Zyrtec)

CONTRAINDICATIONS

Danazol should not be given to children or pregnant women.

PRECAUTIONS

- First-generation drugs may cause drowsiness.
- Second-generation H_1 blockers should be used with caution in pregnancy and the elderly.

DRUG INTERACTIONS

Read drug product information.

OTHER DRUGS

- Doxepin (Sinequan)
- H_2-blockers (cimetidine, ranitidine, etc.) may be helpful in chronic urticaria.
- Corticosteroids (prednisone) for unresponsive nonacute cases

Followup

PATIENT MONITORING

- No followup is necessary after an initial episode of rash.
- See the doctor if symptoms persist or recur.

PREVENTION

If a cause is identified, avoidance is the best solution.

COMPLICATIONS

Severe systemic allergic reaction

WHAT TO EXPECT

About 70% of people with urticaria improve in less than 72 hours. About 30% develop chronic urticaria. Urticaria becomes chronic in 75% of persons with both rash and swelling. About 20% have attacks for more than 20 years.

 ## Medications

OTHER FACTORS

N/A

PEDIATRIC

Isolated acute cases are frequent, but chronic rash is rare.

GERIATRIC

Less likely to occur in this age group

OTHERS

N/A

PREGNANCY

A chronic rash may develop during pregnancy.

FURTHER INFORMATION

N/A

Raynaud's Phenomenon

 ## Basics

DESCRIPTION

Raynaud's phenomenon, or cold intolerance, is a disorder marked by attacks of extreme pallor, then a bluish discoloration of the fingers (rarely, of the toes) brought on by cold exposure. With warming, intense redness develops, followed by swelling, throbbing, and tingling. May accompany emotional upset.

SIGNS AND SYMPTOMS

- Pallor/whiteness of fingertips with cold exposure, followed by a bluish discoloration, then redness and pain with warming
- Ulceration of fingertips, progressing to finger loss in severe, prolonged cases (10–13% of cases)

CAUSES

Unknown

SCOPE

4–10% of population experiences cold intolerance.

MOST OFTEN AFFECTED

Individuals 40 years of age or older; females affected more frequently than males

RISK FACTORS

- Smoking
- Immune or connective tissue disorder

 ## Diagnosis

WHAT THE DOCTOR LOOKS FOR

- The doctor will do a physical examination to discern the signs and symptoms of cold intolerance.
- Numerous other conditions that can cause similar signs and symptoms should be ruled out.

TESTS AND PROCEDURES

- Blood tests
- X-rays
- Special diagnostic tests to assess response to cold may be performed.

 ## Treatment

GENERAL MEASURES

- Dress warmly, wear gloves, avoid cold
- No smoking
- Avoid beta-blockers, amphetamines, ergot alkaloids, and sumatriptan
- Biofeedback training can help increase hand temperature.
- Finger guards over ulcerated fingertips

ACTIVITY

Avoidance of situations in which exposure to cold is likely; avoid vibrating tools

DIET

No special diet

Medications

COMMONLY PRESCRIBED DRUGS

Nifedipine

CONTRAINDICATIONS

Allergy to drug, pregnancy, congestive heart failure

PRECAUTIONS

May cause headache, dizziness, lightheadedness

DRUG INTERACTIONS

Read drug product information.

OTHER DRUGS

- Diltiazem, verapamil, reserpine, methyldopa, prazosin
- Captopril (not FDA approved)
- Prostacyclin
- Nitroglycerin patches may also be helpful, but they may cause severe headache.

 ## Followup

PATIENT MONITORING

The doctor should be seen as often as necessary.

PREVENTION

- Avoid trauma to fingertips
- Avoid exposure to cold
- Smoking cessation

COMPLICATIONS

Gangrene, amputation of fingertips

WHAT TO EXPECT

Cold intolerance usually follows a prolonged course with recurrent attacks and formation of fingertip ulcers.

 ## Miscellaneous

OTHER FACTORS

N/A

PEDIATRIC

N/A

GERIATRIC

Appearance of Raynaud's phenomenom after age 40 almost always indicates an underlying disease.

OTHERS

N/A

PREGNANCY

N/A

FURTHER INFORMATION

N/A

Renal Failure, Acute (ARF)

 Basics

DESCRIPTION

Acute renal failure (ARF) is a syndrome of rapidly deteriorating kidney function with the accumulation of wastes in the bloodstream.

SIGNS AND SYMPTOMS

- Loss of appetite
- Back pain
- Coma
- Delirium
- Diarrhea
- Difficulty breathing
- Bruising
- Swelling
- Brain damage
- Nosebleed
- Fatigue
- Gastrointestinal bleeding
- Headache
- Hiccups
- High blood pressure
- Lethargy
- Muscle cramps, spasm
- Nausea
- Scant urine production
- Rash
- Eye disease
- Seizure
- Sleepiness
- Rapid heart rate
- Rapid breathing rate
- Urine-like odor
- Vomiting
- Weakness
- Dry mouth

CAUSES

- Severe illness (e.g., heart failure, cirrhosis of liver)
- Kidney disease
- Vascular disease
- Urinary tract obstruction

SCOPE

5% of individuals admitted to U.S. hospitals develop acute renal failure.

MOST OFTEN AFFECTED

All ages are affected by ARF, males and females in equal numbers.

RISK FACTORS

- Surgery
- Volume depletion (especially in diabetes)
- Drug side effect
- Medical illness

 Diagnosis

WHAT THE DOCTOR LOOKS FOR

See Causes

TESTS AND PROCEDURES

- Urinalysis
- Blood tests
- A sample of kidney tissue may be obtained by biopsy for laboratory analysis.
- Special radiology procedures that may be performed include angiogram, renal scan, ultrasound, and computed tomography (CT scan).
- The urinary tract may be examined by cystoscopy.

 Treatment

GENERAL MEASURES

Acute renal failure requires hospitalization.

ACTIVITY

As tolerated

DIET

- Restrict fluids.
- Eliminate potassium if serum level increased.
- Increase carbohydrates.

Medications

COMMONLY PRESCRIBED DRUGS

Intravenous (IV) saline solution, mannitol, furosemide (Lasix), and calcium-channel blockers

CONTRAINDICATIONS

N/A

PRECAUTIONS

Read drug product information.

DRUG INTERACTIONS

Read drug product information.

OTHER DRUGS

N/A

 Followup

PATIENT MONITORING

The doctor and other health professionals will be seen as needed.

PREVENTION

See Risk factors

COMPLICATIONS

• Severe, life-threatening infection (leading cause of mortality)
• Convulsions
• Swelling
• Fluid in lungs
• Congestive heart failure
• Paralysis
• Irregular heart rhythms
• Death
• Heart disorders
• Blood poisoning
• Bleeding

WHAT TO EXPECT

Recovery usually occurs in days to 6 weeks. High mortality rate (5–80%) depending on cause, severity, and age.

 Miscellaneous

OTHER FACTORS

N/A

PEDIATRIC

N/A

GERIATRIC

Greater occurrence of ARF among the elderly, especially after surgery

OTHERS

N/A

PREGNANCY

N/A

FURTHER INFORMATION

• National Kidney & Urologic Diseases Information Clearinghouse, Box NKUDIC, Bethesda, MD 20893, (301) 468-6345
• The National Kidney Foundation, Inc., 30 East 33rd Street, NY, NY 10016.

Retinal Detachment

 Basics

DESCRIPTION

A retinal detachment is the separation of the sensory retina (the "screen" at the back of the eye) from the underlying retinal tissue, with an accumulation of fluid between them.

SIGNS AND SYMPTOMS

- Flashes
- Floaters
- Visual field loss (typically, a "curtain" across portion of the visual field)

CAUSES

- Normal aging
- Tumors
- Inflammatory diseases
- Trauma, foreign bodies
- Miscellaneous (uveal effusion, malignant hypertension)

SCOPE

10 persons per 100,000 annually experience retinal detachment without surgery or injury.

PREDOMINANT AGE

- Retinal detachment is rare before age 30 and is seen in 63% of patients over age 70; males and females are affected in equal proportions.

RISK FACTORS

- Near-sightedness
- Absence of lens
- Trauma
- Retinal detachment in other eye
- Retinal degeneration

 Diagnosis

WHAT THE DOCTOR LOOKS FOR

The doctor will examine the eyes to evaluate the status of the retina.

TESTS AND PROCEDURES

N/A

 Treatment

GENERAL MEASURES

- Referral to retina specialist for examination and repair
- Surgery is required.

ACTIVITY

In some cases, bed rest and patching of both eyes

DIET

No special diet

 Medications

COMMONLY PRESCRIBED DRUGS

N/A

CONTRAINDICATIONS

N/A

PRECAUTIONS

N/A

DRUG INTERACTIONS

N/A

OTHER DRUGS

Beta-cyclodextrin beta-decasulfate (experimental)

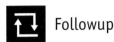 Followup

PATIENT MONITORING

The doctor should be seen as often as necessary.

PREVENTION

Regular eye examination by an ophthalmologist

COMPLICATIONS

Partial or total loss of vision

WHAT TO EXPECT

- Untreated, visual loss progresses and, ultimately, complete blindness results.
- With current techniques, 90–95% of retinal detachments can be repaired.
- Outcome depends on the severity of underlying disorder causing detachment.

 Miscellaneous

OTHER FACTORS

N/A

PEDIATRIC

N/A

GERIATRIC

N/A

OTHERS

N/A

PREGNANCY

N/A

FURTHER INFORMATION

American Academy of Ophthalmology (415) 561-8500

Rhinitis, Allergic

 ## Basics

DESCRIPTION

Allergic rhinitis, or hay fever, is a reaction to airborne allergens. The condition may be seasonal or perennial depending on climate and individual response. Seasonal responses are usually to grasses, trees, and weeds. Perennial responses may be caused by house-dust mites, mold antigens, and animal body products.

SIGNS AND SYMPTOMS

- Nasal stuffiness and congestion
- Sneezing, often in spasms
- Watery eyes
- Dark circles under eyes, "allergic shiners"
- Long eyelashes
- Sensation of plugged ears
- Sleeping difficulties
- Fatigue
- Mouth breathing
- Scratchy throat
- Voice change
- Irritating cough
- Postnasal drip
- Loss or alteration of smell
- Itchy nose, eyes, ears and palate

CAUSES

- Animal and plant proteins: pollens, molds, mite dust, animal danders, dried saliva, and urine
- Insect debris: cockroach, locusts, fish food

SCOPE

Allergic rhinitis affects 8–12% of the U.S. population.

MOST OFTEN AFFECTED

Onset usually before the age of 30; average age of onset is 10; males and females affected in equal proportion

PREDOMINANT SEX

Males and females are affected in equal proportion.

RISK FACTORS

- Family history
- Repeated exposure to offending antigen
- Exposure to multiple allergens
- Presence of other allergies, e.g., asthma, rash
- Noncompliance with therapy

 ## Diagnosis

WHAT THE DOCTOR LOOKS FOR

- The doctor will perform a physical examination to identify the presence of rhinitis.
- Numerous other conditions can produce signs and symptoms similar to rhinitis, including nasal polyps, foreign bodies, drug side effects, and infections.

TESTS AND PROCEDURES

- Blood tests
- Nasal secretions may be sampled for laboratory analysis.
- Allergy testing
- Hearing testing may be performed
- X-ray of head
- The interior of the nose may be examined by rhinoscopy.

 ## Treatment

GENERAL MEASURES

- Rhinitis is managed in the outpatient setting.
- Limit exposure to offending allergen.
- Specific causes should be identified.
- Intensity of treatment is determined by severity of disease.
- Immunotherapy may be beneficial.
- Surgical repair of the nose may be required.

ACTIVITY

No specific restrictions. Avoid activity in areas of allergen exposure.

DIET

No special diet unless food allergies are suspected.

Rhinitis, Allergic

 Medications

COMMONLY PRESCRIBED DRUGS

- Antihistamines: diphenhydramine (Benadryl), clemastine (Tavist), chlorpheniramine, brompheniramine, tripelennamine (PBZ), hydroxyzine (Atarax), promethazine (Phenergan), methdilazine (Tacaryl), astemizole (Hismanal)
- Decongestants: pseudoephedrine, phenylephrine
- Nasal sprays: saline solution, cromolyn sodium (Nasalcrom), beclomethasone (Beconase AQ, Vancenase AQ), flunisolide (Nasalide, AeroBid), triamcinolone (Nasacort), budesonide (Rhinocort)
- Steroids

CONTRAINDICATIONS

Read drug product information.

PRECAUTIONS

The elderly often require less aggressive treatment.

DRUG INTERACTIONS

Numerous interactions; read drug product information.

OTHER DRUGS

N/A

 Followup

PATIENT MONITORING

The doctor should be seen as often as needed.

PREVENTION

- Avoidance: not enough to control symptoms for most people
- Air conditioning and limited outside exposure during season is helpful.
- Housekeeping tactics and control for dust mites in patients sensitive to this allergen
- Minimize exposure to animals. House pets are discouraged.

- Avoid environmental irritants, e.g., smoke and fumes.
- Use an air purifier.
- Use allergy control covers on mattresses and pillows.

COMPLICATIONS

- Infection
- Sinusitis
- Nosebleed
- Impaired lung function
- Changed to appearance

WHAT TO EXPECT

- For many people, symptoms can be well controlled.
- Treatment should be tailored to each individual.
- Symptoms often ease over time.

 Miscellaneous

OTHER FACTORS

N/A

PEDIATRIC

Environmental control may include carpet and drape removal, removal of house plants, pet control, etc.

GERIATRIC

- Increased medication side effects
- Symptoms may decrease among the elderly.

OTHERS

N/A

PREGNANCY

Pregnancy may aggravate rhinitis.

FURTHER INFORMATION

Asthma & Allergy Foundation of America. 1717 Massachusetts Ave., Suite 305, Washington, DC 20036, (800) 7-ASTHMA

Rocky Mountain Spotted Fever

 Basics

DESCRIPTION

Rocky Mountain spotted fever (RMSF) is an acute, potentially fatal illness transmitted by tick bite. The illness is marked by headache, fever, and rash.

SIGNS AND SYMPTOMS

- Fever
- Rash
- Headache
- Nausea, vomiting
- Abdominal pain
- Muscle and joint pain
- Enlarged lymph nodes
- Cough
- Central nervous system dysfunction (stupor, confusion, coma)

CAUSES

RMSF is caused by *Rickettsia rickettsii,* which is transmitted by the bite of ticks.

SCOPE

About 600 new cases are reported each year in the United States. Peak incidence is in late spring and summer.

MOST OFTEN AFFECTED

Highest incidences occur among children and young adults, but all ages are susceptible. RMSF is more common in males than females, due to outdoor activities.

RISK FACTORS

- Outdoor activity during warm months
- Contact with dogs

 Diagnosis

WHAT THE DOCTOR LOOKS FOR

- The doctor will perform a physical examination to identify the presence of illness.
- Numerous other conditions that can cause similar signs and symptoms should be ruled out, such as viral infection, Lyme disease, and other disorders.

TESTS AND PROCEDURES

- Blood tests
- Chest x-ray
- Tissue may be sampled by biopsy for laboratory analysis.

 Treatment

GENERAL MEASURES

- Individuals who are moderately ill are usually hospitalized.
- Individuals with mild disease are treated as outpatients.
- Supportive care as needed

ACTIVITY

Bed rest until symptoms subside.

DIET

Small frequent meals may be necessary to maintain nutritional levels.

Medications

COMMONLY PRESCRIBED DRUGS

- Doxycycline (Vibramycin)
- Tetracycline
- Chloramphenicol

CONTRAINDICATIONS

- Tetrayclines should not be used in children less than 9 years old
- Doxycycline and tetracyclines are contraindicated in pregnancy.

PRECAUTIONS

May cause sensitivity to light; use a sunscreen

DRUG INTERACTIONS

Tetracyclines may interact with milk products, iron preparations, or antacids containing aluminum or magnesium.

OTHER DRUGS

N/A

Followup

PATIENT MONITORING

If not hospitalized, the patient should see the doctor every 2–3 days until symptoms have fully resolved.

PREVENTION

- Wear occlusive clothing.
- Use insect repellants.
- After possible exposure, all body areas should be carefully inspected for ticks, especially legs, groin, belt lines. Risk of infection increases with the duration of tick attachment.
- Ticks should be removed from humans or animals with caution; gloves should be worn or instruments used to minimize direct contact. Place a drop of oil, alcohol, gasoline, or kerosine on the tick first. Hands should be washed thoroughly afterwards.

COMPLICATIONS

- Brain disease, usually temporary
- Seizures
- Kidney failure
- Hepatitis
- Heart failure
- Respiratory failure

WHAT TO EXPECT

- When treated promptly, the usual outcome is excellent with resolution of symptoms over several days and no lasting effects.
- Death is rare with prompt institution of appropriate therapy.
- If complications develop, the course may be more severe and longterm effects may result, such as neurologic disorders.

Miscellaneous

OTHER FACTORS

N/A

PEDIATRIC

N/A

GERIATRIC

Mortality risk higher among the elderly

OTHERS

N/A

PREGNANCY

N/A

FURTHER INFORMATION

N/A

Rosacea

 Basics

DESCRIPTION

Rosacea is a chronic skin eruption with flushing and dilation of small blood vessels in the face, especially nose and cheeks.

SIGNS AND SYMPTOMS

- Skin flushing
- Redness: lower half of nose, sometimes whole nose, forehead, cheeks, chin
- Reddened eyes (sometimes)
- Dusky, reddened skin
- Blood vessels in involved area collapse under pressure
- Acne
- "Spider veins"
- Bulging or overgrowth of nose

CAUSES

No proven cause. Possibilities include:
- Hormone disturbance
- Alcohol, coffee, tea, spiced food overindulgence (unproven)
- Parasite (suspected)
- Exposure to cold, heat, hot drinks
- Emotional stress
- Disorder of the gastrointestinal tract

SCOPE

Rosacea is common in the United States.

MOST OFTEN AFFECTED

Persons 30–50 years of age; females affected more frequently than males

RISK FACTORS

N/A

 Diagnosis

WHAT THE DOCTOR LOOKS FOR

- The doctor will perform a physical examination to assess the presence of rosacea.
- Numerous other conditions that can cause skin eruptions similar to rosacea should be investigated.

TESTS AND PROCEDURES

N/A

 Treatment

GENERAL MEASURES

- Reassurance
- Psychological stress should be treated if present.
- Avoid oil-based cosmetics.
- Treatment of permanently dilated blood vessels
- Surgical repair of nose may be necessary.

ACTIVITY

No restrictions. Physical fitness is encouraged.

DIET

Avoid any food or drink that causes facial flushing, e.g., hot drinks, spiced food, alcohol.

 Medications

COMMONLY PRESCRIBED DRUGS

- Tetracycline
- Alcohol-sulfur (Liquimat), sulfur (Fostril), resorcinol-sulfur (Rezamid), sulfacetamide-sulfur (Sulfacet-R)
- Metronidazole (topical)
- Erythromycin (topical)
- Clindamycin (topical)

CONTRAINDICATIONS

- Tetracycline: not for use in pregnancy or children less than 9 years of age
- Isotretinoin: causes birth defects; not for use in pregnancy or in women of reproductive age who are not using a reliable birth control method

PRECAUTIONS

- Tetracycline: may cause sensitivity to sunlight; use a sunscreen

DRUG INTERACTIONS

- Tetracycline: avoid antacids, dairy products, and iron
- Broad-spectrum antibiotics: may reduce the effectiveness of oral contraceptives

OTHER DRUGS

N/A

 Followup

PATIENT MONITORING

The doctor should be seen as often as needed.

PREVENTION

No preventive measure is known.

COMPLICATIONS

- Thickened, bulbous skin on nose, especially in men
- Conjunctivitis (pink eye)
- Blepharitis
- Keratitis

WHAT TO EXPECT

- Rosacea is usually slowly progressive.
- Sometimes rosacea subsides spontaneously.

 Miscellaneous

OTHER FACTORS

N/A

PEDIATRIC

Uncommon among children

GERIATRIC

Uncommon after age 60

OTHERS

N/A

PREGNANCY

Use of isotretinoin is contraindicated during pregnancy.

FURTHER INFORMATION

American Academy of Dermatology (708) 330-0230

Section S

Salmonella Infection

 Basics

DESCRIPTION

This disease is caused by Salmonella bacteria and produces severe gastrointestinal symptoms. In its most common form, it is transmitted by eating food contaminated with Salmonella.

SCOPE

- There are about 55 outbreaks of salmonella infections reported annually in the United States. The peak frequency occurs in July through November.

MOST OFTEN AFFECTED

- Salmonella infection is most common in individuals younger than 20 or older than 70 years of age.
- Highest incidence occurs in infants younger than 1 year of age.
- Males and females affected equally often

SIGNS AND SYMPTOMS

- Nausea, vomiting, diarrhea
- Abdominal cramps
- Headache, muscle pain
- Fever to 102°F (39°C); may be persistent
- Bone or joint inflammation
- Wound infection
- Inflammation of heart or blood vessels
- Pneumonia
- Shock
- Urinary tract infection

CAUSES

- Ingestion of contaminated food (poultry, meat, eggs, dairy products) or water
- Person-to-person spread
- Contact with infected animal, such as poultry, cows, pigs, birds, sheep, seals, donkeys, lizards, snakes, pets (turtles, cats, dogs, mice, guinea pigs, hamsters)
- Contact with chronic carrier
- Ulcerative colitis
- Systemic lupus erythematosus
- Gallstones
- Kidney stones
- Drugs: antibiotics, purgatives, opiates

RISK FACTORS

- Anemia
- Cancer
- Immune system disorder
- Pets (snakes, iguanas)

 Diagnosis

WHAT THE DOCTOR LOOKS FOR

The doctor will perform a physical examination to identify salmonella poisoning.

TESTS AND PROCEDURES

- Blood tests and culture
- A sample of stool may be obtained for laboratory analysis.
- A radiology procedure, angiography, may be performed on patients over 50 years of age.

 Treatment

GENERAL MEASURES

- Uncomplicated cases of salmonella infection are managed in the outpatient setting; severe cases may require hospitalization.
- Correct fluid and salt imbalances.
- Relief of symptoms (pain, nausea, vomiting)
- Surgery may be required.

ACTIVITY

As tolerated

DIET

Oral rehydration solution during diarrhea phase; advance to normal diet as tolerated

Medications

COMMONLY PRESCRIBED DRUGS

- Ampicillin
- Trimethoprim-sulfamethoxazole (Bactrim, Septra)
- Cefotaxime (Claforan), ciprofloxacin (Cipro), norfloxacin
- Chloramphenicol

CONTRAINDICATIONS

Known drug allergy; read drug product information.

PRECAUTIONS

Read drug product information.

DRUG INTERACTIONS

Read drug product information.

OTHER DRUGS

Ofloxacin (Floxin)

Followup

PATIENT MONITORING

The doctor should be seen as needed; stool culture should be repeated 5 months and 1 year after infection.

PREVENTION

- Maintain proper hygiene during preparation and storage of food. Wash hands, utensils, and surfaces (countertops, serving dishes) thoroughly with soap and hot water after contact with raw meat, especially poultry.
- Keep hot foods hot and cold foods cold during picnics, buffets, etc.
- Do not eat raw eggs or foods prepared with raw or undercooked eggs (e.g., caesar salad, hollandaise sauce).
- Handle animals carefully and avoid contact with animal feces.
- Wash hands thoroughly.

COMPLICATIONS

- Severe colon disorder
- Shock
- Severe infection
- Brain involvement

WHAT TO EXPECT

- Prognosis for gastrointestinal symptoms is excellent. Exceptions include the very young, the very old, and the debilitated and/or hospitalized.
- Prognosis for brain or heart involvement is poor, unless effective treatment is given early.

Miscellaneous

OTHER FACTORS

N/A

PEDIATRIC

Children, especially newborns, are more likely to become chronic carriers.

GERIATRIC

Patients over 60 also have high carrier rate.

OTHERS

Contaminated marijuana is an important source of infection, particularly in young adults.

PREGNANCY

N/A

FURTHER INFORMATION

Food Safety and Inspection Service, Office of Public Awareness, Dept. of Agriculture, Rm. 1165-S, Washington, DC 20205, (202) 447-9351

Scabies

 Basics

DESCRIPTION

Scabies is a contagious disease caused by infestation of the skin by the mite *Sarcoptes scabiei*.

SIGNS AND SYMPTOMS

- Generalized itching
- Itching during sleep hours
- Mites burrow between the fingers, and into the skin of wrists, hands, feet, penis, scrotum, buttocks, and waistline.
- Blisters and welts
- Peeling skin
- Reddening

CAUSES

Skin infestation by *S. scabiei*

SCOPE

Common in the United States

MOST OFTEN AFFECTED

Children and young adults; males and females in equal frequency

RISK FACTORS

- Personal skin-to-skin contact, e.g., sexual promiscuity, crowding, poverty, nosocomial infection
- Immune system disorders
- Eczema

 Diagnosis

WHAT THE DOCTOR LOOKS FOR

The doctor will evaluate for the presence of scabies; numerous other skin conditions may look similar and must be ruled out.

TESTS AND PROCEDURES

A sample of skin may be obtained by biopsy for analysis (rare).

 Treatment

GENERAL MEASURES

- Treat all intimate contacts and close household and family members.
- Wash all clothing, bed linens and towels in a normal wash cycle.

ACTIVITY

Full activity

DIET

No special diet

 Medications

COMMONLY PRESCRIBED DRUGS

- Permethrin (Elimite)
- Lindane (Kwell, Scabene)
- Crotamiton (Eurax)

CONTRAINDICATIONS

Lindane should be avoided in premature, malnourished, or emaciated children, and in individuals with severe skin disease or a history of seizures.

PRECAUTIONS

- Do not overuse the medication when applying it to the skin.
- For medications other than permethrin, use a second application only when specifically advised to do so by the physician.

DRUG INTERACTIONS

N/A

OTHER DRUGS

5% sulfur ointment

 Followup

PATIENT MONITORING

The doctor should be seen weekly only if rash or itching persist.

PREVENTION

N/A

COMPLICATIONS

- Eczema
- Other skin disorders
- Itching
- Scabies nodules

WHAT TO EXPECT

- Lesions begin to heal in 1 to 2 days along with the worst itching.
- Some itching commonly persists for 10 to 14 days and can be treated with topical or oral medication.
- Nodules

 Miscellaneous

OTHER FACTORS

N/A

PEDIATRIC

Infants often have more widespread involvement.

GERIATRIC

The elderly are at greater risk for extensive infestations; they often itch more severely.

OTHERS

N/A

PREGNANCY

Lindane should be used cautiously and no more than twice during pregnancy.

FURTHER INFORMATION

N/A

Schizophrenia

 ## Basics

DESCRIPTION

Schizophrenia is a major psychiatric disorder with symptoms of delusions, hallucinations, disturbed emotion, and impaired thought processes, lasting at least 6 months.

SIGNS AND SYMPTOMS

- Withdrawal from reality
- Delusions, paranoia
- Reference (people or things have unusual significance)
- Patient believes that he or she can hear person's thoughts or put thoughts into another person or control another person
- Grandiose or religious delusions
- Hallucinations, usually auditory
- Flat or inappropriate emotion
- Much speech but conveys little information

CAUSES

Unknown. Schizophrenia is not initiated or maintained by an organic factor. It is probably caused by a complex interaction between inherited and environmental factors.

SCOPE

About 1% of the U.S. population suffers schizophrenia at some point in their lifetime.

MOST OFTEN AFFECTED

Onset before age 45; highest prevalence in lower socioeconomic classes; males and females affected equally often

RISK FACTORS

Relative with schizophrenia

 ## Diagnosis

WHAT THE DOCTOR LOOKS FOR

The doctor will perform an evaluation to arrive at the diagnosis of schizophrenia; mental illnesses are subject to strict definitions.

TESTS AND PROCEDURES

- Blood tests, urinalysis
- Psychological testing may be done.
- Electroencephalogram (EEG) to rule out seizure disorder, brain damage, etc.
- Computed tomography (CT scan) and magnetic resonance imaging (MRI) may be done to assist in diagnosis.
- A sample of spinal fluid may be obtained by lumbar puncture (spinal tap).

 ## Treatment

GENERAL MEASURES

- Management of schizophrenia often involves hospitalization for initial assessment and treatment.
- May be managed in the outpatient setting if the person is not dangerous to self or others, able to cooperate with treatment, and has a supportive family
- Ensure safety of patient and others; the patient may act on delusional thinking.

ACTIVITY

Establish safe environment.

DIET

No special diet

Medications

COMMONLY PRESCRIBED DRUGS

Benzodiazepines and/or neuroleptics: haloperidol (Haldol), lorazepam (Ativan)

CONTRAINDICATIONS

Read drug product information.

PRECAUTIONS

Numerous precautions; read drug product information.

DRUG INTERACTIONS

Read drug product information.

OTHER DRUGS

- Thioridazine (Mellaril)
- Trifluoperazine (Stelazine)
- Thiothixene (Navane)
- Clozapine (Clozaril)
- Risperidone (Risperdal)

 ## Followup

PATIENT MONITORING

The doctor should be seen as often as necessary.

PREVENTION

N/A

COMPLICATIONS

- Drug side effects
- Self-inflicted trauma
- Combative behavior toward others

WHAT TO EXPECT

- Chronic course: good and bad periods
- Guarded prognosis, although 30% recover completely
- The negative symptoms (decreased ambition, energy, and emotional responsiveness) are often the most difficult to treat.

 ## Miscellaneous

OTHER FACTORS

N/A

PEDIATRIC

Unusual before puberty

GERIATRIC

N/A

OTHERS

N/A

PREGNANCY

N/A

FURTHER INFORMATION

Education and support groups for patient and family available from National Alliance for the Mentally Ill (NAMI), 2101 Wilson Blvd., Suite 302, Arlington, VA 22201, (703) 524-7600

Scoliosis

 Basics

DESCRIPTION

Scoliosis is a a curvature of the spine that may
be found in the thoracic, lumbar, or
thoracolumbar spinal segment. It may be
associated with kyphosis (humpback) or lordosis
(swayback). Scoliosis usually causes no other
symptoms.

SIGNS AND SYMPTOMS

CAUSES

- Unknown
- Congenital spine defects
- Musculoskeletal disorders
- Poor posture
- Uneven leg length

SCOPE

N/A

MOST OFTEN AFFECTED

The most common type of scoliosis usually
begins at about 8 to 10 years of age; it is more
common in girls than boys.

RISK FACTORS

N/A

 Diagnosis

WHAT THE DOCTOR LOOKS FOR

The doctor may take several measurements to
determine uneven leg length and may observe
the patient while walking to note spine
curvature.

TESTS AND PROCEDURES

X-rays of the spine may be taken.

 Treatment

GENERAL MEASURES

- Physical therapy and back exercises aimed at
  strengthening back muscles
- Back brace (sometimes worn for several years)
- If legs are of unequal length, a shoe lift for
  the shorter leg
- Surgery to correct the deformity (severe cases
  only).

ACTIVITY

N/A

DIET

N/A

Medications

COMMONLY PRESCRIBED DRUGS
N/A

CONTRAINDICATIONS
N/A

PRECAUTIONS
N/A

DRUG INTERACTIONS
N/A

OTHER DRUGS
N/A

 ## Followup

PATIENT MONITORING
N/A

PREVENTION
N/A

COMPLICATIONS
N/A

WHAT TO EXPECT
N/A

 ## Miscellaneous

OTHER FACTORS
N/A

PEDIATRIC
N/A

GERIATRIC
N/A

OTHERS
N/A

PREGNANCY
N/A

FURTHER INFORMATION
N/A

Seasonal Affective Disorder

 ## Basics

DESCRIPTION

Seasonal affective disorder (SAD) is depression caused by disturbance of circadian rhythms, occuring most often in the winter months. It is believed to be due to a decrease in exposure to sunlight.

SIGNS AND SYMPTOMS

In addition to feelings of sadness and anxiety, symptoms include excessive sleepiness, lethargy, carbohydrate craving, and weight gain.

CAUSES

Decreased exposure to sunlight; exact cause is unknown

SCOPE

N/A

MOST OFTEN AFFECTED

More common in women and individuals living in the northern latitudes

RISK FACTORS

N/A

 ## Diagnosis

WHAT THE DOCTOR LOOKS FOR

The doctor will take a medical history, with particular attention to symptoms of depression.

TESTS AND PROCEDURES

The individual may be asked to chart symptoms.

 ## Treatment

GENERAL MEASURES

- Phototherapy (light therapy)
- Monoamine oxidase (MAO) inhibitor or fluoxetine (Prozac)
- Psychotherapy

ACTIVITY

N/A

DIET

N/A

Medications

COMMONLY PRESCRIBED DRUGS
N/A

CONTRAINDICATIONS
N/A

PRECAUTIONS
N/A

DRUG INTERACTIONS
N/A

OTHER DRUGS
N/A

 Followup

PATIENT MONITORING
N/A

PREVENTION
N/A

COMPLICATIONS
N/A

WHAT TO EXPECT
N/A

 Miscellaneous

OTHER FACTORS
N/A

PEDIATRIC
N/A

GERIATRIC
N/A

OTHERS
N/A

PREGNANCY
N/A

FURTHER INFORMATION
N/A

Seizure Disorders

 Basics

DESCRIPTION

A seizure is a sudden change in behavior, characterized by a sensory perception or motor activity with or without a change in awareness or consciousness. Seizures may involve convulsions. Epilepsy is the name given to a particular group of seizure disorders.

SIGNS AND SYMPTOMS

- Generalized seizures
  - ▶ Absence: loss of consciousness or posture
  - ▶ Myoclonic: repetitive muscle contractions
  - ▶ Tonic-clonic: sustained muscle contraction followed by rhythmic contractions of all four extremities
- Partial seizures
- Febrile seizures (see separate entry on febrile seizures)
  - ▶ Most common in children between 3 months and 5 years of age
  - ▶ Fever without evidence of any other defined cause for seizures

CAUSES

- Brain tumor
- Insufficient oxygen in blood (breath-holding, carbon monoxide poisoning, anesthesia)
- Stroke
- Poisoning (lead, alcohol, strychnine)
- Eclampsia
- Other factors (sound, light, cutaneous stimulation)
- Fever (see entry on febrile seizures)
- Head injury
- Heat stroke
- Infection
- Metabolic disorders
- Withdrawal from, or intolerance of, alcohol

SCOPE

About 1.5 million people in the United States have epilepsy.

MOST OFTEN AFFECTED

All ages; males and females in equal numbers; family history increases risk

RISK FACTORS

Multiple factors

 Diagnosis

WHAT THE DOCTOR LOOKS FOR

The doctor will perform a physical examination to identify the cause of seizures.

TESTS AND PROCEDURES

- Blood tests
- Computed tomography (CT scan) or magnetic resonance imaging (MRI) may be done to assist in diagnosis.
- An electroencephalogram (EEG) may be done to assess brain function.

GENERAL MEASURES

- Protect the person's airway, keeping it free of saliva and other fluids.
- Do not try to restrain person; let seizure run its course.
- Protect person from injury, particularly the head.
- Do not put fingers or any other item between the person's teeth.

ACTIVITY

As tolerated

DIET

Regular

Medications

COMMONLY PRESCRIBED DRUGS

- Phenytoin (Dilantin)
- Phenobarbital
- Carbamazepine (Tegretol)
- Valproic acid (Depakene)
- Divalproex sodium
- Ethosuximide (Zarontin)
- Clonazepam (Klonopin®)

CONTRAINDICATIONS

Read drug product information.

PRECAUTIONS

Read drug product information.

DRUG INTERACTIONS

Read drug product information.

OTHER DRUGS

- Felbamate (Felbatol)
- Gabapentin (Neurontin)
- Lamotrigine (Lamictal)
- Primidone (Mysoline)
- Several additional drugs awaiting FDA approval

 ## Followup

PATIENT MONITORING

The doctor should be seen regularly.

COMPLICATIONS

Drug toxicity

WHAT TO EXPECT

- The outcome depends on the individual circumstances.
- Seizure activity may become less frequent. If a patient has been seizure-free for 2 years, withdrawal of therapy may be considered. Relapse rate after 3 years of being off medications is 33%.

 ## Miscellaneous

OTHER FACTORS

N/A

PEDIATRIC

N/A

GERIATRIC

N/A

OTHERS

N/A

PREGNANCY

Anti-seizure medication may cause birth defects.

FURTHER INFORMATION

Epilepsy Foundation of America, 4351 Garden City Drive, Landover, MD 20785, (800) EFA-1000

Seizures, Febrile

 Basics

DESCRIPTION

A febrile seizure is a seizure occurring with fever in infancy or childhood without evidence of other underlying cause.
- Simple: single episode in 24 hours, lasting less than 15 minutes. Accounts for 85% of febrile seizures.
- Complex: multiple episodes in 24 hours and lasting more than 15 minutes. Accounts for 15% of febrile seizures.

SIGNS AND SYMPTOMS

- Fever usually 102.2°F (39°C) or greater
- Convulsions
  - ▶ Usually occur within hours of fever onset
  - ▶ The seizure is the initial sign of illness in 25% of cases.
  - ▶ Duration is less than 15 minutes with simple seizures; longer with complex episodes.
  - ▶ Average frequency is once in 24 hours with simple seizures; more with complex

CAUSES

- Fever may lower seizure threshold in susceptible children.
- Temperature usually greater than 102.2°F (39°C), but rate of change may be more important than temperature
- Viral illnesses
- Bacterial infections
- Mumps, measles, rubella immunization (MMR) within prior 7 to 10 days or diphtheria, pertussis, tetanus immunization (DPT) within prior 48 hours

SCOPE

Febrile seizures affect 2–5% of all children, comprising 30% of all childhood seizures.

MOST OFTEN AFFECTED

Ninety-five percent of febrile seizures occur in children under 5 years of age; peak incidence at 2 years of age; males affected slightly more frequently than females

RISK FACTORS

Febrile seizure in sibling raises risk 2–3 times

 Diagnosis

WHAT THE DOCTOR LOOKS FOR

- The doctor will perform a physical examination to identify the cause of seizures.
- Seizures can be caused by many disorders.

TESTS AND PROCEDURES

- Blood tests
- Urinalysis
- Spinal fluids may be sampled by lumbar puncture (spinal tap).
- An electroencephalogram (EEG) may be done to evaluate brain function.
- Computed tomography (CT scan) of brain

 Treatment

GENERAL MEASURES

- Febrile seizures require emergency department or extended observation based on health status, seizure type, and other factors.
- Supportive care
- Tepid sponge bath to lower temperature
- If seizure lasts less than 10 minutes, institute supportive measures such as laying individual on side, protecting from injury, and maintaining airway.

ACTIVITY

Bedrest during observation interval

DIET

Nothing by mouth

Medications

COMMONLY PRESCRIBED DRUGS

- Rectal or oral acetaminophen, ibuprofen
- Oxygen

CONTRAINDICATIONS

Allergy to drug

PRECAUTIONS

Read drug product information.

DRUG INTERACTIONS

N/A

OTHER DRUGS

- Phenobarbital
- Phenytoin
- Valproic acid
- Paraldehyde

Followup

PATIENT MONITORING

The doctor should be seen as often as needed based on the severity and origin of the fever.

PREVENTION

- Acetaminophen, ibuprofen for rectal temperature greater than 100.5°F (38°C)

COMPLICATIONS

- Febrile seizures do not cause death, retardation, behavioral problems, or developmental delays.
- Children with febrile seizures are at greater than average risk to develop epilepsy later in life.

WHAT TO EXPECT

- Thirty percent develop recurrent febrile seizures, 50% if first episode occurs before 12 months of age and 45% if two siblings have had febrile seizures.
- Ninety-five percent of recurrences occur within 1 year.
- Epilepsy occurs in 0.5% of the general population but in 3–4% of the population who have had febrile seizure.

Miscellaneous

OTHER FACTORS

N/A

PEDIATRIC

Range is 3 months to 5 years of age; peak incidence occurs at 2 years of age. Ninety-five percent of febrile seizures occur in children 5 years of age or younger.

GERIATRIC

N/A

OTHERS

N/A

PREGNANCY

N/A

FURTHER INFORMATION

N/A

Shingles

Basics

DESCRIPTION

Herpes zoster, or shingles, is a disease usually presenting as a painful eruption of skin blisters on one side of the body. It is caused by the reactivation of varicella zoster (chickenpox) virus that has been dormant in nerves.

SIGNS AND SYMPTOMS

- Prior to rash
  - ▶ Tingling
  - ▶ Itching
  - ▶ Sharp or knife-like pain
- Acute phase
  - ▶ Constitutional symptoms
  - ▶ Fatigue
  - ▶ Malaise
  - ▶ Headache
  - ▶ Low-grade fever
  - ▶ Skin rash
  - ▶ Weakness
  - ▶ Red bumps that evolve into groups of blisters
  - ▶ Vesicles weep pus and/or blood in 3–4 days
  - ▶ Rash resolves in 14–21 days
- Chronic phase
  - ▶ Persistent nerve pain
  - ▶ Weakness of specific nerves (e.g., facial nerves)

CAUSES

Reactivation of dormant varicella zoster (chicken pox) virus

SCOPE

Herpes zoster affects 10–20% of the population at some time.

MOST OFTEN AFFECTED

The incidence of herpes zoster increases with age. 80% of cases occur in persons over 20 years old; males and females are affected in equal proportions.

RISK FACTORS

- Increasing age
- Immune system disorder
- Spinal surgery
- Spinal cord radiation

Diagnosis

WHAT THE DOCTOR LOOKS FOR

- The doctor will perform a physical examination to identify the signs of herpes zoster.
- Other conditions that can cause similar symptoms include skin disorders, gallbladder inflammation, and heart attack.

TESTS AND PROCEDURES

- Blood tests and other procedures are rarely necessary.
- Fluid from a blister may be sampled for laboratory analysis.
- A sample of affected skin may be obtained by biopsy to assist in diagnosis.

GENERAL MEASURES

- Herpes zoster is managed in the outpatient setting except for severe or complicated cases.
- Wet dressings applied for 30–60 minutes 4–6 times per day
- Lotions such as calamine

ACTIVITY

No restrictions

DIET

No special diet

Medications

COMMONLY PRESCRIBED DRUGS

- Antiviral
  - ▶ Acyclovir (Zovirax)
  - ▶ Famciclovir
  - ▶ Valacyclovir
- Pain relievers (acetaminophen, codeine, nonsteroidal anti-inflammatory drugs)
- Silver sulfadiazine (Silvadene)

CONTRAINDICATIONS

Read drug product information.

PRECAUTIONS

Read drug product information.

DRUG INTERACTIONS

Read drug product information.

OTHER DRUGS

- Vidarabine
- Idoxuridine in dimethyl sulfoxide (DMSO)

 ## Followup

PATIENT MONITORING

The physician should be seen as often as needed based on symptoms.

PREVENTION

- None at present
- Individuals with shingles may transmit herpes zoster virus to susceptible persons.
- Chickenpox vaccine does not eliminate virus.

COMPLICATIONS

- Persistent pain
- Eye involvement
- Brain infection
- Severe skin infection
- Hepatitis
- Inflammation of lungs
- Other nerve disorders

WHAT TO EXPECT

- Resolution of rash within 14–21 days
- The incidence of persistent pain (at least 1 month after rash has healed) increases dramatically with age.

 ## Miscellaneous

OTHER FACTORS

N/A

PEDIATRIC

Occurs rarely in children

GERIATRIC

- Increased incidence of herpes zoster
- Increased incidence of persistent pain

OTHERS

N/A

PREGNANCY

Can occur during pregnancy

FURTHER INFORMATION

N/A

Sinusitis

 ## Basics

DESCRIPTION

Sinusitis is an inflammation of the nasal sinuses. It may be acute (of short duration) or chronic (long-lasting) depending on duration of infection. It occurs when pus accumulates in the sinus.

SIGNS AND SYMPTOMS

- Nasal congestion
- Gradual buildup of a feeling of pressure in sinus area with tenderness
- Nasal discharge
- Malaise
- Sore throat (sometimes)
- Headache
- Fever
- Pain over cheeks and upper teeth, worse with bending
- Pain over eyebrows
- Pain over eyes
- Pain behind eyes
- Cough (occasional)
- Postnasal drip
- Swelling around eyes
- Symptoms aggravated by air travel

CAUSES

- Bacterial, viral, or fungal infections
- Preceding upper respiratory infection
- Predisposing factors: chronic nasal swelling, thick mucous, nasal polyps, allergies, sudden temperature changes

SCOPE

Common

MOST OFTEN AFFECTED

All ages; males and females affected equally often

RISK FACTORS

- Allergies
- Immune system supression
- Continuous positive airway pressure
- Air travel during upper respiratory infection
- Tooth abscess
- Swimming in contaminated water

 ## Diagnosis

WHAT THE DOCTOR LOOKS FOR

The doctor will perform a physical examination to identfiy sinusitis; numerous other conditions can cause similar signs and symptoms.

TESTS AND PROCEDURES

- Blood tests
- The sinus may be swabbed for laboratory analysis.
- The sinus may be examined by endoscopy.
- Tissue or fluid from sinus may be obtained to assist in diagnosis.
- X-rays and computed tomography (CT scan) may be used to assess the sinuses.

 ## Treatment

GENERAL MEASURES

- Steam inhalations can aid comfort and draining.
- Avoid smoke and other environmental pollutants if possible.
- Avoid smoking cigarettes.
- Surgery may be required.

ACTIVITY

No restrictions. May need additional rest during acute phase.

DIET

No special diet. Drink plenty of fluids.

Medications

COMMONLY PRESCRIBED DRUGS

- Antibiotics: amoxicillin, trimethoprim-sul-famethoxazole
- Pain relievers
- Decongestants
- Antihistamines

CONTRAINDICATIONS

Read drug product information.

PRECAUTIONS

Read drug product information.

DRUG INTERACTIONS

Read drug product information.

OTHER DRUGS

Decongestant spray

 ## Followup

PATIENT MONITORING

The doctor should be seen until symptoms completely resolve.

PREVENTION

Treat nasal congestion before sinusitis develops.

COMPLICATIONS

- Inflammation of the covering of the brain and spinal cord
- Abscess of brain or related structures
- Bone infection
- Infection around eye
- Unnecessary dental work due to confusion over origin of pain

WHAT TO EXPECT

- Acute: favorable prognosis with timely treatment and avoidance of complications
- Chronic: may improve if cause is removed or drainage is feasible

 ## Miscellaneous

OTHER FACTORS

N/A

PEDIATRIC

N/A

GERIATRIC

- Incidence of sinusitis increases up to age 75 and then decreases.
- Sinusitis is more difficult to heal when it occurs among the elderly.

OTHERS

N/A

PREGNANCY

N/A

FURTHER INFORMATION

Asthma & Allergy Foundation of America, 1717 Massachusetts Avenue, Suite 305, Washington, DC 20036, (800)7-Asthma

Sleep Apnea, Obstructive

 Basics

DESCRIPTION

Sleep apnea consists of episodes of upper airway obstruction during sleep, often depriving the body of oxygen. It is nearly always associated with snoring. Periods of nonbreathing (apnea) often terminate with a snort or gasp. Repeated episodes of apnea disrupts sleep, leading to excessive daytime sleepiness. The usual course is chronic (long-lasting).

SIGNS AND SYMPTOMS

- Excessive daytime sleepiness
- Loud snoring
- Disrupted sleep
- Repeated awakenings with a transient feeling of shortness of breath
- Tired and unrefreshed upon awakening in the morning
- Sleeping partner reports periods of stopped breathing
- Complaints of poor concentration, memory problems, irritability
- Morning headaches
- Short-temperedness
- Decreased libido is also common
- Depression
- High blood pressure

CAUSES

Upper airway narrowing may be due to obesity, enlarged tonsils and uvula, low soft palate, excess tissue in soft palate, large tongue, skull/facial abnormalities, and abnormal control of upper airway muscle or breathing during sleep.

SCOPE

Obstructive sleep apnea affects 4–8% of the U.S. adult population.

MOST OFTEN AFFECTED

Middle-aged individuals; males more frequently than females

RISK FACTORS

- Obesity
- Nasal obstruction
- Hypothyroidism
- Large tongue
- Small jaw
- Acromegaly
- High blood pressure, cardiovascular disease, lung disease

 Diagnosis

WHAT THE DOCTOR LOOKS FOR

- The doctor will obtain a history and perform a physical examination to develop a diagnosis of obstructive sleep apnea.
- Other causes of excessive daytime sleepiness should be investigated, including narcolepsy, inadequate sleep, or depression.
- Other conditions that may be associated with sleep apnea should be assessed, such as asthma, heart failure, lung disease, panic attacks, seizures, or gastroesophageal reflux.

TESTS AND PROCEDURES

- Blood tests
- X-rays of the head and neck
- Echocardiography
- Polysomnogram (nighttime sleep study)
- Magnetic resonance imaging (MRI), computed tomography (CT scan), or fiberoptic evaluation of upper airway

 Treatment

GENERAL MEASURES

- Obstructive sleep apnea is managed in the outpatient setting, except for surgery that involves hospitalization.
- If sleep apnea only occurs when sleeping on the back, then avoid sleeping on the back. Use a tennis ball sewn onto a nightshirt or wear a fanny-pack with tennis balls on the back.
- Surgery may be required for mild to severe obstructive sleep apnea.
- Dental appliances may be of benefit.

- Continuous positive-airway pressure (CPAP) or biphasic positive-airway pressure (BiPAP) may be of benefit.
- Avoid driving if daytime sleepiness is significant.
- No alcohol within 6 hours of bedtime
- Avoid sedatives and sleeping pills.

ACTIVITY

Don't drive motor vehicle or operate heavy equipment injury until treated.

DIET

Obese patients must lose weight. All patients must avoid weight gain and alcohol.

 ## Medications

COMMONLY PRESCRIBED DRUGS

- Protriptyline
- Fluoxetine (Prozac)

CONTRAINDICATIONS

None

PRECAUTIONS

May cause or worsen narrow-angle glaucoma or urinary retention. Use cautiously with rapid heart rate conditions.

DRUG INTERACTIONS

Read drug product information.

OTHER DRUGS

- Medroxyprogesterone
- Acetazolamide (Diamox)

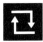 ## Followup

PATIENT MONITORING

The doctor should be seen as often as needed for the management of snoring, excessive daytime sleepiness, or sleep disruption.

PREVENTION

- Excess weight is one of the most common causes of obstructive sleep apnea; in many cases losing weight is the best cure.

- Avoid the use of alcohol, sedatives, or depressants.

COMPLICATIONS

- Untreated, obstructive sleep apnea is associated with high blood pressure, irregular heart rhythms, and heart failure.
- Excessive daytime sleepiness is a significant cause of death and injury.

WHAT TO EXPECT

- With appropriate control of apnea, excessive daytime sleepiness dramatically improves quickly.
- All therapy other than surgery and weight loss in obese patients are methods of control, rather than cure. Lifelong compliance with weight loss or nasal CPAP are necessary.
- Untreated, obstructive sleep apnea will get worse.

 ## Miscellaneous

OTHER FACTORS

N/A

PEDIATRIC

- Obstructive sleep apnea is not as common in pediatric age group.
- If present, it is often due to enlarged tonsils, craniofacial abnormalities, or diseases such as cerebral palsy or spinal muscular atrophy. Response to tonsil removal surgery is often good.

GERIATRIC

Obstructive sleep apnea appears to increase in frequency after middle age and after the menopause in women. It often coexists with other health problems in the elderly.

OTHERS

N/A

PREGNANCY

Rare

FURTHER INFORMATION

N/A

Snakebite

Basics

DESCRIPTION

There are two types of poisonous snakes in the United States: coral snakes and pit vipers, the latter including rattlesnakes and water moccasins. Many other varieties of poisonous snakes are maintained as pets.

- Rattlesnakes and water moccasins characteristically have triangular-shaped heads, eyes with elliptical pupils, and small heat-sensing facial pits located between the nostril and the eye. They are most commonly found in southeastern and southwestern United States.
- Coral snakes have a characteristic rounded head with round pupils. Coloration is important. In the United States, poisonous coral snakes have broad rings of red and black that are separated by narrow rings of yellow. ("Red on yellow, kill a fellow; red on black, venom lack.") Coral snakes are found in Arizona, Texas, Arkansas, Louisiana and the Southeastern United States.

SIGNS AND SYMPTOMS

- Signs and symptoms vary by species.
- Fang marks; one or two punctures; may be shallow or appear as a scratch
- Pain out of proportion to size of puncture wound
- Swelling of site; swelling progresses up the extremity
- Weakness, dizziness
- Numbness/tingling in extremity, mouth, tongue
- Bruising of skin
- Rapid heart rate
- Double vision
- Nausea/vomiting
- Muscle twitching, spasms
- Mental status changes including coma

CAUSES

- Contact with poisonous snake
- Coral snakes are nocturnal and timid; therefore, they rarely bite humans. They must be deliberately provoked to bite.

SCOPE

There are at least 8,000 snakebites annually in the United States; and 20 to 25 % of these bites do not result in envenomation (injection of venom).

MOST OFTEN AFFECTED

Individuals 19–30 years of age; males affected more often than females

RISK FACTORS

- Risk-taking behaviors
- Judgement impaired by alcohol or drug intoxication

Diagnosis

WHAT THE DOCTOR LOOKS FOR

The doctor will perform a physical examination to determine whether a wound is a snake bite, whether it was a venomous snake, and to identify the species of snake involved.

TESTS AND PROCEDURES

- Blood tests
- Urinalysis

Treatment

GENERAL MEASURES

- True envenomations and resulting signs/symptoms demand immediate emergency department evaluation, with hospital admission if necessary.
- Provide emergency first aid as needed, including rescue breathing and cardiopulmonary resuscitation (CPR).
- Provide reassurance to victim.
- Remove rings and constrictive items between site of envenomation and body.
- Place affected injured part at level of heart.
- Do NOT attempt to cut the snakebite wound and suck out the venom.

ACTIVITY

Bed rest with elevation of extremity. Physical therapy may be needed in severe cases of envenomation.

DIET

Nothing by mouth initially

 # Medications

COMMONLY PRESCRIBED DRUGS

- Antivenin is not available for all poisonous snakes.
- Polyvalent Crotalidae antivenin: pit vipers (rattle snakes, water moccasins)
- Micrurus fulvius antivenin: North American coral snake

CONTRAINDICATIONS

History of allergy to horse serum

PRECAUTIONS

N/A

DRUG INTERACTIONS

N/A

OTHER DRUGS

N/A

 # Followup

PATIENT MONITORING

- The doctor should be seen within 48 hours, then as needed.
- Physical therapy referral should be made early for optimal outcome.

PREVENTION

- Use of preventive measures if handling snakes
- In snake-infested areas:
  - ▶ Wear protective shoes and clothing when walking
  - ▶ Do not insert hands or feet into cracks or crevices or hollow logs
  - ▶ Carry a flashlight if walking at night

COMPLICATIONS

- Serum sickness from antivenin therapy
- Local wound infection
- Pneumonia

WHAT TO EXPECT

- If properly treated, death is rare.
- Death can occur even with antivenin therapy.
- Deterioration may progress despite antivenin; complete paralysis can occur.
- Muscle strength may not return to normal for 4 to 6 weeks.
- Long-term illness is rare.

 # Miscellaneous

OTHER FACTORS

N/A

PEDIATRIC

Course may be more severe.

GERIATRIC

Course may be more severe.

OTHERS

N/A

PREGNANCY

N/A

FURTHER INFORMATION

N/A

Sore Throat

 Basics

DESCRIPTION

Sore throat, or pharyngitis, is an inflammation most commonly caused by acute infection.

SIGNS AND SYMPTOMS

- Sore throat
- Enlarged tonsils
- Enlarged lymph nodes in neck
- Absence of cough, hoarseness, or lower respiratory symptoms
- Fever over 102.5°F (39.1°C)
- Rash
- Loss of appetite
- Chills
- Malaise
- Headache
- Reddened eyes

CAUSES

- Bacterial or viral infection
- Chronic (long-lasting): noninfectious; chemical irritation; smoking; cancer

SCOPE

An estimated 30 million cases of sore throat are diagnosed yearly in the United States.

MOST OFTEN AFFECTED

Pharyngitis occurs in all age groups; males and females affected in equal proportions

RISK FACTORS

- Epidemics
- Age (young are more susceptible)
- Family history
- Close quarters, such as in new military recruits
- Immune system disorders
- Fatigue
- Smoking
- Excess alcohol consumption
- Oral sex
- Diabetes mellitus
- Recent illness

 Diagnosis

WHAT THE DOCTOR LOOKS FOR

- The doctor will evaluate the status of the throat.
- The cause of sore throat should be identified and treated.

TESTS AND PROCEDURES

The throat may be swabbed for laboratory analysis.

 Treatment

GENERAL MEASURES

- Salt-water gargles
- Acetaminophen
- Dyclonine lozenges
- Cool-mist humidifier

ACTIVITY

As tolerated

DIET

No restrictions. Extra fluids are encouraged.

Medications

COMMONLY PRESCRIBED DRUGS

- Penicillin
- Erythromycin
- Cephalexin

CONTRAINDICATIONS

Allergy to specific antibiotic

PRECAUTIONS

Read drug product information.

DRUG INTERACTIONS

Read drug product information.

OTHER DRUGS

N/A

 Followup

PATIENT MONITORING

Contact the doctor by telephone as needed for the duration of the illness.

PREVENTION

Avoid contact with infected people.

COMPLICATIONS

- Rheumatic fever
- Kidney inflammation
- Abscess of tonsil
- Systemic infection
- Ear infection
- Rhinitis
- Sinusitis
- Pneumonia

WHAT TO EXPECT

- Sore throat often lasts 5–7 days; fever peaks at 2 to 3 days.
- Symptoms will resolve spontaneously without treatment, but complications are possible.
- Severe complications may require surgery.

 Miscellaneous

OTHER FACTORS

N/A

PEDIATRIC

N/A

GERIATRIC

N/A

OTHERS

N/A

PREGNANCY

N/A

FURTHER INFORMATION

N/A

Sprains & Strains

 Basics

DESCRIPTION

A sprain is an injury to a ligament. A strain is a partial or complete disruption of the muscle or tendon. Strains usually are associated with overuse injuries, whereas sprains usually result from trauma (falls, twisting injuries, or motor vehicle accidents).

SIGNS AND SYMPTOMS

- Swelling
- Pain
- Reddening or bruising
- Tenderness
- Gait disturbances if severe
- Decreased range of motion of joint and joint instability

CAUSES

- Falls
- Motor vehicle accident
- Trauma
- Excessive exercise or inadequate warm-up and stretching prior to activity
- Poor conditioning

SCOPE

At one time or another, almost 80% of persons experience a sprain or strain.

MOST OFTEN AFFECTED

- Sprains: any age in which patient is physically active
- Strains: usually individuals 15–40 years of age
- Males are affected more frequently than females.

RISK FACTORS

- Change in or improper shoe gear, protective gear, or environment (e.g., surface)
- Inappropriate increase in training schedule

 Diagnosis

WHAT THE DOCTOR LOOKS FOR

- The doctor will perform a physical examination to assess for the presence of sprain or/and strain.
- Other musculoskeletal disorders should be ruled out, including fractures, tendonitis, bursitis, and other conditions (tendonitis, bursitis, bony injuries).
- Rarely, muscle hematomas account for some of the signs and symptoms of strains.

TESTS AND PROCEDURES

- X-rays
- Computed tomography (CT scan) or magnetic resonance imaging (MRI) may be done.
- The joint may be examined by arthroscopy in some cases.

 Treatment

GENERAL MEASURES

- RICE therapy: Rest, Ice, Compression, Elevation
- Elastic bandage wrap (Ace) is comfortable.
- Splint for pain relief and stability
- Crutches and gait training
- After initial treatment, rehabilitation may be recommended.

ACTIVITY

- Bed rest for acute injuries
- Physical therapy for more severe injuries
- Elevate joint while sleeping.

DIET

Weight loss if obese

Medications

COMMONLY PRESCRIBED DRUGS

Nonsteroidal anti-inflammatory drugs (NSAID's)

CONTRAINDICATIONS

Read drug product information.

PRECAUTIONS

Read drug product information.

DRUG INTERACTIONS

Read drug product information.

OTHER DRUGS

- Pain relievers
- Analgesic balms
- Capsaicin cream

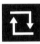 ## Followup

PATIENT MONITORING

The doctor should be seen as often as necessary.

PREVENTION

- Maintain a reasonable level of physical fitness.
- Avoid excessive physical stresses.
- Wear exercise gear (particularly shoes).
- Use proper equipment for the activity.
- Know the risks associated with the intended activity.
- Appropriate conditioning and warm-up and cool-down exercises

COMPLICATIONS

- Chronic joint instability
- Arthritis

WHAT TO EXPECT

With appropriate treatment and rest, recovery takes 6–8 weeks or longer, depending on severity of injury.

 ## Miscellaneous

OTHER FACTORS

N/A

PEDIATRIC

N/A

GERIATRIC

More likely to see associated bone injuries due to decreased joint flexibility and prevalence of osteoporosis

OTHERS

N/A

PREGNANCY

N/A

FURTHER INFORMATION

N/A

Stroke (Brain Attack)

 Basics

DESCRIPTION

Stroke, or cerebrovascular accident (CVA), is the sudden onset of a neurological deficit resulting from a loss of blood circulation to a portion of the brain, either by blood clot (infarction) or bleeding (hemorrhage). Stroke rehabilitation involves restoration of function after medical and neurologic stability have been achieved.

SIGNS AND SYMPTOMS

- The signs and symptoms of stroke vary depending on what part of the brain is affected.
- Paralysis or loss of sensation on one side of the body
- Visual disturbances
- Paralysis of the facial muscles on one side
- Dizziness, difficulty walking or moving
- Difficulty speaking, understanding language
- Altered level of consciousness
- Sudden headache, nausea, vomiting, and incoordination

CAUSES

- Coronary artery disease
- High blood pressure
- Blockage of arteries in brain
- Formation of clots within the heart or blood vessels
- Foreign body in bloodstream
- Frequently, the combination of gout, diabetes, and hypertension that has been untreated for 5 to 10 years can contribute to the onset of a stroke.
- Blood vessel disorders
- Blood-clotting disorders
- Other causes: trauma, drug use, other diseases

SCOPE

There are about 160 cases of stroke per 100,000 persons in the United States.

MOST OFTEN AFFECTED

The risk of stroke increases in people over age 45 and is highest in individuals 60–80 years of age; more common in males than females

RISK FACTORS

- Increasing age
- High blood pressure
- Heart disease
- Smoking
- Diabetes
- Family history
- Many risk factors are lifestyle-oriented and preventable, such as coffee consumption, obesity, inactivity, hyperactivity to the point of exhaustion, mood swings, sexual hyperactivity, starvation, antidepressant or diet reduction medication, alcohol or recreational drug habituation, and unusual stress states.

Stroke (Brain Attack)

 Diagnosis

WHAT THE DOCTOR LOOKS FOR

- The doctor will perform a physical examination to determine the severity and extent of damage caused by stroke.
- Conditions that can appear similar to stroke include epilepsy, migraine, tumor, diabetes, infection, and trauma.
- The doctor should also identify and treat conditions known to be associated with stroke, such as heart disease, high blood pressure, bleeding disorders, and other diseases.
- Different types of stroke disorders can occur in one person.

TESTS AND PROCEDURES

- Blood tests
- Urinalysis
- The carotid arteries may be evaluated by ultrasound.
- Cerebral angiography
- An electrocardiogram (ECG) and echocardiogram may be done.
- Computed tomography (CT), magnetic resonance imaging (MRI) and positron emission tomography (PET) may be done to assist in diagnosis.
- A sample of spinal fluid may be obtained by lumbar puncture (spinal tap).
- Special senory and neurologic tests may be done to assess recovery.

 Treatment

GENERAL MEASURES

- Immediately after stroke:
  - ▶ Provide emergency first aid as needed, including rescue breathing and cardiopulmonary resuscitation (CPR)
  - ▶ Call 9-1-1
  - ▶ Seek medical attention as soon as possible
- In many cases, thrombolytic (clot-busting) therapy may restore circulation if given promptly after stroke.
- During the acute phase, management of stroke requires hospitalization.
- Recovery of stroke may require a rehabilitation center or special care facility; or, stroke may be managed on an outpatient basis.
- A full-service rehabilitation center and rehabilitation medicine team can make the difference between independence and dependency
- Full-service rehabilitation center characteristics include closed units; regular team meetings to discuss long- and short-term objectives; quality assurance system in place; accreditation by Commission on Accreditation of Rehabilitation Facilities.
- Surgery may be recommended.

Stroke (Brain Attack)

ACTIVITY

- Walking as soon as possible
- Physical therapy, occupational therapy, speech pathology, psychology, and nursing therapy should be provided for at least 3 hours per day during hospitalization.
- While most rehabilitative efforts take place within a very short time after stroke, successful rehabilitative efforts have taken place as long as 5 years later.

DIET

- Depends upon other medical conditions
- Diet as tolerated (no added salt if hypertensive)

 ## Medications

COMMONLY PRESCRIBED DRUGS

- Thrombolytics (clot-busting drugs)
- Enteric coated aspirin (EC ASA)
- Ticlopidine (Ticlid)

CONTRAINDICATIONS

- EC ASA: peptic ulcer disease, allergy to aspirin or other nonsteroidal anti-inflammatory drugs (NSAIDs)
- Ticlopidine: known hypersensitivity to the drug, blood disorders, severe liver failure

PRECAUTIONS

EC ASA therapy may aggravate peptic ulcer disease, may worsen asthma.

DRUG INTERACTIONS

Read drug product information.

OTHER DRUGS

- Nimodipine, nicardipine

Stroke (Brain Attack)

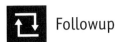 Followup

PATIENT MONITORING

The doctor should be seen 1 month after stroke, every 3 months for first year, then yearly.

PREVENTION

- Stroke is usually an unnecessary illness; major risk factors are nearly all preventable.
- Stop smoking.
- Control blood pressure, diabetes, and dietary fats.
- Daily aspirin to reduce clots (only with doctor's permission)
- Use alcohol in moderation, if at all.
- Regular exercise
- Maintain positive psychological outlook.
- Maintain weight control.
- The progressive physical and mental deterioration noted with high blood pressure and heart disease is not inevitable.
- Family support may help the patient to become interested in his or her health and may assist the patient in maintaining health
- Disuse will add subsequent complications and long-term effects.
- Surgery (endarterectomy) may prevent stroke.

COMPLICATIONS

- Muscle and joint disorders
- Depression

WHAT TO EXPECT

- The outcome varies depending on severity and location of stroke.
- Overall, the outcome is generally good, although pneumonia, respiratory failure, heart failure, and heart attack occur more frequently after stroke.

 Miscellaneous

OTHER FACTORS

N/A

PEDIATRIC

N/A

GERIATRIC

N/A

OTHERS

N/A

PREGNANCY

Hypertension in pregnancy can lead to stroke.

FURTHER INFORMATION

National Stroke Association, 300 East Hampden Ave., Suite 240, Englewood, CO 80110-2622

Stye

 Basics

DESCRIPTION

A stye, or hordeolum, is an inflammation or infection of the eyelid margin, often involving the hair follicles of the eyelashes.

SIGNS AND SYMPTOMS

- Redness of the edge of the eyelid with peeling, weeping
- Inflammation of the eyelashes
- Itching or peeling of the eyelids, chronic redness, eye irritation leading to tenderness and pain

CAUSES

- The most common cause of stye is a staphylococcal infection, although other organisms may also be involved.
- Seborrhea can predispose to infections of the eyelid.

SCOPE

Extremely common

MOST OFTEN AFFECTED

Stye can affect all age groups; males and females with equal frequency

RISK FACTORS

- Predisposing eyelid infection
- Poor eyelid hygiene
- Contact lens wear
- Application of make-up

 Diagnosis

WHAT THE DOCTOR LOOKS FOR

The doctor will perform a physical examination to identify the presence of a stye.

TESTS AND PROCEDURES

N/A

 Treatment

GENERAL MEASURES

- Warm compresses to the area of inflammation can help increase blood supply and promote healing.
- Clean the eyelids using a solution of tap water and baby shampoo or a commercially prepared hypoallergenic cleanser.
- The stye should not be squeezed.
- Good personal hygiene should be maintained, with attention to cleansing the eyelids on a daily basis to prevent recurrent infections.
- Apply an antibiotic ointment (such as erythromycin) to the margin of the eyelid after proper cleansing (except children under 12 years of age or in cases in which there is a risk of vision problems). The antibiotic helps reduce bacterial growth.
- Minor surgery may be required to drain infection.

ACTIVITY

No restrictions

DIET

No special diet

Medications

COMMONLY PRESCRIBED DRUGS

- Erythromycin ophthalmic ointment
- Aminoglycoside ophthalmic ointment (gentamicin)

CONTRAINDICATIONS

None

PRECAUTIONS

None

DRUG INTERACTIONS

None

OTHER DRUGS

None

 Followup

PATIENT MONITORING

The doctor should be seen within several weeks to assess the effectiveness of therapy.

PREVENTION

Eyelid hygiene

COMPLICATIONS

None expected.

WHAT TO EXPECT

Styes usually resolve with treatment but tend to recur in some patients.

 Miscellaneous

OTHER FACTORS

N/A

PEDIATRIC

N/A

GERIATRIC

N/A

OTHERS

N/A

PREGNANCY

N/A

FURTHER INFORMATION

N/A

Sudden Infant Death Syndrome (SIDS)

 Basics

DESCRIPTION

This syndrome is defined as the sudden death of an infant under 1 year of age that remains unexplained after a thorough case investigation, including performance of a complete autopsy, examination of the death scene, and review of the clinical history.

- Apparent Life-Threatening Event (ALTE), such as apnea that sometimes but not always precedes SIDS, is a related entity.

SIGNS AND SYMPTOMS

SIDs infants generally appear healthy or may have had a minor upper respiratory or gastrointestinal infection in the last 2 weeks of life.

CAUSES

- There are many theories about the cause of SIDS. There may be subtle developmental abnormalities resulting from brain injury.
- Possible causes:
  - ▶ Abnormal respiratory control
  - ▶ Upper airway obstruction
  - ▶ Nervous system abnormalities
  - ▶ Irregular heart rhythms
  - ▶ Carbon dioxide rebreathing in face-down position on soft surface
  - ▶ SIDS may occur when a combination of factors coincide; such triggers may include infectious agents, climatic changes, or environmental factors.

SCOPE

There are about 4,700 cases of SIDS annually in the United States.

MOST OFTEN AFFECTED

SIDS is rare in the first month of life. Peak incidence occurs in infants between 2 and 4 months of age; 90% of deaths occur by 6 months of age; more common in males than females

RISK FACTORS

- Most SIDS deaths occur in children who are "low-risk." However, there are several risk factors associated with SIDS:
  - ▶ Race: Native-Americans and African-Americans have highest incidence.

- ▶ Season: late fall and winter months
- ▶ Time of day: between midnight and 6 AM
- ▶ Activity: during sleep
- ▶ Low birth weight
- ▶ Poverty
- Maternal factors: teenage mothers; maternal use of cigarettes or drugs (cocaine, opiates) during pregnancy; large number of children; maternal anemia during pregnancy
- Respiratory or gastrointestinal infection in recent past
- Sleep practices: prone sleep position, heavier clothing and bedding, soft bedding
- Lack of breast-feeding
- Passive cigarette smoke exposure after birth

 Diagnosis

WHAT THE DOCTOR LOOKS FOR

The doctor will perform a physical examination to rule out an identifiable cause of distress or death, including suffocation, metabolic disorders, child abuse, homicide, or other conditions.

TESTS AND PROCEDURES

- For apparent life-threatening events:
  - ▶ Arterial blood may be drawn for laboratory analysis.
  - ▶ X-rays
  - ▶ An electrocardiogram (ECG) may be done.
  - ▶ A electroencephalogram (EEG) may be done to monitor brain activity.
  - ▶ Other tests may be done to assist in diagnosis.

 Treatment

GENERAL MEASURES

- Because a SIDS death is sudden and the cause is unknown, SIDS cannot be "treated." However, there are some measures that may be effective in preventing SIDS:
  - ▶ Maternal avoidance of cigarette and illicit drug use during pregnancy
  - ▶ Breast-feeding

Sudden Infant Death Syndrome (SIDS)

▶ Avoid letting the baby sleep on his or her stomach.

▶ Avoid excessive bed clothing and soft bedding.

▶ Avoid passive cigarette smoke exposure.

• Recent studies suggest significant risk reduction when baby is placed on the back or side for sleep. Because infants placed on their side may turn over during sleep onto their stomach, it is now believed that back position is best.

ACTIVITY

N/A

DIET

N/A

 Medications

COMMONLY PRESCRIBED DRUGS

N/A

CONTRAINDICATIONS

N/A

PRECAUTIONS

N/A

DRUG INTERACTIONS

N/A

OTHER DRUGS

N/A

 Followup

PATIENT MONITORING

Some authorities recommend monitoring of siblings of prior SIDS victims.

PREVENTION

see General Measures

COMPLICATIONS

N/A

WHAT TO EXPECT

• SIDS deaths have a powerful impact on families and their functioning. Health care providers can play an important role in providing immediate information about SIDS and sensitive counseling to limit parents' misinformation and feelings of guilt.

• Counseling needs of families vary from short-term to long-term; support groups are helpful to many couples. Providers should be familiar with resources available in their communities to help families mourning a SIDS death. Parents need to be counseled about subsequent pregnancies.

• Followup counseling, including review of the autopsy report with the family after some time has passed, will be important to help with understanding this condition and to clear the tremendous guilt these families experience.

 Miscellaneous

OTHER FACTORS

N/A

PEDIATRIC

Occurs in infants only

GERIATRIC

N/A

OTHERS

N/A

PREGNANCY

N/A

FURTHER INFORMATION

• American Sudden Infant Death Syndrome Institute, (800) 232-SIDS in Atlanta, Georgia

• National SIDS Alliance/National SIDS Foundation, Columbia, MD, (800) 221-SIDS

• Back to Sleep Information Line, (800)505-CRIB (sponsored by the U.S. Public Health Service)

• National SIDS Resource Center, (703)821-8955, ext. 249

Sunburn

 Basics

DESCRIPTION

A sunburn is an acute reaction to the toxic effects of ultraviolet (UV) in sunlight.

SIGNS AND SYMPTOMS

- Mild reddening with subsequent peeling
- Pain
- Swelling
- Skin tenderness
- Blisters
- Fever, chills, weakness
- Shock
- Secondary infections

CAUSES

- Exposure to sunlight (or other ultraviolet light source) following administration of photosensitivity-producing drugs.
- Overexposure to ultraviolet rays; danger increases proportionately to higher altitudes

SCOPE

Common

MOST OFTEN AFFECTED

All ages

RISK FACTORS

N/A

 Diagnosis

WHAT THE DOCTOR LOOKS FOR

N/A

TESTS AND PROCEDURES

None required

 Treatment

GENERAL MEASURES

- Avoid additional exposure until well.
- Use tap-water compresses.
- Avoid topical anesthetic lotions and ointments.

ACTIVITY

N/A

DIET

N/A

Medications

COMMONLY PRESCRIBED DRUGS

Prednisone

CONTRAINDICATIONS

Read drug product information.

PRECAUTIONS

Read drug product information.

DRUG INTERACTIONS

Read drug product information.

OTHER DRUGS

N/A

 Followup

PATIENT MONITORING

N/A

PREVENTION

- Prevention with sunscreens rated SPF (sun-protection factor) 15 or better
- Avoid sun exposure during "peak tanning hours," approximately 11:00am to 2:00pm.

COMPLICATIONS

Usually none

WHAT TO EXPECT

- Longterm risks include:
  - ▶ Melanoma and other skin cancers
  - ▶ Skin aging

 Miscellaneous

OTHER FACTORS

N/A

PEDIATRIC

Children at high risk

GERIATRIC

N/A

PREGNANCY

N/A

FURTHER INFORMATION

N/A

Swimmer's Ear

 ## Basics

DESCRIPTION

Otitis externa, or swimmer's ear, is an inflammation of the external ear canal. It may be caused by infection with bacteria or fungus.

SIGNS AND SYMPTOMS

- Itching
- Plugging of the ear
- Pain
- Reddening
- Discharge of pus
- Eczema of ear

CAUSES

- Trauma
- Infection (bacterial, fungal)
- Skin disorders (e.g. eczema, seborrhea)

SCOPE

Unknown; incidence is higher in the summer months

MOST OFTEN AFFECTED

All ages; males and females affected in equal numbers

RISK FACTORS

- Trauma of external ear canal
- Swimming
- Hot humid weather
- Use of a hearing aid
- Advancing age
- Diabetes
- Debilitating disease

 ## Diagnosis

WHAT THE DOCTOR LOOKS FOR

The doctor will evaluate the ear and identify the cause of inflammation.

TESTS AND PROCEDURES

- Fluid from the ear may be sampled for laboratory analysis
- X-rays of the head, rarely

 ## Treatment

GENERAL MEASURES

- Otitis externa is managed in the outpatient setting, except for severe cases that require hospitalization.
- The external ear canal should be thoroughly cleaned.
- Pain relievers
- Anti-itch and antihistamine medication

ACTIVITY

No restrictions

DIET

No restrictions

Medications

COMMONLY PRESCRIBED DRUGS

- Topical therapy for approximately 10 days
- Pain relievers
- 2% acetic acid
- Antibiotics, antifungal medications

CONTRAINDICATIONS

Allergies to prescribed drugs; read drug product information.

PRECAUTIONS

Read drug product information.

DRUG INTERACTIONS

Read drug product information.

OTHER DRUGS

N/A

Followup

PATIENT MONITORING

- The doctor should be seen 48 hours after treatment begins to assess improvement and at the end of therapy.
- For chronic otitis externa, the doctor should be seen every 2–3 weeks for repeated cleansing of ear canal.

PREVENTION

- Avoid prolonged exposure to moisture.
- Use preventive antiseptics.
- Treat skin conditions.
- Eliminate trauma to canal.
- Diagnose and treat underlying medical conditions.

COMPLICATIONS

Inflammation may spread.

WHAT TO EXPECT

- Acute otitis externa rapidly responds to therapy with total resolution.
- In the case of chronic otitis externa, most cases resolve with repeated cleansing and antibiotic therapy. Occasionally, surgery may be required.

Miscellaneous

OTHER FACTORS

N/A

PEDIATRIC

N/A

GERIATRIC

N/A

OTHERS

N/A

PREGNANCY

N/A

FURTHER INFORMATION

N/A

Syphilis

 Basics

DESCRIPTION

Syphilis is a sexually transmitted disease that is characterized by sequential stages. After the initial period of symptoms, the disease can remain latent, flaring up years later. Syphilis can also occur congenitally, passed from mother to baby during pregnancy.

SIGNS AND SYMPTOMS

- A chancre or lesion usually found on genitalia, which heals in 3 to 6 weeks; 75% have no further symptoms.
- Latent phase may be marked by rash, frequently on palms and soles; bald patches on scalp, eyebrows, and beard; moist lesions on genital area; generalized flu-like symptoms of aches and malaise; may be accompanied by more severe symptoms
- Tertiary syphilis: symptoms involving cardiovascular and bone disease, dementia, and other severe symptoms

CAUSES

- Exposure through sexual contact
- Exposure to infected body fluids
- Congenital (passed to fetus during pregnancy)

SCOPE

There are about 20 cases of syphilis per 100,000 persons in the United States. In some groups, the rate is 6 times higher; reported cases are rising rapidly.

MOST OFTEN AFFECTED

Sexually active individuals; males affected more frequently than females

RISK FACTORS

- Multiple sexual partners
- Intravenous (IV) drug use
- Male homosexuality

 Diagnosis

WHAT THE DOCTOR LOOKS FOR

The doctor will perform a physical examination to identify the presence of syphilis.

TESTS AND PROCEDURES

- Blood tests
- A sample of spinal fluids may be obtained by lumbar puncture (spinal tap).
- A sample of skin may be obtained by biopsy for laboratory analysis.

 Treatment

GENERAL MEASURES

- Syphilis is usually managed in the outpatient setting.
- All sexual contacts must be traced and treated.
- Keep followup appointments to monitor success of therapy.
- Avoid intercourse until treatment is complete.
- Local health department can provide literature and contact tracing.

ACTIVITY

- Full activity, but no sexual contacts until cured

DIET

No special diet

Syphilis

 ## Medications

COMMONLY PRESCRIBED DRUGS

Penicillin

CONTRAINDICATIONS

Allergy to penicillin

PRECAUTIONS

Read drug product information.

DRUG INTERACTIONS

None

OTHER DRUGS

Erythromycin, tetracyclines, ceftriaxone (Rocephin)

 ## Followup

PATIENT MONITORING

Blood tests should be repeated for 3 months, then annually. Blood tests may be more frequent for individuals also infected with human immunodeficiency virus (HIV).

PREVENTION

- Safe sex practices
- Mutually monogamous relationship
- Use of condoms

COMPLICATIONS

- Cardiovascular disease
- Central nervous system disease
- Kidney disease
- Irreversable organ damage
- Many other disorders

WHAT TO EXPECT

The prognosis is excellent in all cases, except late syphilis complications and a few HIV-infected patients.

 ## Miscellaneous

OTHER FACTORS

N/A

PEDIATRIC

Must consider possible child abuse

GERIATRIC

N/A

OTHERS

N/A

PREGNANCY

Early detection is imperative; all expectant mothers should have testing as part of routine prenatal care.

FURTHER INFORMATION

N/A

Systemic Lupus Erythematosus (SLE)

 ## Basics

DESCRIPTION

Systemic lupus erythematosis (SLE) is an autoimmune disorder involving the inflammation of many body systems, characterized by a fluctuating, chronic course. SLE varies from mild to severe and may be lethal.

SIGNS AND SYMPTOMS

- Arthritis
- Fever
- Loss of appetite
- Malaise
- Weight loss
- Skin lesions
- Mouth ulcers
- Eye pain and/or redness
- Chest pain and/or shortness of breath
- Pallor
- Nausea, vomiting, diarrhea
- Muscle tenderness, aching, and stiffness
- Headaches and visual problems
- Psychosis, delirium

CAUSES

- Most cases have unknown causes.
- Drugs

SCOPE

SLE affects about 20 out of 100,000 persons in the United States.

MOST OFTEN AFFECTED

All ages; most common in individuals 30–50 years of age; females affected about 10 times more often than males

RISK FACTORS

- Race: African-Americans, Hispanics, Asians, and Native-Americans have higher prevalence than Caucasians.
- Genetic factors

 ## Diagnosis

WHAT THE DOCTOR LOOKS FOR

The doctor will do a physical examination to identify the signs and symptoms of SLE.
- Many other disorders mimic SLE, such as rheumatoid arthritis, connective tissue diseases, scleroderma, cancer, fever, and many skin rashes.

TESTS AND PROCEDURES

- Blood tests
- Urinalysis
- Chest x-ray
- Echocardiography
- Samples of skin, kidney, or nerves may be obtained by biopsy for laboratory analysis.
- Blood vessels of the brain may be examined by a radiological procedure, cerebral angiography.
- Magnetic resonance imaging (MRI) may be done to assist with diagnosis.

 ## Treatment

GENERAL MEASURES

- Protect skin from ultraviolet light by using sunscreens, hats, etc.
- Early intervention when infections occur
- Conserve energy.
- Stress avoidance/management

ACTIVITY

- As active as possible
- Individuals with arthritis may be limited by their pain, but active exercises are encouraged.

DIET

No special diet unless complications such as kidney failure are present

Systemic Lupus Erythematosus (SLE)

Medications

COMMONLY PRESCRIBED DRUGS

- No one drug of choice available. Treatment is aimed at symptom relief.
- Immunosuppressants
- Nonsteroidal anti-inflammatory drugs (NSAIDs)
- Hydroxychloroquine
- Prednisone
- Cyclophosphamide
- Methotrexate
- Immune globulin, intravenous (IVIG)

CONTRAINDICATIONS

Read drug product information.

PRECAUTIONS

Read drug product information.

DRUG INTERACTIONS

Read drug product information.

OTHER DRUGS

N/A

Followup

PATIENT MONITORING

- Individuals with acute flares should be seen frequently by the doctor (weekly to monthly) for adjustment of medication.
- In the absence of acute attack, the doctor should be seen as often as necessary.

PREVENTION

- Avoiding sun exposure is only necessary for approximately one-sixth of SLE patients (those who self report such sensitivity).
- Routine vaccinations are safe and appropriate for SLE patients.
- Drugs known to induce SLE in normal individuals are not necessarily contraindicated in patients who have idiopathic SLE.

COMPLICATIONS

Fever, inflammation of blood vessels, muscle disorders, bone disorders, lung disease, heart disease, nerve disorders, blood-clotting disorders, and numerous other conditions.

WHAT TO EXPECT

- Most patients with SLE follow a course of remissions and acute episodes. Many experience spontaneous permanent remission.
- Treatment of kidney lupus (the most serious form) has increased the five-year life expectancy to over 90%. For patients surviving the first two years of disease, life expectancy is essentially normal.
- In patients with drug-induced SLE, symptoms should gradually decrease upon discontinuation of the suspected agent.

Miscellaneous

OTHER FACTORS

N/A

PEDIATRIC

N/A

GERIATRIC

Higher percentage of males affected by SLE among the elderly

OTHERS

N/A

PREGNANCY

- Onset of SLE and flares are more common during pregnancy.
- Fetal loss is increased for mothers with SLE.
- Newborns of mothers who have SLE are more likely to have irregular heart rhythms.
- Consultation with a specialist during pregnancy is recommended.

FURTHER INFORMATION

- Arthritis Foundation, 1314 Spring Street N.W., Atlanta, GA 30309, (404)872-7100
- Lupus Foundation of America, 1717 Massachusetts Avenue, NW, Suite 203, Washington, DC 20036, (800)558-0121

Section T

Temporomandibular Joint (TMJ) Syndrome

 Basics

DESCRIPTION

Temporomandibular joint (TMJ) syndrome is characterized by pain and tenderness in the jaw muscles and sound and/or pain over the joint, with limitation of jaw movement.

SIGNS AND SYMPTOMS

- Facial pain
- Pain of the temporomandibular joint of the jaw
- Locking or catching of the jaw
- Jaw clicking, grinding, popping
- Headache
- Earache
- Neck pain

CAUSES

- TMJ disorders
- Grinding of the teeth
- Chewing muscle spasm
- Trauma
- Poorly fitting dentures

SCOPE

Up to half the U.S. population has symptoms or signs of TMJ syndrome, but only 5 to 25% seek treatment.

MOST OFTEN AFFECTED

More common among individuals 30–50 years of age; more common in females than males

RISK FACTORS

- Chronic habits such as clenching or grinding of the teeth
- Osteoarthritis, rheumatoid arthritis
- Dental problems
- Psychosocial stress

 Diagnosis

WHAT THE DOCTOR LOOKS FOR

- The doctor will perform a physical examination to identify TMJ syndrome.
- Other conditions that can cause similar signs and symptoms should be investigated, such as fracture or dislocation, nerve disorders, dental disorders, or cancer.

TESTS AND PROCEDURES

- Tests may be done to assess jaw function.
- X-rays, magnetic resonance imaging (MRI), and other radiology procedures may be done to assist in diagnosis.
- The jaw may be examined by arthroscopy.

 Treatment

GENERAL MEASURES

- Jaw rest
- Local heat therapy
- Anti-inflammatory medications
- Muscle relaxants
- Pain relievers
- Correction of dental problems
- Stress reduction
- Behavior modification to eliminate oral habits that may contribute to TMJ syndrome

ACTIVITY

Jaw rest

DIET

Soft diet to reduce chewing

Temporomandibular Joint (TMJ) Syndrome

 Medications

COMMONLY PRESCRIBED DRUGS

Nonsteroidal anti-inflammatory drugs (NSAIDs).
No single drug is more effective than another.

CONTRAINDICATIONS

- History of severe allergy to aspirin
- Peptic ulcer disease
- Renal insufficiency

PRECAUTIONS

- Peptic ulcers, gastritis, or gastrointestinal bleeding may occur with chronic use of NSAIDs.
- Kidney disorders

DRUG INTERACTIONS

Numerous interactions; read drug product information.

OTHER DRUGS

Analgesic agents; muscle relaxants

 Followup

PATIENT MONITORING

The doctor should be seen as often as needed to assess level of discomfort and the effect of therapy.

PREVENTION

- Be aware of any teeth-clenching or grinding habits, and relax the jaw by disengaging the teeth.
- Avoid wide, uncontrolled opening of the mouth, such as yawning.
- Stress management; behavioral modification counseling may be helpful

COMPLICATIONS

- Degenerative joint disease
- Chronic TMJ dislocation
- Loss of joint range of motion
- Depression and chronic pain syndromes

WHAT TO EXPECT

- With conservative therapy, symptoms resolve in 75% of the cases within 3 months.
- The most benefit is received from a comprehensive treatment approach including correction of dental problems, restoration of normal muscle function, pain control, stress management, and behavior modification.

 Miscellaneous

OTHER FACTORS

N/A

PEDIATRIC

N/A

GERIATRIC

N/A

OTHERS

N/A

PREGNANCY

No association

FURTHER INFORMATION

N/A

Tendinitis

 Basics

DESCRIPTION

Tendinitis is an inflammation of the tendon, which may affect adjacent areas.

SIGNS AND SYMPTOMS

- Pain over the point of inflammation. Tendinitis is usually worsened by active motion but may be present at rest.
- Tenderness over the affected tendon
- Mild reddening and increased heat of overlying skin

CAUSES

Usually related to repetitive activity or trauma, but can be without obvious cause

SCOPE

Common

MOST OFTEN AFFECTED

All ages; males affected slightly more frequently than females

RISK FACTORS

Professional athletes and manual laborers are especially prone to tendinitis due to repetitive use.

 Diagnosis

WHAT THE DOCTOR LOOKS FOR

- The doctor will perform a physical examination to identify the presence and severity of tendinitis.
- Other conditions can cause symptoms similar to tendinitis, such as tendon injury, bursitis, arthritis, or infection.

TESTS AND PROCEDURES

Ultrasound, computed tomography (CT scan), and magnetic resonance imaging (MRI) may be done to assist with diagnosis.

 Treatment

GENERAL MEASURES

Treatment goals are to relieve pain, reduce inflammation, and rest the joint.

ACTIVITY

- In acute phases, the involved muscle and tendon should be rested. Use slings and splints for the upper extremity. Use braces, canes, and/or crutches for the lower limbs.
- Physical therapy, once patient is free of pain

DIET

No special diet

Medications

COMMONLY PRESCRIBED DRUGS

- Nonsteroidal anti-inflammatory drugs (NSAIDs)
- Corticosteroids: injected

CONTRAINDICATIONS

Read drug product information.

PRECAUTIONS

Read drug product information.

DRUG INTERACTIONS

Read drug product information.

OTHER DRUGS

N/A

 Followup

PATIENT MONITORING

Symptoms will usually subside within a few days after treatment.

PREVENTION

After adequate rest and treatment, prevention of recurrences is important. Circular bands for forearm extension tendinitis or knee tendinitis may be useful.

COMPLICATIONS

- Tendon rupture, fractures
- Repeated bouts of pain

WHAT TO EXPECT

The great majority of cases subside without complications.

 Miscellaneous

OTHER FACTORS

N/A

PEDIATRIC

Osgood-Schlatter disease is seen in adolescents, especially during a growth spurt.

GERIATRIC

N/A

OTHERS

N/A

PREGNANCY

N/A

FURTHER INFORMATION

N/A

Tinea

 Basics

DESCRIPTION

Tinea is a fungal infection of the skin. It may cause bright red, sharply defined rings of dry skin affecting the face, trunk, or extremities (ring worm). It may affect the head (tinea capitis), the groin (tinea cruris, or jock itch), or the feet (tinea pedis, or athlete's foot).

SIGNS AND SYMPTOMS

- Rash
- Itching
- Bright red, sharply defined circular areas of dry skin
- Patient may experience intense itching
- May affect groin (jock itch)
- May affect area between toes (athlete's foot)
- Changes in skin pigmentation

CAUSES

Fungal infection

SCOPE

Fairly common

MOST OFTEN AFFECTED

All ages; males and females affected with equal frequency

RISK FACTORS

- Warm climates
- Day care centers or schools
- Institutionalization
- Poor hygiene
- Wearing wet clothing or socks
- Obesity
- Direct contact with an active lesion on a human, an animal, or rarely from soil
- Working with animals
- Immune system suppression

 Diagnosis

WHAT THE DOCTOR LOOKS FOR

The doctor will perform a physical examination to identify the presence of tinea.

TESTS AND PROCEDURES

The affected area may be swabbed for laboratory analysis.

 Treatment

GENERAL MEASURES

- Proper hygiene
- Careful hand washing
- Launder towel, clothing, and head wear of infected individual.
- Check other family members.
- Topical medications

ACTIVITY

Avoid contact sports, e.g., wrestling, for 2 days after starting treatment

DIET

Unrestricted diet

 Medications

COMMONLY PRESCRIBED DRUGS

- Miconazole (Monistat-Derm, Micatin)
- Clotrimazole (Lotrimin, Mycelex)
- Ketoconazole (Nizoral, Nizoral Shampoo)
- Econazole (Spectazole)
- Naftifine (Naftin, Lamisil)
- Griseofulvin (Gris-PEG)
- Iitraconazole, itraconazole (Sporanox)
- Ciclopirox (Loprox)
- Haloprogin (Halotex)
- Tolnaftate (Tinactin)
- Undecylenic acid (Desenex)

CONTRAINDICATIONS

Known allergy to agent

PRECAUTIONS

Read drug product information.

DRUG INTERACTIONS

Numerous interactions; read drug product information.

Followup

PATIENT MONITORING

The doctor should be seen as often as necessary.

PREVENTION

- Avoid risk factors.
- Avoid contact with suspicious lesions.
- Good personal hygiene
- Don't share head wear, brushes, or combs.
- Wear rubber or wooden sandals in community showers or bathing places.
- Careful drying between the toes after showering or bathing
- Change socks frequently.
- Apply drying or dusting powder.

COMPLICATIONS

- Bacterial super-infection
- Generalized, invasive infection
- Scarring
- Hair loss
- Spread of disease

WHAT TO EXPECT

Resolution without complications within 1 to 2 weeks of therapy

Miscellaneous

OTHER FACTORS

N/A

PEDIATRIC

N/A

GERIATRIC

N/A

OTHERS

N/A

PREGNANCY

N/A

FURTHER INFORMATION

N/A

Toxic Shock Syndrome

 Basics

DESCRIPTION

Toxic shock syndrome (TSS) is an acute, multisystem illness caused by the bacterium *Staphylococcus aureus*. TSS is characterized by the sudden onset of high fever, peculiar skin rash, and shock.

- Menstrual TSS: associated with menstruation and tampon use
- Nonmenstrual TSS: more common than the menstrual form; associated with surgical wounds, barrier contraception, etc. Can occur in children, men, and women.

SIGNS AND SYMPTOMS

- Almost always present
  - ▶ Temperature above 102°F (38.9°C)
  - ▶ Reddened skin
  - ▶ Rash
  - ▶ Peeling skin a few days after rash appears
  - ▶ Shock, fainting
  - ▶ Nausea or vomiting
- Common
  - ▶ Headache
  - ▶ Confusion or agitation
  - ▶ Acute respiratory distress syndrome
  - ▶ Sore throat
  - ▶ Vaginitis or vaginal discharge
  - ▶ Reddened eyes
  - ▶ Swelling around the eyes
  - ▶ Swelling
  - ▶ Muscle and joint ache
  - ▶ Scant urine production
  - ▶ Diarrhea
- Rare
  - ▶ Arthritis
  - ▶ Enlarged lymph glands
  - ▶ Heart disease
  - ▶ Visual sensitivity to light
  - ▶ Seizure

CAUSES

Toxins produced by *S. aureus*

SCOPE

There are 0.22–1.23 cases of toxic shock syndrome per 100,000 persons annually in the United States.

MOST OFTEN AFFECTED

All ages, but especially individuals 30–60 years of age; females affected more frequently than males

RISK FACTORS

- Infection with *S. aureus*
- Continuous use of super-absorbency tampons during menstruation
- Use of regular-absorbency tampons during menstruation
- Use of contraceptive sponge

 Diagnosis

WHAT THE DOCTOR LOOKS FOR

- The doctor will perform an examination to identify the presence of TSS.
- Other conditions that may appear similar to TSS should be investigated, such as scarlet fever, drug reactions, Rocky Mountain spotted fever, Kawasaki disease, and other infections.

TESTS AND PROCEDURES

- Blood tests
- Blood, nose, vagina, wound, or other body areas may be swabbed for laboratory analysis.

Toxic Shock Syndrome

 Treatment

GENERAL MEASURES

- Treatment of TSS requires hospitalization.
- Removal of tampon or other vaginal foreign bodies
- Intravenous (IV) fluids
- Management of kidney or heart failure
- Mechanical ventilation may be necessary.
- Surgery may be required.

ACTIVITY

Bed rest throughout acute illness

DIET

As tolerated

 Medications

COMMONLY PRESCRIBED DRUGS

- Fluid replacement
- Dopamine
- Oxacillin, nafcillin

CONTRAINDICATIONS

Penicillin allergy

PRECAUTIONS

Read drug product information.

DRUG INTERACTIONS

Read drug product information.

OTHER DRUGS

- Clindamycin
- Vancomycin
- Immune globulin, intravenous (IVIG)

 Followup

PATIENT MONITORING

The doctor and other health care professionals will be seen continuously during hospitalization.

PREVENTION

- Avoid continuous tampon use during menstruation.
- Avoid super-absorbency tampons.
- Frequent tampon changes during the day are encouraged.
- Use sanitary napkins at night.
- Early medical attention to infected wounds

COMPLICATIONS

- Acute kidney failure
- Adult respiratory distress syndrome
- Excessively heavy menstrual flow
- Loss of hair
- Nail loss
- Other complications

WHAT TO EXPECT

- Death rate is 3 to 9%.
- Recurs in 10 to 15% of cases

 Miscellaneous

OTHER FACTORS

N/A

PEDIATRIC

May occur as a complication of chickenpox

GERIATRIC

May result from cellulitis or surgical wound infections

OTHERS

None

PREGNANCY

May result from infections after birth, especially cesarean section wound infection or episiotomy infections

FURTHER INFORMATION

N/A

Toxoplasmosis

Basics

DESCRIPTION

Toxoplasmosis is an infection with the protozoan *Toxoplasma gondii*. There are four types:
- Congenital toxoplasmosis: acute infection of mother during gestation that is passed to fetus.
- Ocular toxoplasmosis: eye infection, usually resulting from congenital exposure but remaining latent until the second or third decade of life
- Acute toxoplasmosis in person with normal immune system: acute, self-limiting infection in normal host
- Acute toxoplasmosis in person with immune deficiency: a life-threatening infection involving many organ systems such as heart, lung, liver, but especially the central nervous system

SIGNS AND SYMPTOMS

- No symptoms in 80 to 90% of cases
- Fever, malaise, night sweats, muscle ache
- Sore throat
- Rash
- Brain inflammation
- Paralysis of half the body, seizures, mental status changes
- Visual changes
- Heart, lung inflammation

CAUSES

- *T. gondii*
- Congenital disease is passed from newly infected mother to fetus during pregnancy.
- Other syndromes may result from newly acquired infection or reactivation of latent infection.
- Ingestion of meats or foods containing eggs present in cat feces
- Infection can be transmitted by blood transfusion or organ transplantation.

SCOPE

- Up to 70% of healthy adults in the United States have been exposed to *T. gondii*.
- Toxoplasmosis affects more than 3500 newborns in the United States each year.

MOST OFTEN AFFECTED

All ages can be affected by toxoplasmosis, males and females in equal proportions

RISK FACTORS

- Immune system disorders, such as AIDS
- Risk of transmission to fetus is greatest during third trimester.

Diagnosis

WHAT THE DOCTOR LOOKS FOR

The doctor will perform a physical examination to identify the presence of toxoplasmosis.

TESTS AND PROCEDURES

- *T. gondii* may be isolated from blood, body fluids, or tissue.
- Blood tests
- Spinal fluid may be obtained by lumbar puncture (spinal tap).
- If pregnancy is involved, amniocentesis and fetal ultrasound may be done.
- Computed tomography (CT scan) or MRI of head may be performed.
- A sample of lymph node or brain tissue may be obtained by biopsy for laboratory analysis.

Treatment

GENERAL MEASURES

- Toxoplasmosis is managed in the outpatient setting except for severe disease that requires hospitalization.
- Usually no treatment in individuals without symptoms except in child under 5 years of age
- Symptomatic patients should be treated until immunity is assured.

ACTIVITY

Level of activity depends on severity of disease and organ systems involved.

DIET

No special diet

Medications

COMMONLY PRESCRIBED DRUGS

- Sulfadiazine (Microsulfon)
- Pyrimethamine (Daraprim)
- Leucovorin (folinic acid)

CONTRAINDICATIONS

- Pyrimethamine should not be used in first trimester of pregnancy.
- Known hypersensitivity to pyrimethamine or sulfadiazine

PRECAUTIONS

Numerous precautions; read drug product information.

DRUG INTERACTIONS

Read drug product information.

OTHER DRUGS

- Spiramycin
- Clindamycin
- Corticosteroids
- Atovaquone (Mepron), azithromycin (Zithromax), clarithromycin (Biaxin)

 ## Followup

PATIENT MONITORING

- The doctor should be seen every 2 weeks until stable, then monthly during therapy.
- Repeat blood tests monthly.

PREVENTION

- Avoid eating raw meat, unpasteurized milk, and uncooked eggs.
- Avoid contact with cat feces.
- Pregnant women should not empty litter boxes.

COMPLICATIONS

- Seizure disorder
- Brain damage
- Partial or complete blindness
- Many complications may occur with congenital toxoplasmosis, including mental retardation, seizures, deafness, and blindness.

WHAT TO EXPECT

- Individuals with immune system disorders often relapse if treatment is stopped.
- Treatment may prevent the development of complications in infants with congenital toxoplasmosis.

 ## Miscellaneous

OTHER FACTORS

N/A

PEDIATRIC

N/A

GERIATRIC

N/A

OTHERS

None

PREGNANCY

- Take extra precautions to avoid contact with cats.
- Do not eat raw meat; wash all fruits and vegetables carefully.
- For toxoplasmosis infection during pregnancy, a specialist should be seen.

FURTHER INFORMATION

National Institute of Allergy and Infectious Disease, Dept. of Health and Human Services, Bldg. 31, Rm 7A-32, 9000 Rockville Pike, Bethesda, MD 20892, (301) 496-5717

Transient Ischemic Attack (TIA)

 ## Basics

DESCRIPTION

Transient ischemic attack, called TIA or "mini-stroke," is the sudden onset of neurological deficit due to a lack of oxygenated blood being delivered to the brain. A TIA lasts less than 24 hours.

SCOPE

There are about 160 new cases of TIA per 100,000 persons annually in the United States.

MOST OFTEN AFFECTED

Risk increases over age 45 and is highest among individuals 60 to 70 years of age; males affected more often than females

SIGNS AND SYMPTOMS

- Paralysis of one side of the body, loss of sensation on one side of the body, difficulty speaking, visual disturbances
- Less often: headaches, seizures, amnesia, confusion
- Double vision, vertigo, incoordination, paralysis of facial muscles, difficulty swallowing, difficulty moving

CAUSES

- Atherosclerotic plaques in the carotid artery that lead to formation of blood clots
- High blood pressure
- Heart disease: valve disorders, heart attack, irregular heart rhythm (atrial fibrillation)
- Blood-clotting disorders
- Other causes: spontaneous TIA, trauma

RISK FACTORS

- Age
- High blood pressure
- Heart disease
- Smoking
- Diabetes
- Family history

 ## Diagnosis

WHAT THE DOCTOR LOOKS FOR

- The doctor will perform a physical examination to identify TIA.
- Other possible causes of similar signs and symptoms should be investigated, such as migraine, seizures, and other disorders

TESTS AND PROCEDURES:

- Blood tests
- Ultrasound may be used to assess carotid arteries.
- Blood vessels in the brain may be imaged with a radiology procedure, called cerebral angiography.
- The electrocardiogram (EKG) will be monitored.
- Computed tomography (CT scan) may be used to assist in diagnosis.

 ## Treatment

GENERAL MEASURES

- TIA is managed in the outpatient setting except for surgery or procedures requiring hospitalization.
- Strict control of medical risk factors, e.g., diabetes, hypertension, hyperlipidemia, cardiac disease
- Cessation of smoking
- Surgery (endarterectomy) may be required.

ACTIVITY

No restrictions

DIET

As appropriate to underlying medical problems (diabetic diet, low-fat diet, low-salt diet etc.)

Transient Ischemic Attack (TIA)

 Medications

COMMONLY PRESCRIBED DRUGS

- Enteric-coated aspirin
- Ticlopidine

CONTRAINDICATIONS

Many contraindications; read drug product information.

PRECAUTIONS

Aspirin may worsen peptic ulcer or asthma.

SIGNIFICANT POSSIBLE INTERACTIONS

Read drug product information.

OTHER DRUGS

N/A

 Followup

PATIENT MONITORING

The doctor should be seen every 3 months for first year, then yearly.

PREVENTION

- Stop smoking
- Control blood pressure, diabetes, high lipids in bloodstream.
- Aspirin, ticlopidine
- Low fat diet

COMPLICATIONS

- Stroke
- Seizure
- Trauma if patient experiences sudden fall due to weakness

WHAT TO EXPECT

Individuals with TIA have a 5 to 20% risk of stroke within 1 year. Risk is cumulative thereafter. Risk increases with addition of multiple risk factors and severity of carotid narrowing.

 Miscellaneous

OTHER FACTORS

N/A

PEDIATRIC

N/A

GERIATRIC

Atrial fibrillation is a frequent cause of TIA among the elderly.

OTHERS

N/A

PREGNANCY

Clotting disorders leading to mini-strokes are associated with pregnancy and birth.

FURTHER INFORMATION

National Stroke Association, 300 East Hampden Ave., Suite 240, Englewood, CO 80110-2622

Tuberculosis

 ## Basics

DESCRIPTION

Tuberculosis (TB) is an increasingly common bacterial infection. After organisms take residence in the lung, TB can lead to involvement of multiple areas of the body including middle ear, bones, joints, brain, heart, and skin. Organisms can survive many years in the body. The highest risk for active disease is within the first 2 years after exposure.

SCOPE

The incidence of TB varies greatly; there may be 32–100 cases per 100,000 persons in the United States.

MOST OFTEN AFFECTED

TB can affect all ages; more common in males than females

SIGNS AND SYMPTOMS

- Cough
- Spitting of blood
- Fever and night sweats
- Weight loss
- Decreased activity
- Enlarged lymph glands
- Chest pain

CAUSES

Mycobacterium tuberculosis, Mycobacterium bovis, and Mycobacterium africanum.

RISK FACTORS

- Urban, homeless, minority
- Institutionalization (e.g., correctional facility)
- Immune system disorders
- Cancer
- Diabetes
- Chronic kidney failure
- Malnutrition
- Chronic high dose steroids
- Close contact with an infected individual

 ## Diagnosis

WHAT THE DOCTOR LOOKS FOR

- The doctor will perform a physical examination to identify the presence of tuberculosis.
- Conditions that can appear similar to TB should be ruled out, including pneumonia, cancer, and fungal infections.

TESTS AND PROCEDURES

- Blood tests
- Special tests for tuberculosis, including sputum culture
- Chest x-ray
- Spinal fluid may be sampled by lumbar puncture (spinal tap).
- A sample of bone marrow may be obtained by biopsy for laboratory analysis.

 ## Treatment

GENERAL MEASURES

- TB is managed in the outpatient setting.
- TB requires careful evaluation and monitoring to make sure medication is taken properly and public health authorities are notified.

ACTIVITY

- As tolerated
- Coughing children may be contagious.
- After a few days of treatment, coughing persons are usually not contagious.

DIET

No restrictions

 ## Medications

COMMONLY PRESCRIBED DRUGS

- Isoniazid
- Rifampin
- Pyrazinamide
- Streptomycin

CONTRAINDICATIONS

Read drug product information.

PRECAUTIONS

Read drug product information.

DRUG INTERACTIONS

- Rifampin: colors urine, tears, and secretions orange and can permanently stain contact lenses. May inactivate birth control pills.
- Isoniazid: peripheral nerve inflammation and allergy possible

OTHER DRUGS

- Ethambutol
- Steroids

 Followup

PATIENT MONITORING

- The doctor should be seen every 2–3 months for duration of treatment.
- Repeat x-ray at 2- to 3-month intervals.

PREVENTION

- TB screening at 15 months of age and annually for individuals who are in close contact with people with TB
- Careful tracking to identify and treat contagious persons is mandatory. The public health department should be notified of all confirmed cases.

COMPLICATIONS

- Progression of disease outside the lungs to other systems
- Spread of disease
- Drug resistance

WHAT TO EXPECT

Generally few complications and full resolution if drugs are taken regularly as prescribed for full course

 Miscellaneous

OTHER FACTORS

N/A

PEDIATRIC

N/A

GERIATRIC

Symptoms may be more subtle in the elderly and may be attributed to aging or other health problems.

OTHERS

N/A

PREGNANCY

N/A

FURTHER INFORMATION

N/A

Section U

Ulcerative Colitis

 ## Basics

DESCRIPTION

Ulcerative colitis, also called idiopathic proctocolitis, is one of a group of inflammatory bowel diseases of unknown cause characterized by periodic acute episodes of rectal bleeding and various constitutional symptoms.

SIGNS AND SYMPTOMS

- Bloody diarrhea
- Abdominal pain
- Fever
- Weight loss
- Joint pain
- Inflammation of the backbone
- Eye diseases
- Painful nodes on the lower extremities
- Chronic ulcers of the skin
- Mouth ulcers
- Liver and gallbladder disease
- Blood clotting disorders

CAUSES

The basic cause of ulcerative colitis is unknown. Genetic, infectious, immunologic, and psychological factors have been suggested.

SCOPE

Ulcerative colitis affects 70–150 per 100,000 persons. 6–8 new cases per 100,000 population occur annually in the United States.

MOST OFTEN AFFECTED

Ulcerative colitis most often affects those between 15 and 35 years of age. It also affects individuals in their 80s. The disease occurs with equal frequency in males and females. Ulcerative colitis tends to run in families; about 8–11% have a family history of the disease. It is more common in Jews than other ethnic groups.

RISK FACTORS

- None known
- Higher incidence in Jews and those with a family history
- Lower risk associated with smoking

 ## Diagnosis

WHAT THE DOCTOR LOOKS FOR

- Other sources of rectal bleeding including hemorrhoids, Crohn's disease, diverticula, cancer, infection, antibiotic usage
- The colon may be visually inspected by sigmoidoscopy or colonoscopy.

TESTS AND PROCEDURES

- Blood tests to detect inflammation and anemia, and to asses liver function
- A barium enema may be performed to evaluate the large colon.
- A sample of intestinal tissue obtained by biopsy may be examined.

 ## Treatment

GENERAL MEASURES

- The overall goal of treatment is to control inflammation, prevent complications, and replace nutritional losses and blood volume.
- Ulcerative colitis is usually managed on an outpatient basis except for severe episodes which may require hospitalization.
- Complications or disease that does not respond to medical treatment may require surgery.

ACTIVITY

Full activity as tolerated

DIET

No specific diet; milk products do not need to be avoided unless the person is lactose intolerant.

 ## Medications

COMMONLY PRESCRIBED DRUGS

- Sulfasalazine is the treatment of choice for mild flare-ups and management of ulcerative colitis.
- Limited disease may be treated with enemas and suppositories.

- Oral or parenteral corticosteroids are used for more severe flare-ups.
- Approximately 10% of patients have chronic disease activity and require continuous steroid doses.
- Immunomodulators such as azathioprine, mer-captopurine, methotrexate, levamisole, and cyclosporine are controversial in a disease potentially curable by surgery. However, these drugs have been shown to be effective in patients for whom surgery is not an option.
- Antimicrobial agents are sometimes useful in Crohn's disease but not in ulcerative colitis.
- Antidiarrheal agents: diphenoxylate-atropine and loperamide may be used to help control diarrhea.

CONTRAINDICATIONS

- Allergy to any of the above medications
- Read drug product information.

PRECAUTIONS

Use of antidiarrheal agents in severe disease could cause a serious colon condition.

DRUG INTERACTIONS

Read drug product information.

OTHER DRUGS

N/A

 Followup

PATIENT MONITORING

- Regularly scheduled appointments are important to evaluate for disease activity, appearance of complications, and psychological and social well-being.
- Colonoscopy should be performed every 1–2 years after the disease has been present for 7–8 years.
- The liver should be evaluated annually.
- The gallbladder may be evaluated by cholangiography to assess the flow of bile.

PREVENTION

Regular check-ups with primary care provider for physical exams and colonoscopy

COMPLICATIONS

- Perforation of the intestine
- Other intestinal disorders
- Liver disease
- Colon cancer. Cancer may affect up to 30% of those with colitis for 25 years.

WHAT TO EXPECT

- The course of the disorder is extremely variable. About 75–85% of patients have a repeat episode of acute illness, and up to 20% may eventually require surgery.
- The risk of death from an initial attack is relatively low (about 5% of patients).
- Colon cancer risk is the single most important risk factor affecting long-term prognosis.

 Miscellaneous

OTHER FACTORS

N/A

PEDIATRIC

- Approximately 20% of patients are 21 years of age or younger.
- Cancer surveillance is important.

GERIATRIC

Having an initial attack if over 60 years of age is linked with a higher risk of death.

OTHERS

N/A

PREGNANCY

- Outcome of pregnancy is similar to general population.
- Treatment with sulfasalazine does not seem to affect pregnancy.
- Person with ulcerative colitis should delay pregnancy until time when disease is inactive.

FURTHER INFORMATION

National Foundation for Ileitis and Colitis 444 Park Avenue S., 11th Floor, New York, NY 10016-7374, (800)343-3637

Urinary Incontinence

 Basics

DESCRIPTION

Urinary incontinence is the involuntary loss of urine from the bladder. It can occur while asleep or awake. The amount of urine lost can vary greatly. The condition becomes a medical issue when it is perceived to be a social and/or health problem by the patient or family.

SIGNS AND SYMPTOMS

- Involuntary loss of urine
- Urinary urgency
- Burning with urination
- Irritation of the perineal region

CAUSES

- Pelvic muscle weakness
- Urethral sphincter weakness
- Bladder irritation (cystitis, tumors, stones, etc.)
- Neurological disorders (stroke, dementia, spinal injury, multiple sclerosis, etc.)
- Anatomic obstruction (prostate disorders, scarring, etc)

SCOPE

- About 10 million persons in the United States have urinary incontinence.
- Affects 5–15% elderly living at home, 50% of nursing home residents

MOST OFTEN AFFECTED

Urinary incontinence primarily affects the elderly (65 years of age or older). Incidence increases with age. Women are affected more often than men.

RISK FACTORS

- Increasing age
- Estrogen deficiency (women)
- Prostatic hypertrophy (men)
- Multiple births (women)
- Dementia
- Diabetes
- Spinal cord injury
- Multiple sclerosis
- General debilitated condition
- Stroke

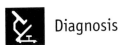
Diagnosis

WHAT THE DOCTOR LOOKS FOR

- The diagnosis of urinary incontinence is generally made on the basis of the patient history.
- Physical examination of men should include examination of the abdomen, digital rectal exam to assess the prostate, and neurological examination.
- Physical examination of women should include examination of the abdomen, pelvic examination, and neurologic examination.
- The doctor may ask the patient to reproduce the activities (e.g., coughing, sneezing, laughing) that result in loss of urine.
- The doctor should seek causes of loss of bladder control, such as urinary tract infection or a side effect of diuretics or other medication.

TESTS AND PROCEDURES

- Urinalysis and culture
- Blood test for prostate-specific antigen (PSA)
- The urinary system may be visually assessed by a radiology procedure called intravenous pyelogram (IVP).
- Special procedures may be done to assess bladder function, such as cystometry, voiding cystourethrogram, and cystometrogram.
- Ultrasound may be used to assess the urinary system or prostate.

TREATMENT

GENERAL MEASURES

- Urinary incontinence is usually managed on an outpatient basis.
- All conditions relating to urinary incontinence should be identified and treated (e.g., urinary tract infection, bladder tumors, prostatic hypertrophy).
- Patient should be taught proper toilet hygiene.
- Patient may be taught pelvic floor (Kegel) exercises or biofeedback/behavioral training.
- Some patients may require catheterization or incontinence pads.
- Some patients with incontinence due to prostatic hypertrophy may benefit from transurethral resection of the prostate (TURP).
- Some patients with stress incontinence may benefit from bladder surgery.

Urinary Incontinence

ACTIVITY

Full activities should be encouraged.

DIET

- No special diet
- In situations where access to bathroom facilities is limited, a person with incontinence may want to avoid high-volume fluid intake and reduce intake of caffeine or alcohol-containing beverages.

 Medications

COMMONLY PRESCRIBED DRUGS

- Detrusor instability: oxybutynin, popantheline (Pro-Banthine), dicyclomine (Bentyl), flavoxate (Urispas), imipramine (Tofranil)
- Sphincter incompetence: pseudoephedrine (Sudafed), phenylpropanolamine, imipramine (Tofranil)
- Overflow/atonic bladder: bethanechol (Urecholine)
- Overflow/prostatic enlargement: prazosin (Minipress), finasteride (Proscar)

CONTRAINDICATIONS

- Read drug product information.
- May be contraindicated in patients with glaucoma or prostatic hypertrophy

PRECAUTIONS

- The smallest dose possible should be used in elderly patients.
- Common side effects include dry mouth, blurred vision, constipation, low blood pressure upon standing, and mental confusion.

DRUG INTERACTIONS

Varies for each drug; read drug product information.

OTHER DRUGS

- Oral or topical estrogens for stress incontinence associated with vaginitis
- Prostaglandin inhibitors (experimental)
- Calcium antagonists (experimental)
- Desmopressin (DDAVP) nasal spray for bed-wetting

Urinary Incontinence

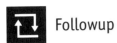 Followup

PATIENT MONITORING

- Patient should be seen every other week while exercises are being learned and medication dosage is being adjusted.
- Patient should be seen every 3 months once incontinence is under control and medication doses are stable.
- Patient should be evaluated for side effects of medication.
- Intraocular pressure may be tested in high-risk patients.
- Patient should have periodic urinalysis to detect early urinary tract infection.

PREVENTION

- Women should routinely use Kegel exercises following childbirth.
- Women should have regular pelvic exams to detect disease early.
- Men should have regular rectal exams to identify prostatic disease early and receive treatment for hypertrophy.

COMPLICATIONS

- Urinary tract infection
- Kidney disease
- Adverse drug reactions

WHAT TO EXPECT

Prognosis is generally good. Most patients can achieve an increase in bladder control with appropriate medical management.

 Miscellaneous

OTHER FACTORS

N/A

PEDIATRIC

N/A

GERIATRIC

Urinary incontinence is most common in the aging population.

OTHERS

N/A

PREGNANCY

Stress incontinence can occur during pregnancy.

FURTHER INFORMATION

N/A

Urinary Tract Infection in Men

 Basics

DESCRIPTION

Lower urinary tract infection (UTI) is usually caused by bacteria. It is also called cystitis.

SIGNS AND SYMPTOMS

- Frequent urination
- Difficult urination
- Urinary urgency
- Hesitancy
- Slow urinary stream
- Dribbling of urine
- Frequent urination during sleep hours
- Discomfort in the lower abdomen
- Low back pain
- Blood in the urine
- Systemic symptoms (chills, fever) present with coexisting kidney or prostate disease

CAUSES

Bacterial infection

SCOPE

Urinary tract infection in men is not common in the United States.

MOST OFTEN AFFECTED

Urinary tract infection is uncommon in men under 50 years of age, with about 8 infections per 10,000 men 21–50 years old. Incidence increases with age.

RISK FACTORS

- Benign prostatic hypertrophy (BPH)
- Cognitive impairment
- Fecal incontinence
- Urinary incontinence
- Anal intercourse
- Recent urologic surgery, catheterization or other procedures
- Infection of the prostate or kidney
- Immune system disorders

 Diagnosis

WHAT THE DOCTOR LOOKS FOR

- Anatomical or functional conditions that may be causing symptoms
- Other infections of the genitourinary system
- Patients with UTI often have associated conditions, including kidney and prostate disease.

TESTS AND PROCEDURES

- Urinalysis and culture for microbiologic evaluation
- A radiological procedure called intravenous pyelography may be done to assess the urinary tract.
- Ultrasound may be used to evaluate the urinary system.
- The bladder may be visually examined by the doctor with a cystoscope.

 Treatment

GENERAL MEASURES

- Urinary tract infection is managed on an out-patient basis, except for acute illness with toxicity or kidney failure.
- The patient should be given fluids and pain relief as required.
- Discontinue sexual activity until cured.

ACTIVITY

Activity as tolerated

DIET

No special diet

Medications

COMMONLY PRESCRIBED DRUGS

- For acute UTI , first infection, no risk factors for treatment: 7–10 days of oral antibiotics
- For complicated or repeated UTI: 14–21 days of antibiotics

CONTRAINDICATIONS

Read drug product information.

PRECAUTIONS

Read drug product information.

SIGNIFICANT POSSIBLE INTERACTIONS

Read drug product information.

OTHER DRUGS

N/A

 Followup

PATIENT MONITORING

- The doctor should follow all individuals with UTI closely until the infection is cured.
- Urinalysis should be periodically repeated.

PREVENTION

- Predisposing factors should be promptly treated.

COMPLICATIONS

- Kidney disorders
- Infection may get worse
- Recurring infection

WHAT TO EXPECT

Infections usually clear up with appropriate antibiotic treatment.

 Miscellaneous

OTHER FACTORS

N/A

PEDIATRIC

UTI is usually associated with obstruction to normal flow of urine.

GERIATRIC

Bacteria is commonly found in the urine of an elderly person. If there are no symptoms, treatment is not necessary. Giving antibiotics may allow the growth of resistant microbes.

OTHERS

N/A

PREGNANCY

N/A

FURTHER INFORMATION

National Kidney Foundation, 30 E. 33rd Street, Suite 1100, New York, NY 10016, (212) 889-2210

Urinary Tract Infection in Women

 Basics

DESCRIPTION

Urinary tract infection (UTI) is also called cystitis. UTI causes inflammation of the bladder. UTI is caused by bacteria.

SIGNS AND SYMPTOMS

Any or all of the following may be present:
- Burning during urination
- Pain during urination
- Urgency (sensation of need to urinate frequently)
- Sensation of incomplete bladder emptying
- Blood in urine
- Lower abdominal pain or cramping

CAUSES

Bacterial infection

SCOPE

Between 3–8% of women have bacteria in their urine at any given time. About 43% of women between 14 and 61 years of age have had at least one episode of UTI. It is the cause of 7 million doctor visits a year.

MOST OFTEN AFFECTED

Young adult and older females

RISK FACTORS

- Previous urinary tract infection
- Diabetes mellitus
- Pregnancy
- More frequent or vigorous sexual activity than usual
- Use of spermicide or diaphragm
- Underlying condition of the urinary tract such as tumors or stones

 Diagnosis

WHAT THE DOCTOR LOOKS FOR

- Vaginitis
- Sexually transmitted diseases
- Other causes of blood in the urine, such as kidney stones or cancer
- Psychological dysfunction

TESTS AND PROCEDURES

- Urinalysis and culture for microbiologic evaluation
- Urine may be obtained by catheterization of the bladder.
- X-rays, ultrasound, or endoscopic imaging may be employed to assess the urinary tract.
- Special procedures such as voiding cystourethrogram may be done .

 Treatment

GENERAL MEASURES

- UTI is managed on an outpatient basis, except for complicated or upper urinary tract infections.
- The patient should maintain good fluid intake.
- One-fourth of women with UTI have another infection within 6 months. Women with repeated UTI and no underlying urinary tract abnormality may receive long-term antibiotic treatment.
- Patients with chronic indwelling urinary catheters always have infections. UTI should not be treated unless the patient has fever, sepsis, or other systemic symptoms.

ACTIVITY

Avoid sexual intercourse when symptoms are present.

DIET

No special diet

Urinary Tract Infection in Women

 Medications

COMMONLY PRESCRIBED DRUGS

- Antibiotics
  - ▶ Sulfamethaxazols/trimethoprim (Septra, Bactrim)
  - ▶ Ampicillin
  - ▶ Nitrofurantoin (Macrodantin)
- Urinary analgesics
  - ▶ Phenazopyridize (Pyridium)

CONTRAINDICATIONS

Read drug product information. Some drugs should not be used during pregnancy.

PRECAUTIONS

Read drug product information.

DRUG INTERACTIONS

Read drug product information.

OTHER DRUGS

Antibiotic therapy may be changed based on microbiological assessment.

 Followup

PATIENT MONITORING

- The patient should return to the doctor if symptoms are not resolved or markedly improved within 48 hours.
- The patient should return to the doctor if fever, chills, or flank pain develop.
- First or rare UTI: A young or middle-aged, nonpregnant adult woman requires no follow-up if a single dose of antibiotic clears the infection.
- If UTI is not resolved within 2 to 3 days after single dose therapy, urine should be cultured for microbiological evaluation. Antibiotic therapy may be changed.
- All other patients should have urine culture repeated after treatment to make sure the infection has been cleared.

PREVENTION

- Maintain good fluid intake.
- Women with frequent or intercourse-related UTI should empty bladder immediately before and following intercourse and consider post-coital antibiotic treatment.

COMPLICATIONS

Kidney disease

WHAT TO EXPECT

Symptoms resolve within 2–3 days after starting treatment in almost all patients

 Miscellaneous

OTHER FACTORS

N/A

PEDIATRIC

Infants and young children at higher risk of kidney disease

GERIATRIC

- Elderly may have bacteria in their urine but may not have symptoms. This condition generally does not require treatment if urinary tract is otherwise normal.
- Elderly are more apt to have underlying urinary tract abnormality.
- Acute UTI is often associated with incontinence in the elderly.

OTHERS

N/A

PREGNANCY

UTI during pregnancy always requires culture and usually requires 10–14 days of antibiotic treatment. After treatment of acute infection, pregnant women often receive antibiotics for the remainder of pregnancy.

FURTHER INFORMATION

N/A

Section V

Vaginal Bleeding During Pregnancy

 Basics

DESCRIPTION

Vaginal bleeding during pregnancy has many causes. The bleeding can range in severity from mild (with normal pregnancy outcome) to life threatening for both infant and mother. Bleeding can vary from light to heavy, from brown to bright red, and can be painless or painful.

SIGNS AND SYMPTOMS

- Bleeding can vary from light to heavy.
- Color of blood varies from brown to bright red.
- May be painless or painful

CAUSES

- Vaginal infection or trauma
- Disorders of the cervix
- Complications of pregnancy
- "Bloody show" (bloody discharge that normally precedes labor)
- Unknown: No cause is found in 50% of first trimester bleeding.

SCOPE

Vaginal bleeding is common in the United States.

MOST OFTEN AFFECTED

Females of childbearing age

RISK FACTORS

Varies, based on individual causes

 Diagnosis

WHAT THE DOCTOR LOOKS FOR

- Vaginal or cervical causes of bleeding can occur throughout pregnancy.
- The doctor will perform a thorough pelvic examination.
- A sample of fluid may be withdrawn from the womb.

- The patient may be visually examined by minimally invasive laparoscopy.

LABORATORY

- Blood tests, including clotting studies and hormone tests
- Ultrasound: Several ultrasounds may be required in early pregnancy to make diagnosis.

 Treatment

GENERAL MEASURES

- During the first trimester, most patients with bleeding can be managed on an outpatient basis.
- During late pregnancy, most patients with bleeding need to be hospitalized for observation.
- In late pregnancy bleeding, the amount of bleeding and the status of mother and baby indicates whether urgent cesarean section is performed or whether conservative measures are appropriate.
- Threatened abortion: bed rest and nothing by vagina (no intercourse or douching). If bleeding is severe, hospitalization and close observation are needed.
- Surgery may be necessary for ectopic pregnancy, incomplete miscarriage, etc.
- Grief counseling is appropriate if pregnancy loss is inevitable.

ACTIVITY

Bed rest, no intercourse, no douching

DIET

No restrictions

Vaginal Bleeding During Pregnancy

 Medications

COMMONLY PRESCRIBED DRUGS

None

CONTRAINDICATIONS

N/A

PRECAUTIONS

N/A

SIGNIFICANT POSSIBLE INTERACTIONS

N/A

OTHER DRUGS

N/A

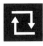 Followup

PATIENT MONITORING

- The doctor should be seen daily to weekly depending on diagnosis and severity of bleeding.
- Any increase in the amount and frequency of bleeding should be reported to the doctor.
- Seek immediate care if abdominal pain occurs or bleeding suddenly increases.
- Bring any tissue that is passed vaginally for examination.

PREVENTION

N/A

COMPLICATIONS

- Anemia
- Shock
- Fetal or maternal death
- Infection
- Premature delivery of baby with associated complications
- Bleeding disorders

WHAT TO EXPECT

The outcome depends on the cause of vaginal bleeding, the severity of bleeding and how promptly it is diagnosed and treated. About 1 in 826 ectopic pregnancies (pregnancy in which the embryo implants in the fallopian tube instead of the uterus) result in the death of the mother.

 Miscellaneous

OTHER FACTORS

N/A

PEDIATRIC

N/A

GERIATRIC

N/A

OTHERS

N/A

PREGNANCY

A complication of pregnancy

FURTHER INFORMATION

American College of Obstetricians & Gynecologists (ACOG), 409 12th St., SW, Washington, DC 20024-2188, (800) 762-ACOG

Vaginal Yeast Infection

 Basics

DESCRIPTION

Candidal vulvovaginitis is a vaginal infection caused by a yeast (Candida). It causes itching and/or burning of the vulva, often with abnormal vaginal discharge.

SCOPE

- 16% of nonpregnant premenopausal women are carriers of infection without symptoms.
- 40% of vaginal infections are caused by Candida.

MOST OFTEN AFFECTED

Women from their first menstrual period until menopause

SIGNS AND SYMPTOMS

- Intense itching of the vulva
- Thick curd-like vaginal discharge
- Painful or difficult urination
- Reddened, inflamed skin on vulva
- Reddening, pain, and itching of perineal area or upper thigh
- Thick, white patches on vaginal skin

CAUSES

Overgrowth of Candida in vagina

RISK FACTORS

- Pregnancy
- Diabetes mellitus
- Antibiotic therapy
- Steroid therapy
- Immune system disorders
- Synthetic underpants and undergarments
- Hypothyroidism
- Oral contraceptive medications (low-dose contraceptive pills usually do not cause an increased infection risk)
- Anemia
- Zinc deficiency

 Diagnosis

WHAT THE DOCTOR LOOKS FOR

- Other possible genitourinary infections, such as trichomonas or gonorrhea
- Possible allergic reactions

TESTS AND PROCEDURES

- Culture for microbiological analysis
- Pap smear

 Treatment

GENERAL MEASURES

- Vulvovaginitis is managed on an outpatient basis.
- Any foreign body should be removed if present.
- Consider providone iodine douche relief of symptoms until specific therapy is effective.
- If urination causes burning:
  - ▶ Urinate through a tubular device such as a toilet-paper roll or plastic cup with the end cut out.
  - ▶ Pour warm water over vaginal area while urinating.
- Diabetes must be strictly controlled if the patient is diabetic.

ACTIVITY

- Avoid overexertion, heat, and excessive sweating.
- Delay sexual intercourse until symptoms clear.

DIET

Limit sweets and dairy products in recurrent infections.

 Medications

COMMONLY PRESCRIBED DRUGS

- Fluconazole (Diflucan)
- Miconazole nitrate (Monistat)
- Butoconazole nitrate (Femstat)

- Terconazole (Terazol)
- Clotrimazole (Gyne-Lotrimin)

CONTRAINDICATIONS

N/A

PRECAUTIONS

Read drug product information.

SIGNIFICANT POSSIBLE INTERACTIONS

Read drug product information.

OTHER DRUGS

- A different drug may be used if the infection recurs.
- Oral nystatin
- Topical gentian violet
- Boric acid

 Followup

PATIENT MONITORING

- No specific followup is generally needed.
- See doctor if symptoms persist.
- If infection recurs, sexual partner(s) may require treatment as well.

PREVENTION

- Keep the genital area clean. Use plain unscented soap.
- Take showers rather than tub baths.
- Wear cotton underpants with a cotton crotch.
- Avoid clothing made from nonventilating materials, including most synthetic under-clothing.
- Avoid tight-fitting jeans or slacks.
- Sleep in loose gown without underpants.
- Don't sit around in wet clothing, especially a wet bathing suit.
- Avoid frequent douches.
- After urinating or bowel movements, cleanse by wiping or washing from front to back.
- Lose weight, if obese.

COMPLICATIONS

Bacterial infections of the vagina or vulva

WHAT TO EXPECT

- Vigorous treatment usually results in a complete cure.
- Infections often recur.

 Miscellaneous

OTHER FACTORS

N/A

PEDIATRIC

Less common before puberty

GERIATRIC

N/A

OTHERS

N/A

PREGNANCY

Common during pregnancy

FURTHER INFORMATION

American College of Obstetricians & Gynecologists (ACOG), 409 12th St., SW, Washington, DC 20024-2188, (800) 762-ACOG

Varicose Veins

 ## Basics

DESCRIPTION

Varicose veins are elongated, enlarged veins that primarily affect the legs where blood flow is restricted.

SIGNS AND SYMPTOMS

- Sometimes has no symptoms
- Leg muscular cramps, aches
- Enlarged, tortuous superficial veins, mostly in the legs
- Swelling of affected limb
- Fatigue
- Symptoms worse during menstruation
- Pain if varicose ulcer develops

CAUSES

- Faulty valves in one or more lower leg veins
- Deep thrombophlebitis
- Increased pressure in the veins
- In many individuals, no cause is identified.

SCOPE

Varicose veins affect about 20% of adults in the United States.

MOST OFTEN AFFECTED

Persons of middle age. Varicose veins are five times more common in women than in men.

RISK FACTORS

- Pregnancy
- Occupations requiring prolonged standing or restrictive clothing (e.g., tight girdles)

 ## Diagnosis

WHAT THE DOCTOR LOOKS FOR

- Diagnosis of varicose usually is made by physical examination.
- The doctor should consider other conditions that may appear similar, such as nerve disorders or arthritis.

TESTS AND PROCEDURES

The patient may be evaluated on a tilting table or bed.

 ## Treatment

GENERAL MEASURES

- Varicose veins are usually managed on an out-patient basis.
- Conservative methods:
  - ▶ Frequent rest periods with legs elevated
  - ▶ Lightweight, elastic compression hosiery. Best put on before getting out of bed.
  - ▶ Avoidance of girdles and other restrictive clothing
  - ▶ If ulcers develop, use warm, wet dressings.
- Spider veins may be treated by injection.
- Surgery and other methods:
  - ▶ Surgery may be done if pain, recurrent phlebitis, or skin changes are present or for cosmetic improvement for severe cases.
  - ▶ Ligation and stripping
  - ▶ Injections
  - ▶ For extensive scarring: The entire area may be surgically removed, followed by skin graft.

Varicose Veins

ACTIVITY

- Avoid long periods of standing.
- Appropriate exercise routine as part of conservative treatment
- Walking regimen after therapy is important to help promote healing.
- Apply elastic stockings before lowering legs from the bed.
- Never sit with legs hanging down.

DIET

- No special diet
- Weight loss diet recommended if obesity is a problem.

Medications

COMMONLY PRESCRIBED DRUGS

N/A

CONTRAINDICATIONS

N/A

PRECAUTIONS

N/A

SIGNIFICANT POSSIBLE INTERACTIONS

N/A

OTHER DRUGS

Antibiotics for infected ulcers

Followup

PATIENT MONITORING

- The patient should be followed by the doctor until surgery or conservative therapy brings maximal benefit.
- Treatment or surgery may not prevent development of varicose veins. Procedures may need to be repeated in later years.

PREVENTION/AVOIDANCE

See Activity

COMPLICATIONS

- Bleeding
- Chronic swelling
- Infection
- Varicose ulcers
- Skin color changes
- Eczema
- Recurrence after surgical treatment
- Scarring or nerve damage from stripping technique

WHAT TO EXPECT

- Varicose veins usually become chronic.
- The outcome can be favorable with appropriate treatment.

Miscellaneous

OTHER FACTORS

N/A

PEDIATRIC

Varicose veins are uncommon in children.

GERIATRIC

Recommended therapy is elastic support hose and frequent rests with legs elevated rather than stripping.

OTHERS

N/A

PREGNANCY

Varicose veins are a frequent problem of pregnancy. Use of elastic stockings is recommended for women who have a history of varicose veins or when activities involve a great deal of standing.

FURTHER INFORMATION

National Heart, Lung & Blood Institute, Communications & Public Information Branch, National Institutes of Health, Building 31, Room 41-21, 9000 Rockville Pike, Bethesda, MD 20892, (301) 496-4236

Vitamin Deficiency

 Basics

DESCRIPTION

Vitamin deficiency develops slowly and is difficult to diagnose. Multiple deficiencies of vitamins occur more frequently than deficiency of a single vitamin.

SIGNS AND SYMPTOMS

- Vitamin A (retinol)
  - ▶ Night blindness
  - ▶ Dandruff, dry scaly skin
  - ▶ Dry eyes
  - ▶ Growth retardation, loss of appetite, and anemia commonly found in children
- Vitamin B1 (thiamine)
  - ▶ Beriberi
  - ▶ Wernicke-Korsakoff syndrome
- Vitamin B2 (riboflavin)
  - ▶ Inflammation at the corners of the mouth
  - ▶ Dry, peeling lips
  - ▶ Corneal disease
  - ▶ Diminished vision in one eye
  - ▶ Dermatitis
  - ▶ During pregnancy, deficiency leads to fetal skeletal abnormalities such as shortened bones and deformed growth.
- Vitamin B3 (niacin [nicotinic acid], niacinamide)
  - ▶ Pellagra
- Vitamin B6 (pyridoxine)
  - ▶ Convulsions in infants
  - ▶ Anemia
  - ▶ Nerve disorders
  - ▶ Seborrhea-like skin lesions
- Vitamin B12 (cobalamin)
  - ▶ Nerve disorders
  - ▶ Anemia
  - ▶ Some psychiatric syndromes
- Vitamin C (ascorbic acid)
  - ▶ Scurvy (loose teeth, gingivitis, hemorrhages)
- Vitamin D
  - ▶ Rickets
  - ▶ Softening of the bone
- Vitamin E (alpha-tocopherol)
  - ▶ Blood disorders
- Vitamin K
  - ▶ Bleeding

SCOPE

Unknown

Vitamin Deficiency

MOST OFTEN AFFECTED

The elderly are most often affected. Men and women are affected in equal proportion. Some forms of vitamin deficiency are inheritable.

CAUSES

- Inadequate dietary intake
- Impaired absorption or storage of vitamins

RISK FACTORS

- Alcoholism
- Malabsorption
- Gallbladder disease
- Dialysis
- Chronic malnutrition
- Deficiencies of other vitamins
- Drug interactions
- Infants
- Elderly
- Lower socioeconomic status
- Laxative abuse
- Genetic disorder
- Prolonged lactation (vitamin C)
- Intestinal parasites
- Drug abuse
- Food faddism or bizarre nutritional practices
- Gastrointestinal surgery

 Diagnosis

WHAT THE DOCTOR LOOKS FOR

- The doctor will take a history of the patient and perform a thorough physical examination.
- The doctor should consider other causes of similar signs and symptoms, such as neurological, intestinal, or skin diseases.

TESTS AND PROCEDURES

- Blood test to measure vitamin levels

Vitamin Deficiency

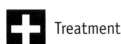 Treatment

GENERAL MEASURES

- The patient with vitamin deficiency is usually managed on an outpatient basis.
- Severe cases may require hospitalization for observation.
- Any underlying causes should be treated.
- Therapy involves replacing vitamins.
- Maintenance vitamin supplement as required
- For vitamin D deficiency: adequate exposure to sunlight
- The doctor may refer the patient to social service agencies if socioeconomic factors contribute to vitamin deficiency.
- The patient may need help with alcohol or smoking cessation.

ACTIVITY

As tolerated

DIET

- For dietary deficiencies: nutritional counseling with emphasis on appropriate foods and the proper methods for preparation
- Abstain from alcohol.

 Medications

COMMONLY PRESCRIBED DRUGS

Appropriate vitamins as needed

CONTRAINDICATIONS

Read drug product information.

PRECAUTIONS

Read drug product information.

DRUG INTERACTIONS

Read drug product information.

OTHER DRUGS

N/A

Followup

 Miscellaneous

PATIENT MONITORING

The doctor should be seen as needed depending on severity of problem.

PREVENTION

- Proper nutrition
- Supplemental vitamins if needed
- Compliance with vitamin supplementation regimens is important to health.
- Reduce risk factors that lead to deficiency where possible.
- Vitamin D deficiency: Adequate exposure to sunlight (30 minutes several times a week)

COMPLICATIONS

- Vitamin A deficiency: Risk of death is high in advanced cases; eye lesions are a threat to vision.
- Vitamin B1 deficiency: May be fatal if untreated
- Vitamin B6 deficiency: Chronic deficiency may increase risk of kidney stones.
- Vitamin D deficiency: Skeletal deformities, greenstick fractures, bone pain
- Excessive synthetic vitamin K may lead to anemia and jaundice in infants

WHAT TO EXPECT

With proper diagnosis and therapy, full recovery without complications can be expected.

OTHER FACTORS

N/A

PEDIATRIC

- Vitamin D deficiency rickets is now rare in the United States, but may occur in breast-fed infants who do not receive a vitamin D supplement, or in infants fed a formula with a nonfortified milk base.
- Vitamin E deficiency in infants usually results from formulas high in polyunsaturated fatty acids that are fortified with iron but not vitamin E.
- Vitamin K deficiency: common among newborns

GERIATRIC

The elderly are more likely to have multiple risk factors that can lead to vitamin deficiencies.

OTHERS

N/A

PREGNANCY

Pregnant women should take a supplemental multivitamin tablet that contains at least 60 milligrams (mg) of elemental iron and 1.0 mg of folic acid.

FURTHER INFORMATION

N/A

Vulvovaginitis, Estrogen Deficient

 Basics

DESCRIPTION

Estrogen-deficient vulvovaginitis is a thinning and atrophy of female genital tissue. It is caused by decreased blood flow resulting from changes in the levels of estrogen. It is often associated with urinary incontinence.

SIGNS AND SYMPTOMS

- Vaginal dryness
- Decreased vaginal secretions
- Difficult or painful urination
- Itching

CAUSES

- Menopause (surgical or natural)
- Ovarian surgery
- Radiation of the pelvis

SCOPE

Will affect all women, to some degree, unless estrogen replacement therapy is provided

MOST OFTEN AFFECTED

Predominantly a problem of the postmenopausal woman

RISK FACTORS

- Metabolic disorders caused by estrogen deficiency
- Vaginal infections with bacteria and fungi

 Diagnosis

WHAT THE DOCTOR LOOKS FOR

Other conditions that may be causing symptoms, such as cancer

TESTS AND PROCEDURES

- Blood tests, including hormone levels
- Urinalysis and culture
- Cells from urine or vaginal swab may be microscopically analyzed.

 Treatment

GENERAL MEASURES

- Estrogen-deficient vulvovaginitis is managed in an outpatient setting.
- Estrogen replacement therapy (ERT) will relieve and reverse symptoms.
- Relief of symptoms as needed, e.g., cool baths or compresses

ACTIVITY

No restriction

DIET

No special diet

Vulvovaginitis, Estrogen Deficient

 Medications

COMMONLY PRESCRIBED DRUGS

A wide variety of estrogen preparations are available.

CONTRAINDICATIONS

- ERT should not be given to those with a history of breast cancer or estrogen-positive tumor receptors.
- ERT may not be given if the patient has a history of uterine malignancy.

PRECAUTIONS

Read drug product information.

SIGNIFICANT POSSIBLE INTERACTIONS

Read drug product information.

OTHER DRUGS

N/A

 Followup

PATIENT MONITORING

Symptoms should resolve within 30–60 days. See the doctor if symptoms do not resolve.

PREVENTION

N/A

COMPLICATIONS

Complications are those associated with ERT; e.g., bleeding, nausea, headache, libido changes, clotting disorders.

WHAT TO EXPECT

The outcome of estrogen-deficient vulvovaginitis is excellent. The vast majority of symptoms are relieved with ERT.

 Miscellaneous

OTHER FACTORS

N/A

PEDIATRIC

N/A

GERIATRIC

N/A

OTHERS

N/A

PREGNANCY

The lactating mother of a newborn may have low levels of estrogen. Lubrication may help relieve symptoms of difficult urination. Symptoms will resolve when breast-feeding is stopped.

FURTHER INFORMATION

American College of Obstetricians & Gynecologists (ACOG), 409 12th St., SW, Washington, DC 20024-2188, (800) 762-ACOG

Section W

Warts

 Basics

DESCRIPTION

Warts are painless, benign skin tumors characterized by an area of well-defined thickening of the skin. They are caused by a virus passed by direct contact with an infected person or from recently shed virus kept intact in a moist, warm environment. There are many types of warts, with different appearances and growth patterns. Plantar warts are individual or groups of warts that occur on the sole of the foot.

SIGNS AND SYMPTOMS

- Rough-surfaced, raised, skin-colored bumps 1–10 millimeter in diameter
- Warts may occur individually, in a line, or in a cluster.
- Some warts are a taller, flexible mass of skin resembling cauliflower.
- Some warts are flat and reddish.
- Signs and symptoms of plantar warts include:
  - ▶ Individual or grouped warts on the sole of the foot
  - ▶ Foot pain
  - ▶ Formation of callus
  - ▶ Pain in the foot, leg, or back due to distortion of normal posture

SCOPE

Warts affect 7–10% of the United States population, primarily young adults and children. Plantar warts are widespread, affecting about 2% of the population.

WHO MOST AFFECTED

Warts can affect persons of any age, but are more common among children and young adults. They are more common among women than men.

CAUSES

Human papillomavirus (HPV)

RISK FACTORS

- Acquired immune deficiency syndrome (AIDS) or other immune system disorder
- Immunosuppressive drug use
- Dermatitis
- Locker room use
- Skin trauma

 Diagnosis

WHAT THE DOCTOR LOOKS FOR

- The doctor will consider other conditions that may appear similar, such as corns, calluses or scar tissue.
- Visual inspection usually confirms the diagnosis of warts.

TESTS AND PROCEDURES

A biopsy of tissue may be obtained for pathological examination.

 Treatment

GENERAL MEASURES

- Warts are managed on an outpatient basis.
- Spontaneous remissions are common and are probably related to the normal immune response.
- If warts cause no symptoms, no treatment is necessary. However, warts may spread.
- Conservative, non-scarring treatments are preferred.
- Treatment is associated with a 60–70% cure rate.
- Warm soaks followed by peeling the top layer of skin on repeated occasions may speed disappearance.
- Over-the-counter remedies containing salicylic acid may help. Read and follow directions carefully.
- Other measures include use of a heel bar or appropriate padding to relieve pressure points where warts tend to aggregate.
- Occlusion: the easiest and least expensive treatment. The wart is covered with a waterproof tape for a week. The tape is removed and left open for 12 hours, then re-taped if the wart is still present. The environment under the tape hinders viral growth.
- Surgical measures include:
  - ▶ Cryotherapy: Freezing of warts is often preferred because scar formation is minimized; usually requires several treatments.

- ► Excision with electrocautery, laser, or curettage
- ► Blunt dissection: a simple surgical procedure that is effective and usually nonscarring; involves separating wart and normal skin with a blunt instrument

ACTIVITY

Plantar warts occasionally cause discomfort, requiring a decrease in activity.

DIET

N/A

 ## Medications

COMMONLY PRESCRIBED DRUGS

- No effective antiviral wart medications currently exist.
- All treatments begin by paring the wart as closely as possible, then soaking the area in warm water to moisten the wart.
- Chemotherapy:
  - ► Topical retinoids: tretinoin (retinoic acid, Retin-A)
  - ► Salicylic acid (Trans-Ver-Sal, Mediplast, Duofilm, Keralyt)

CONTRAINDICATIONS

Read product information for specific drugs. Vascular disorders may be contraindicated for some treatments. Infection may be a contraindication.

PRECAUTIONS

Avoid normal skin when using topical chemicals. Treatment may cause the formation of scars.

OTHER DRUGS

- Chemotherapy:
  - ► Benzoyl peroxide
  - ► Other chemotherapy: dichloroacetic acid, trichloroacetic acid, podophyllin, 5-fluorouracil, silver nitrate, idoxuridine (Herplex Liquifilm)
  - ► Bleomycin: expensive and causes severe pain, but has a 75% cure rate
- Vesicants containing cantharidin (Cantharone, Verrusol)
- Immunotherapy:
  - ► Dinitrochlorobenzene (DNCB)
  - ► Interferon

 ## Followup

PATIENT MONITORING

Up to one-third of warts may become malignant.

PREVENTION

- Warts are infectious and can be transmitted to others. Warts should be covered during treatment to avoid being transmitted to healthy skin or other people.
- Avoid the wound fluid after cryotherapy.
- Use personal footwear in locker room settings.

POSSIBLE COMPLICATIONS

- Warts may spread to healthy skin.
- Removal of plantar warts may cause chronic pain and formation of scar.
- Warts of the nail bed may cause deformity of fingernails.

WHAT TO EXPECT

The outcome of warts varies. Many times, warts completely resolve with or without treatment. The course of plantar warts is highly variable. Most resolve spontaneously in weeks to months.

 ## Miscellaneous

OTHER FACTORS

N/A

PEDIATRIC

Warts are more common in children. The duration of plantar warts is generally shorter in children than in adults.

GERIATRIC

Less common in non-immunocompromised adults

OTHERS

N/A

PREGNANCY

N/A

FURTHER INFORMATION

American Academy of Dermatology (708) 330-0230.

Index

Contraception, 114–117

Contraindications for drugs (*see* Drug precautions/interactions)

COPD (chronic obstructive pulmonary disease), 100–101

Corticosteroids (*see* Drug precautions/interactions; Steroids)

Crib death (SIDS, sudden infant death syndrome), 454–455

Cromolyn sodium, 45 (*see also* Anti-asthma drugs)

Croup, 120–121

Curvature of spine (scoliosis), 428–429

Cutaneous (skin) diseases (*see* Skin problems)

Cutaneous (skin) drug reactions, 122–123

Cyanocobalamin (vitamin B12) deficiency, 24–25

Cystic fibrosis, 124–127

Deafness (*see* Ear problems)

Decongestants, 108, 415 (*see also* Antihistamines)

Dehydration, 130–131, 180
in cholera, 97

Dementias, 132–133
Alzheimer's disease, 18–19, 132–133
multi-infarct (from multiple strokes), 132–133
in Parkinson's disease (parkinsonism), 367

Dental problems
gingivitis (gum inflammation), 194–195
halitosis (bad breath), 206–207 (*see also* Gingivitis)
temporomandibular joint (TMJ) syndrome, 466–467

Depression, 73, 134–135 (*see also* Mood disorders)
in alcoholism, 8, 9
in dementia, 133

Dermatitis (*see also* Skin problems)
allergic, 136
contact, 136–137
diaper (diaper rash), 144–145
primary, 136

Desipramine (Norpramin, Pertofrane) (*see* Antidepressants)

Dexfenfluramine (Redux), 353

Diabetes mellitus, 20
drug precautions in, 238
insulin-dependent (IDDM, type I diabetes, juvenile-onset diabetes), 138–141
non-insulin-dependent (NIDDM, type II diabetes, adult-onset diabetes), 142–143

Diaper rash, 144–145

Diaphragm (contraceptive), 115

Diarrhea (*see also* Gastrointestinal problems; Irritable bowel syndrome (spastic colon))
acute viral, 146
protozoal, 146
travelers', 146

Didanosine, 230

Diethylpropion, 353

Dieting (for obesity), 352–353

Digestive problems (*see* Eating disorders; Gastrointestinal problems)

Dihydroergotamine mesylate, 209

Dilantin (phenytoin), 433 (*see also* Seizure disorders)

Diltiazem (*see* Calcium channel blockers)

Diphenhydramine (Benadryl) (*see* Antihistamines)

Diphtheria, tetanus, pertussis (DPT) immunization, 250

Disk (lumbar disk, spinal disk) disorders, 300–301

Dissociative amnesia, 148

Dissociative disorders, 148–149

Dissociative fugue, 148

Dissociative identity disorder, 148

Diuretics ("water pills")
in essential hypertension, 238
in glomerulonephritis (kidney inflammation), 199

Dizziness (vertigo), 260

Doxepin (Adapin, Sinequan) (*see* Antidepressants)

DPT (diphtheria, tetanus, pertussis) immunization, 250

Droperidol, 149

Drug allergy, 203

Drug poisoning (*see also* Drug precautions/interactions)
acetaminophen (Tylenol), 2–3
imipramine, 57

Drug precautions/interactions
in alcohol detoxification, 10
allopurinol, 203
amantadine, 258
anti-acne drugs, 5
anti-asthma drugs, 46
antibiotics, 5, 373, 419, 479
antidepressants, 133, 135, 384
antidiarrheals, 147
antifungal drugs, 13, 81
antihistamines, 108, 137
antipsychotic drugs, 133
antiviral drugs, 381
aspirin, 258, 259, 317
Bellergal (ergotamine-belladonna-phenobarbital), 312
benzodiazepines, 34, 268, 269
beta blockers, 145, 238
bismuth compounds (Pepto-Bismal), 147, 186
calcium channel blockers, 238